Working in Mental Health

A paradigm shift is taking place in the ways in which mental health services are delivered, both for service users and for professional mental health care workers. A more influential service user movement, a range of new community-based mental health care programmes delivered by an increasing plurality of providers, and new mental health policy and legislation are all changing the landscape.

Written by a team of experienced authors, and drawing on their expertise in policy and clinical leadership as well as user perspectives, this textbook explains how mental health services and their staff can operate and contribute in this new environment. Divided into three parts, the first focuses on the socio-political environment, incorporating service user perspectives. The second part goes on to look at current themes and ways of working in mental health, including chapters on recovery, the Improving Access to Psychological Therapies (IAPT) programme and mental health care for specific vulnerable populations. The final part explores new and future challenges, such as changing professional roles and commissioning services. The book focuses throughout on the importance of public health approaches to mental health care.

This important text will be of interest to all those studying and working in mental health care, whether from a nursing, medical, social work or allied health background.

Peter Phillips is Senior Lecturer in Addiction at City University London and Honorary Lecturer in Social and Community Mental Health at University College London.

Tom Sandford is Executive Director of services across England for the Royal College of Nursing. His previous roles in the organisation include five years as a mental health policy adviser and three years as London Regional Director.

Claire Johnston is the Director of Nursing for Camden and Islington NHS Foundation Trust, which provides mental health and substance misuse services in central London.

Working in Mental Health

Practice and policy in a changing environment

**Edited by Peter Phillips, Tom Sandford
and Claire Johnston**

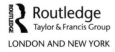

LONDON AND NEW YORK

First published 2012
by Routledge
2 Park Square, Milton Park, Abingdon, Oxon, OX14 4RN

Simultaneously published in the USA and Canada
by Routledge
711 Third Avenue, New York, NY 10017

Routledge is an imprint of the Taylor & Francis Group, an informa business

British Library Cataloguing in Publication Data
A catalogue record for this book is available from the British Library

Library of Congress Cataloging-in-Publication Data
Working in mental health : practice and policy in a changing
environment / edited by Peter Phillips, Tom Sandford, and Claire
Johnston.
   p. ; cm.
  Includes bibliographical references.
  I. Phillips, Peter, 1968- II. Sandford, Tom. III. Johnston, Claire,
MSc RGN.
  [DNLM: 1. Mental Health Services–trends–Great Britain. WM
30 FA1]
  362.1–dc23   2011043603

ISBN: 978-0-415-69109-3 (hbk)
ISBN: 978-0-415-69110-9 (pbk)
ISBN: 978-0-203-12091-0 (ebk)

Typeset in Bembo
by HWA Text and Data Management

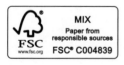

MIX
Paper from
responsible sources
FSC
www.fsc.org FSC® C004839

Printed and bound in Great Britain by
TJ International Ltd, Padstow, Cornwall

Contents

List of contributors   vii

Acknowledgements   xv

Foreword   xvi
Jo Brand

Foreword   xvii
Michael Parsonage

PART I
Mental health care and the socio-political environment   **1**

1   UK mental health policy development: a framework for meaningful change   3
     Andrew McCulloch and Simon Lawton-Smith

2   UK mental health policy development: a counter-argument deriving
     from users' experiences   14
     Rachel E. Perkins

3   Collaborative partnerships with service users: models that work   25
     Alan Simpson

4   The care pathway approach: a contemporary, inclusive and
     outcome-focused rationale for service provision   39
     Sylvia Tang

PART II
Characteristics of new mental health services   **49**

5   Home treatment for mental health crises: presenting the evidence and
     potential for improvement   51
     Fiona Nolan

6   Contemporary rehabilitation   61
     Helen Killaspy

7   Recovery: a journey of discovery for individuals and services   71
     Julie Repper and Rachel E. Perkins

8   Drugs, drink and mental health: the impact and consequences of dual
    diagnosis for mental health service delivery   81
    LIZ HUGHES AND PETER PHILLIPS

9   Gender-specific mental health care: the case for women-centred care   90
    LOUISE PHILLIPS AND ANN JACKSON

10 Race, ethnicity and mental health care   104
    HÁRI SEWELL

11 Age-specific service lines   116
    CHRIS FOX, SIOBHAN REILLY, STEVE ILIFFE AND JILL MANTHORPE

12 Improving access to psychological therapies: practice and policy in a
    changing environment   129
    JOHN CAPE AND CAROLINE HUMPHRIES

PART III
The new territory   **147**

13 Delivering new services: changes in professional roles   149
    SALLY HARDY AND NEIL BRIMBLECOMBE

14 Delivering physical health care in modern mental health services: what
    works and why we all have to bother   159
    DAVID P. OSBORN

15 Commissioning new mental health services   170
    DAVID JOBBINS

16 Working in mental health: practice and policy in a changing environment –
    conclusions   180
    TOM SANDFORD, CLAIRE JOHNSTON AND PETER PHILLIPS

    Index   184

Contributors

The editors

Peter Phillips PhD MSc RMN PGCAP FHEA FRSA

Dr Peter Phillips is Senior Lecturer in Addiction at City University London, and Honorary Lecturer/Researcher in Social & Community Mental Health at University College London (UCL) Medical School, and Camden and Islington NHS Foundation Trust. Peter trained as a mental health nurse at High Royds Hospital in Leeds and, after qualifying, worked in the Alcohol Unit at the Maudsley Hospital (London), and later in other specialist mental health, drug and alcohol and harm reduction services in London. He worked as a dual diagnosis nurse specialist in Tower Hamlets (Harm Reduction Services), prior to obtaining a research fellowship at UCL Medical School in 1998, where he completed a PhD on the motivations for, and social context of, drug use amongst the mentally ill. In 2003, Peter received a Band Trust scholarship to investigate dual diagnosis in Northern India. During his time at UCL Peter maintained a clinical link with Camden and Islington National Health Service (NHS) Mental Health Services where he implemented and later evaluated interventions to reduce heroin overdose deaths. Peter is active in the drug policy reform movement, and is a strong proponent of public health in the area of harm reduction approaches to drug and alcohol problems. Peter is an advisory board member for *Mental Health and Substance Use: dual diagnosis*, and an editorial board member of *Advances in Dual Diagnosis*.

Tom Sandford FRCN BSc (Hons) Dip N RGN RMN

Tom Sandford is employed by the Royal College of Nursing (RCN) as the executive director of their services across England. His previous roles in the organisation include five years as a mental health policy adviser and three years as London regional director. Before joining the RCN Tom was general manager of mental health services across the London boroughs of Camden and Islington. Tom trained as a general nurse and a mental health nurse at the London Hospital in Whitechapel. He has held a variety of clinical nursing posts in the fields of family therapy, acute psychiatry and liaison psychiatry. He was Head of Professional Development in Bloomsbury Health Authority and was a member of the ministerial task force coordinating the development of the NHS mental health national service framework. He has served on several public untoward incident inquiries and has taught multi-professional mental health service integration programmes at universities in Frankfurt and Irsee in Germany, and case management programmes in the Nursing Faculty at the University of Barcelona in Spain. He writes on mental health issues and his recent book with Peter Phillips and Olive McKeown, *Dual Diagnosis – practice in context*, was published in January 2010 by Wiley Blackwell.

Claire Johnston MSc RGN

Claire Johnston is the Director of Nursing for Camden and Islington NHS Foundation Trust, which provides mental health and substance misuse services in central London. Claire has worked as a Trust Director for over a decade and remains passionate about the contribution of mental health nurses to providing flexible, effective, user-focused services. Claire has held previous roles as a national nursing advisor at the Royal College of Nursing, as well as serving on the Department of Health's social care task force. Claire is on the editorial board of the Nursing and Midwifery Council's (NMC) journal, *NMC Review*.

The authors

Neil Brimblecombe RN PhD

Dr Neil Brimblecombe is Chief Operating Officer for a mental health trust in central England and visiting professor at Nottingham University. He has worked in clinical, managerial and professional leadership roles, including as Director of Mental Health Nursing for the English Department of Health. His research interests include crisis services, the history of mental health and international health issues.

John Cape BA MPhil PhD FBPsS

Dr John Cape is Head of Psychological Therapies, Camden and Islington NHS Foundation Trust and Visiting Professor, Division of Psychology and Language Sciences, University College London. He has a long-standing interest in improving mental health in primary care and in the organisation of mental health services between primary and secondary care.

Chris Fox MD MRCPsych MMedSci BSc MB BS

Dr Chris Fox is Clinical Senior Lecturer in Old Age Psychiatry at Norwich Medical School University of East Anglia. He is also Eastern Region Director of Dementia Research at the Dementias and Neurodegenerative Diseases Research Network. He has a long-standing interest in health service research and has worked in the NHS on modernisation and innovation of services and has ongoing US and European collaborations in service research in dementia care. His current studies cover rehabilitation in dementia, screening for memory problems, medication management and collaborative care in dementia.

Sally Hardy EdD ACHEP MSc BA(Hons) RMN RN

Sally Hardy is Professor of Mental Health and Practice Innovation, School of Health Sciences, City University, London; Adjunct Associate Professor, Monash University, Melbourne, Australia; Visiting Professor Canterbury and Christchurch University, Kent. Since starting nurse training at Guy's Hospital London and then moving into mental health nursing at the Maudsley, through to an academic role, Sally has maintained an interest in how nursing contributes and enhances individual experience of health care, for service users, carers and practitioners. Working at the Royal College of Nursing Institute, and as Director of Research and Practice Development at the Royal Children's Hospital Melbourne, Australia, Sally's interest and experience remains active in promoting nursing, balancing her academic role at City University and associate posts to further integrate practice-based wisdom with academic advancements.

Liz Hughes PhD BSc Dip HE

Dr Liz Hughes is a senior lecturer in Mental Health in the Department of Health Sciences at the University of York and is involved in both research and teaching related to mental health and nursing. Liz first obtained a BSc in Psychology in 1989, and then went on to train as a mental health nurse. She has worked in both acute inpatient settings as well as in inpatient and community addictions treatment services. Her first academic post was at the Institute of Psychiatry, Kings College London where she was a research nurse for seven years, and was involved in two trials of dual diagnosis training. She obtained a PhD in 2008. Liz has significantly contributed to the Department of Health Dual Diagnosis programme, producing a range of national resources to assist the workforce development for dual diagnosis, in particular *Closing the Gap: a capability framework for effective working with people who have combined mental health and substance use problems*. Her main research interests include dual diagnosis of mental health and substance use; sexual health and relationships in people with serious mental health problems; and workforce development in mental health.

Caroline Humphries BA MA

Caroline Humphries is a Churchill Fellow of the Winston Churchill Memorial Trust, researching the role of social enterprise in the delivery of health services in the developing world. She was previously the Improving Access to Psychological Therapies Programme Manager for Islington Primary Care Trust (NHS Islington). She has a keen interest in improving health service delivery, with a career background of policy development and NHS performance management at the Department of Health.

Steve Iliffe FRCGP FRCP

Steve Iliffe was a general practitioner in inner London from 1978 to 2007, and is currently Professor of Primary Care for Older People at University College London. His research interests are in health and ageing, particularly health promotion and the care of patients with dementia. He is also an associate director of the Dementia and Neurodegenerative Diseases Research Network (DENDRON) and associate editor of *Aging & Mental Health*.

Ann Jackson RMN BA (Hons) Health studies MA

Ann Jackson's clinical background is in acute inpatient mental health care on a ward run as a modified therapeutic community in 1984–1992. She has twenty year's experience working in practice development and research; working with teams as external facilitator to systematically review practice and integrate with best evidence and policy. She was recently appointed as the Associate Director of Healthcare at St. Andrew's Healthcare, the largest UK charitable provider of specialist mental health services. She is primarily responsible for leading and supporting the Heads of Professions and strategic clinical developments across the Charity. Ann was previously at the Royal College of Nursing for sixteen years and gained a wealth of experience working across national policy and practice agendas. Secondments to the Department of Health (Offender Health) and Leicestershire Partnership NHS Trust afforded the opportunity to lead policy making and practice specifically around women's mental health. Ann represented the RCN on multiple forums over the years, most notably the Department of Health Taskforce for the Health Aspects of Violence against Women; the Women's Mental Health Programme Board and the subsequent National Mental Health Development Unit (NMHDU) Equalities

Programme Board. She now sits on the Ministerial Working Group for Mental Health and Equalities. Ann's academic and policy interests include women's mental health – in relation to gendered violence; women in the criminal justice system; and intersectional approaches. Other interests include socially inclusive practice: equality, diversity and human rights as applied within the workplace and in clinical practice. She is currently the Chair of the Board of Directors of Women's Aid Leicestershire Limited.

David Jobbins MSc

David Jobbins has worked in the NHS in London for most of the last twenty-five years. This has included a range of commissioning and strategic change roles that have included roles as Head of Modernisation and Director of Strategy in two south London Primary Care Trusts (PCTs). Many of these roles have included commissioning and service development responsibilities for mental health but he has also had lead responsibilities for other service areas including primary care, long-term conditions and substance misuse. Currently David is working as Associate Director – Mental Health at London Health Programmes. David also worked as Health Access Adviser for the Refugee Council for two years in the 1990s and has been Chair of a borough-based Mind organisation in north-east London for the last ten years. He also holds an MSc in Social Analysis.

Helen Killaspy MBBS PhD FRCPsych

Dr Helen Killaspy is reader and honorary consultant in rehabilitation psychiatry at University College London Medical School and Camden and Islington NHS Foundation Trust in London. She is Chair of the Faculty of Rehabilitation and Social Psychiatry of the Royal College of Psychiatrists. Dr Killaspy's research focuses on the evaluation of interventions and services for people with longer term, complex mental health needs. She led the international study that developed the Quality Indicator for Rehabilitative Care and she is leading a national programme of research into the clinical and cost-effectiveness of contemporary mental health rehabilitation services in England.

Simon Lawton-Smith

Simon Lawton-Smith is Head of Policy at the Mental Health Foundation, the leading UK charity working in mental health and learning disabilities. He is author/co-author of a range of reports and articles on mental health. From 2003 to 2008, Simon was Senior Fellow in Mental Health at the King's Fund, where he led the mental health work programme, linking policy development with service development and research projects. From 1997 to 2003 Simon was Head of Public Affairs at national service provider mental health charity Together. Previously he spent seventeen years in the civil service, at the Department of Health, the Northern Ireland Office and the Cabinet Office.

Andrew McCulloch MA PhD MBPS

Dr Andrew McCulloch has been Chief Executive of the Mental Health Foundation for nine years. Prior to his appointment, he was Director of Policy at the Sainsbury Centre for Mental Health for six years where he established a reputation as a leading authority on mental health policy. He was formerly a senior civil servant in the Department of Health for sixteen years and was head of mental health and learning disabilities policy from 1992 to 1996. He has spoken and published widely on mental health issues. Andrew's other experience has included being a school governor, the non-executive director of an NHS Trust, a Trustee of the UK Council for Psychotherapy and the Chair of Mental Health Media, a charity dedicated to giving people with mental health problems and learning disabilities a voice. He has chaired or served on a range of national advisory committees. He has a PhD in the psychology of old age from the University of Southampton.

Jill Manthorpe

Jill Manthorpe is Professor of Social Work at King's College London and Director of the Social Care Workforce Research Unit. She is also Associate Director of the National Institute for Health Research (NIHR) School for Social Care Research. She has a long-standing interest in mental health practice and policy and has undertaken research on dementia care, safeguarding, risk and student suicide. Her current studies cover carers' support, personalisation and social care workforce changes.

Fiona Nolan RMN BSc PhD

Dr Fiona Nolan is a mental health nurse, and trained in the old psychiatric institutions in Surrey (Horton and Banstead Hospitals) prior to completing a BSc in Political Science. She has since then worked in a variety of inpatient and community services, including a generic community mental health team, an assertive outreach team and most recently as team manager of a crisis resolution team. She has been involved in mental health services research since 1999, and recently was awarded a PhD in Social and Community Psychiatry from University College London. Fiona currently holds a joint clinical academic position with UCL and Camden and Islington NHS Foundation Trust, representing the first nursing post of its kind between these partners. She works as a nurse consultant in clinical research for the Foundation Trust with a focus on developing nursing capacity and activity in research. She is chief investigator on one Research for Patient Benefit funded study and co-applicant on several other NIHR studies. She presents at several national and international conferences annually.

David P. Osborn MBBS MSc MA DSHTM PhD MRCPsych FHEA

Dr David P. Osborn is Senior Lecturer in Psychiatry and Honorary Consultant Psychiatrist. David trained in medicine and social and political sciences at Cambridge University and UCL. He has worked at UCL as a clinical academic since 2003, with a research expertise in psychiatric epidemiology and the interface between physical and mental health. He has been awarded research grants from a range of funding bodies, to explore and improve the physical health of people with severe mental illnesses. He works half the week as a consultant psychiatrist in acute adult mental health, within the Camden and Islington NHS Foundation Trust, North London. This includes work in a crisis team, a six-bedded crisis house and an acute, multidisciplinary day service.

Michael Parsonage

Michael Parsonage is an economist who since 2003 has been working as a Senior Policy Adviser at the Centre for Mental Health (formerly the Sainsbury Centre for Mental Health), where he has produced a number of reports based on the application of economic analysis to mental health issues. He has also worked on a consultancy basis for a number of other organisations in the mental health field, including the Mental Health Foundation, the Scottish Association for Mental Health, the Northern Ireland Association for Mental Health and the All Wales Mental Health Promotion Network, and is a Visiting Senior Fellow at the London School of Economics and Political Science. He was previously employed as a senior economist in the Department of Health and in Her Majesty's Treasury.

Rachel E. Perkins PhD OBE

Professor Rachel E. Perkins was Director of Quality Assurance and User Experience at South West London and St. George's Mental Health NHS Trust. She is now a freelance consultant and Chair of Equality 2025 (the cross Government strategic advisory group on issues relating to disabled people hosted by the UK Department of Work and Pensions). In this capacity she is a member of the Mental Health Strategy Ministerial Advisory group and co-chairs the Ministerial Working Group on Equality A member of the 'Implementing Recovery – Organisational Change' project team (a programme to help organizations to develop recovery-focused practice commissioned by the Department of Health and delivered by a partnership between the NHS Confederation and Centre for Mental Health). She is also a long-term user of mental health services and a trustee of Mind. In 2009 she was commissioned by the Secretary of State for Work and Pensions to lead an independent review into how Government might better support people with mental health problems to gain work and prosper in employment (*Realising Ambitions: better employment support for people with a mental health condition*, DWP, December 2009). She has written and spoken widely about recovery and social inclusion for people with mental health conditions and has pioneered the UK development of programmes to help people with mental health difficulties to access employment and education based on the 'Individual Placement with Support' approach, including one designed to increase employment opportunities within mental health services for people who have themselves experienced mental health problems. In 2010 she was awarded an OBE for services to mental health and voted Mind Champion of the Year. Her latest book, written with Julie Repper, is *Social Inclusion and Recovery: a model for mental health practice* (2003, Balliere Tindall).

Louise Phillips PhD RMN BA (Hons) PGDip Academic Practice FHEA

Dr Louise Phillips is the Senior Lecturer in Women's Mental Health, School of Health Sciences, City University, London. Louise is a mental health nurse and before starting her academic career, she practised in a variety of settings including elderly care, the voluntary sector and the NHS, and worked for a number of years as a Community Psychiatric Nurse in the King's Cross area of London. In addition to her nursing qualification she has a PhD on approaches to the body and mental illness which became a book entitled *Mental Illness and the Body: beyond diagnosis,* published by Routledge (2006). Louise has undertaken and published research in the areas of staff who work with women patients in acute mental health care, and the support of student mental health nurses witnessing suicide and suicidal behaviours. She is currently developing her research profile in the areas of perinatal mental health and the experiences of motherhood.

Siobhan Reilly BSc (Hons), PhD

Dr Siobhan Reilly is Research Fellow at NIHR School for Primary Care Research, Health Sciences Research Group, University of Manchester. She gained a PhD in 2000 in health service research from Liverpool John Moores University. The title of her PhD was *Addressing the Health Problems of the Homeless: a systematic review and a controlled trial*. She has methodological expertise in systematic reviews, the design and analysis of projects and programme evaluations at both national and local, and organisational and practice levels, quantitative methods in health and social care research and the use of routine health service data in research. In October 2010, Siobhan was awarded a three-year NIHR School for Primary Care Research Training Fellowship. Her current research interests are focused upon improving the interface between specialist mental health and specialist dementia services and primary care; collaborative care approaches and case management in mental health services; and homelessness and the integration of health and social care.

Julie Repper

Dr Julie Repper is Recovery Lead in Nottinghamshire Healthcare Trust, Associate Professor of Recovery and Social Inclusion at University of Nottingham, Director of two service user led voluntary sector groups and she is working on the Department of Health funded 'Implementing Recovery in Organisational Contexts' project two days per week. She works collaboratively with people who have lived experience to develop innovative training, research and service developments and is currently Director of the Nottingham Recovery Education Centre and leading the development of the Peer Support Workers' training and employment in her local services.

Hári Sewell

Hári Sewell is founder and Director of HS Consultancy and is a former executive director of health and social care in the NHS. He is a writer and speaker in his specialist area of ethnicity, race and culture in mental health. Hári is honorary Senior Visiting Fellow at University of Central Lancashire and also at Buckinghamshire New University. He has worked as an expert panellist with the Department of Health and the Royal College of Psychiatrists. Hári is joint editor of the journal *Ethnicity and Inequalities in Health and Social Care* and is on the editorial board of *Journal of Integrated Care*. He was the founder and chair of the national Social Care Strategic Network (Mental Health) until November 2010. Hári was part of the Marmot Review of Health Inequalities Post-2010. His book, *Working with Ethnicity Race and Culture in Mental Health: a handbook for practitioners*, was published in October 2008. He has had various articles and book chapters published, and new material emerges regularly.

Alan Simpson PhD PG Cert (Academic Practice) PG Cert (Research Methods) PG Diploma (Counselling) BA (Hons) (Social Psychology) RMN

Alan Simpson is Professor of Collaborative Mental Health Nursing in the School of Health Sciences, City University, London and Chair of Mental Health Nurse Academics UK. He leads on mental health nursing research with a special focus on service user and carer involvement. Currently leading a trial of peer support for people being discharged from mental health hospitals, he is also involved in a study of 'protected engagement time' on acute inpatient wards. He has previously conducted a number of research studies in community and inpatient mental health settings, advised and evaluated the highly successful Star Wards initiative and has led evaluations of several innovative educational projects. Alan supervises PhD and Masters Degree students and teaches pre-registration students and post-registration student staff. Alan is a mental health nurse and a member of the Joint Institute of Mental Health Nursing established by East London NHS Foundation Trust and City University, London. He previously worked as a Community Mental Health Nurse for homeless people with mental health problems; a drug and alcohol liaison nurse; staff nurse in mental health day hospital and acute care settings; and is a qualified counsellor.

Sylvia Tang MB BS FRCPsych

Dr Sylvia Tang has been the Medical Director at Camden and Islington NHS Foundation Trust since 2006, and was previously the associate Medical Director. She continues to work as a Consultant Psychiatrist in General Adult Psychiatry in Islington, which remains the main driver for her work. She has led the programme of service line management implementation at Camden and Islington, and the associated reorganisation of services and mental health PbR (Payment by Results) in the trust. The clinical strategy is based around the implementation of clinical care pathways that drive operational services. The process of implementation of the acute care pathway, setting out common aims, outcomes and addressing interface issues has led to two phases of bed reductions over the last five years, which have now resulted in the closure of two hospital sites, with a third to follow shortly. She has also established with the Darzi fellow, the clinical leadership programme for higher trainees, which has seen thirty medical trainees and other multi-professional staff participating in management projects and attending training at Middlesex University in the last years. She also does some advisory and educational work with a local charity providing bereavement counselling.

Acknowledgements

As editors we are very grateful for the work of our contributors. We set out to produce a collection of chapters written by some of the most distinguished doctors, clinical academics, nurses, service user commentators and policists on mental health in the United Kingdom.

We asked all our contributors to write in as accessible a way as possible, while introducing complex issues in a succinct and pithy style. Mental health authors are no different from other authors, however: some write sharply and clearly, while others are more difficult to follow and pack difficult ideas together. This book reflects the range of styles of writing and the array of mental health practice and policy positions that readers are likely to encounter. All the chapters, of course, can only provide a short summary of wide range of issues and information about the authors' specialisms and expertise.

We hope that we will encourage readers to investigate further and read and discuss more widely the ideas, thinking and standpoint of our commentators.

We as editors have made the difficult and contentious decisions about what should be left out, what should be included, and who should be asked to write the chapters. We should like to thank Grace McInnes and James Watson at Routledge for their support in the production of this book as well as the anonymous reviewers who all gave us such helpful advice. Any shortcomings, however, are our responsibility. We hope that what we have produced is worthy of all this support and that this book will make a valuable contribution to the mental health and social care community, and that above all you will find it an enjoyable and thought-provoking read.

Foreword

Jo Brand

I am probably not the best person to provide a short foreword for this book, given that I left my job as a Senior Charge Nurse in a 24-hour psychiatric emergency clinic in south-east London in 1988 to pursue what I assumed would be a short-lived career in stand-up comedy. The emergency clinic is no more and, 24 years later, I am still in comedy. I keep in touch with friends from the job I did, but although I am aware of changes broadly speaking, from reading the newspapers, the finer points of how mental health services have moved on are somewhat of a mystery to me. And you may not be surprised to learn that on a night out with old friends we tend not to spend much time on mental health policy.

So, in many ways, as an ex-professional in mental health services, this book is exactly what I need. Written in clear and concise language with mercifully few buzzwords and phrases (a real bête noire of mine) it lays out accessibly what has been done, how things are, and what needs to be done in the vast and complex arena of mental health services. The political impact on all NHS services is, of course, something that we cannot ignore and the impossible task of adequately funding mental health services and making them count is something I found usefully addressed in this book, too. Personally, as a staunch Labour voter, I fear the future of the NHS is in shaky hands, although one hopes that the services and all the good work achieved up to this point will not be completely abandoned. And just for the record, my perfect mental health care worker is a combination of instinctive intelligence, kindness and humour ... something that I hope to see in our services as they progress towards the future.

Foreword

The economic context shaping the development of mental health services

Michael Parsonage

Public expenditure on mental health services for adults of working age more than doubled in the ten years following publication of the National Service Framework for Mental Health in 1999 (Department of Health, 1999). The actual increase was 142 per cent in cash terms (based on data in Healthcare Commission (2008) for the years 1999/2000–2001/02 and Mental Health Strategies (2010) for the years 2001/02–2009/10), equivalent to average growth of 9.2 per cent a year. Rising prices accounted for some of this increase, but – even after allowing for general inflation – spending rose by no less than 90 per cent in real terms over the period, or 6.6 per cent a year on average.

The increase in expenditure for mental health was almost exactly the same as for other services in the National Health Service (NHS), with total health spending rising in cash terms by 143 per cent in the ten years to 2009/10 (HM Treasury, 2010a). While the comparative figures do not suggest any particular prioritisation of mental health, they do at least imply that the sector shared fully in the extra provision made available to the NHS, which was underpinned by strong economic growth during much of the period in question.

The additional resources for mental health meant that:

- many more staff were employed, including for example nearly 50 per cent more consultant psychiatrists and a trebling of the numbers of staff professionally qualified in psychotherapy (NHS Information Centre, 2011a);
- more patients were treated, with the number of adults using secondary mental health services increasing by around 3 per cent a year on average (NHS Information Centre, 2011b); and
- new community-based services were introduced, including more than 700 teams providing specialist crisis resolution, assertive outreach and early intervention services (Department of Health, 2007).

Looking ahead, the prospects for all health services including mental health are very different. Public expenditure will be severely constrained for some years to come, because of the need for deficit reduction alongside a general expectation that recovery from the recession starting in 2009 is likely to be slow and protracted. The Coalition Government has pledged not to reduce NHS spending in real terms, but any increases in the foreseeable future are likely to be very modest, as shown by the settlement in the 2010 public spending review, which will result in NHS expenditure growing by a total of just 0.4 per cent in real terms over the next three years (HM Treasury, 2010b).

In the face of continuing pressures from demographic change, new technology and the tendency of health costs to increase more rapidly than general inflation, it will be possible to maintain the quantity and quality of existing services only by making very substantial improvements in efficiency. The NHS is already committed to generating up to £20 billion of annual savings by 2014/15 through the Quality, Innovation, Productivity and Prevention (QIPP) programme. There is no precedent for making efficiency improvements on this scale, particularly at a time when the health service will be in the throes of structural reorganisation.

Another feature of the economic context particularly affecting mental health is that there will be upward pressures on the demand for services just as budgets become increasingly constrained. One reason for this is the persistence of high unemployment, which is well established as a risk factor for mental ill health, as are other aspects of a weak labour market such as job insecurity, debt problems and housing repossessions. Unemployment increased by nearly half between 2008 and 2009, to around 8 per cent of the economically active population, and, according to forecasts published by the Office for Budget Responsibility in advance of the 2011 budget, is expected to remain at or around this level well into 2013, and even by 2015 will still be above the level experienced at any time in the ten years up to 2009 (Office for Budget Responsibility, 2011). Additional demands on mental health services are also likely to arise from the knock-on effects of cuts in other public spending programmes such as social care, welfare benefits, housing and criminal justice.

The combination of severely constrained budgets and continuing cost and demand pressures clearly creates a difficult environment for the development of mental health services and not surprisingly this is a recurring theme throughout the chapters of this book. In helping to formulate an appropriate response, here are a few very brief pointers from an economic perspective:

- It is an important feature of mental ill health that its consequences reach far and wide, affecting many different aspects of people's lives and imposing costs that fall on many different budgets. As a corollary, effective treatment can yield economic benefits that go well beyond the mental health sector, including savings elsewhere in the NHS (because of the strong links between mental health and physical health), savings in other parts of the public sector (including social security, social services and – in some cases – criminal justice) and benefits to the wider economy (mainly because of improved employability). Budget cuts which reduce the availability of evidence-based treatments will often be a false economy in terms of their overall impact on NHS costs, the public finances and economic activity.
- Another risk is that resources will be disproportionately diverted from prevention and early intervention, where the potential benefits and cost savings are less immediate than in the case of services for existing clients. Such short-termism is again likely to be a false economy, as there is now an increasingly strong body of evidence to show that many interventions in this area are good value for money, in some cases outstandingly so (Knapp *et al.*, 2011).
- Mental health services should always be ready to discuss the scope for rationalisation and efficiency savings, particularly where these can be achieved through the spread of best practice rather than the introduction of new and untried solutions. For example, the Audit Commission has shown that there is wide variation between providers in the use of mental health inpatient beds, even after adjusting for the needs of local populations, and that if all trusts could achieve the median rate of bed days, the number of beds required would be reduced by 15 per cent, at a saving of well over £200 million a year (Audit Commission, 2010).
- Finally, in the development of new models of service delivery, it is particularly important in the present economic climate that close attention is always given to the scope for potential

efficiency savings. For example, there is some evidence from research that the use of peer support workers can reduce admissions to hospital and shorten inpatient stays (Lawn *et al.*, 2008), a finding that is directly relevant to the design and implementation of recovery-oriented services.

In summary, even at a time of financial stringency there remains a good economic case for improving mental health, because of the multiple potential benefits.

References

Audit Commission (2010) *Maximising resources in adult mental health.* Available at http://www.audit-commission.gov.uk/nationalstudies/health/financialmanagement/Pages/100623maximisingresources.aspx.

Department of Health (1999) *Mental health national service framework.* London: Department of Health.

Department of Health (2007) *Mental health ten years on: progress on mental health care reform.* Available at http://www.dh.gov.uk/en/Publicationsandstatistics/Publications/PublicationsPolicyAndGuidance/DH_074241.

Healthcare Commission (2008) *Bringing value for money to mental health.* London: Healthcare Commission.

HM Treasury (2010a) *Public expenditure statistical analyses 2010.* Cm 7890. London: HM Treasury.

HM Treasury (2010b) *Spending review 2010.* Cm 7942. London: HM Treasury.

Knapp, M., McDaid, D. and Parsonage, M. (2011) *Promoting mental health and preventing mental illness: the economic case.* London: Department of Health.

Lawn, S., Smith, A. and Hunter, K. (2008) Mental health peer support for hospital avoidance and early discharge: an Australian example of consumer driven and operated service. *Journal of Mental Health,* 17, 498–508.

Mental Health Strategies (2010) *2009/10 National survey of investment in adult mental health services.* Available at http://www.dh.gov.uk/en/Publicationsandstatistics/Publications/PublicationsPolicyAndGuidance/DH_117488.

NHS Information Centre (2011a) *NHS staff 2000–2010.* Available at http://www.ic.nhs.uk/statistics-and-data-collections/workforce/nhs-staff-numbers.

NHS Information Centre (2011b) *Mental health bulletin 2010.* Available at http://www.ic.nhs.uk/statistics-and-data-collections/mental-health.

Office for Budget Responsibility (2011) *Economic and fiscal outlook – March 2011.* Cm 8036. London: TSO.

Part I
Mental health care and the socio-political environment

1   UK mental health policy development

A framework for meaningful change

Andrew McCulloch and Simon Lawton-Smith

This chapter seeks to give an overview of English mental health policy over the last few decades, focusing particularly on the period 1997 to the present day, and on future challenges. It will also seek to explain what mental health policy is, and to give a little of the history before 1997. The aim is to draw out the key components for those actually involved in or affected by mental health policy and practice.

What is mental health policy?

Policy itself is often misunderstood. Koontz and Weihrich usefully define it as 'General statements or understandings which guide thinking on decision making' (Koontz and Weihrich, 1988). As such it breaks down into primary and secondary legislation (law), explicit administrative policy (e.g. published Government statements) and unwritten policy (e.g. verbal briefings by Ministers and civil servants to, for example, senior health service managers). At the coalface policy is only one factor in decision making and often a secondary one to clinical or resource issues (Muijen and McCulloch, 2009).

National mental health policy per se is specific to mental health, e.g. mental health legislation or a mental health white paper. However, mental health services and mentally ill people are of course impacted by generic policies on health, welfare, housing and others and these impacts are often more important than that of specialist policy. This must always be borne in mind when considering mental health policy. Each part of the UK has its own mental health policies although there is some sharing of legislation to which Scotland is an exception and Northern Ireland is becoming so. It is too complicated within a short chapter to deal with UK mental health policy so we have focused on England. It is generally, however, considered that Scotland is in advance of England in its development of public mental health and perhaps legislation (for example, Scottish mental health legislation on compulsory treatment takes account of a person's capacity to make decisions about their own care; English legislation does not). In England service development has been very much to the fore.

Mental health policy until 1979

Modern mental health policy started with the introduction of legislation to control the governance of lunatic asylums in early Victorian times and has evolved from there. After the First World War more modern approaches such as psychotherapy started to evolve and after the Second World War charitable and local authority mental health services, mainly asylum based, were mostly incorporated into the NHS. These started to decline in size in the 1950s and this policy direction was explicitly acknowledged in Enoch Powell's 'water tower' speech in the 1960s. Almost all of the old asylums are now closed, depending on how closure is defined. During the 1970s more detailed and explicit mental health policies began to emerge dealing with the establishment of acute psychiatric units in general hospitals and the beginnings of community care. However, many would argue that during the initial period of the decline of asylums the needs of people with severe and enduring mental illness, especially those with deteriorating conditions, were not well addressed in policy perhaps because there was an assumption that some of these conditions were caused by institutionalisation.

Mental health policy from 1979 to 1997

Mental health policy during the Conservative administration of this period was primarily about the process of discovering the consequences of the closure of the old asylums. In 1983 an excellent new Mental Health Act was introduced that consisted essentially of a substantial update of the landmark 1959 Act. Reforms included the creation of a Mental Health Act Commission to defend the rights of detained patients.

In the latter part of the 1980s it became increasingly clear that the model of providing care via hospital beds and undifferentiated community services would not succeed in meeting the needs of a core group of people with severe and enduring mental illness. Much of policy from this point on was about addressing the needs of this group and responding to inquiries into homicides by people with severe mental illness (McCulloch and Parker, 2004). The inquiry into the killing of a social worker by a patient at Bexley Hospital (Sharon Campbell) was one such event that led to the introduction of obligatory care planning for people requiring secondary mental health care. Other changes included the introduction of supervision registers, conditional discharge and compulsory inquiries into serious incidents. This created a new risk management industry, some of it perhaps beneficial and some certainly not.

Alongside this, however, there was also a healthy emphasis on public mental health in documents such as the Health of the Nation mental illness key area, and also on developing services for groups such as children and homeless people. Some of this activity set the scene for the major development programme that was introduced under Labour.

Policy under New Labour

The National Service Framework

When the National Service Framework for Mental Health (NSFMH) (Department of Health, 1999) was launched, the Sainsbury Centre for Mental Health commented: 'For the first time, Government has set out a comprehensive agenda for mental health services which acknowledges that the whole system of mental health care must be made to work if we are to succeed in modernising care' (Sainsbury Centre for Mental Health, 1999).

Whilst the NSFMH was radically new in terms of its comprehensiveness and ambition it can be located within a general attempt to develop health care policy on a more comprehensive, evidence-based way (McCulloch, Glover and St John, 2003) – although it should be noted that the NSFMH was for adults of working age, and that standards for the mental health of older people was covered in the NSF for older people (2001) and for children in the NSF for children and young people (2004).

The NSFMH set out seven 'standards', which are really key areas for service and practice development, and these are summarised in Box 1.1.

Inevitably with such a comprehensive document there were some confusions and contradictions and there was a subsequent debate about differing emphases on safety and compulsion as opposed to care and choice, for example. However, there seem to be six readily definable core aims that can be deduced from the document (McCulloch, Glover and St John, 2003).

1   Modernising primary, secondary and tertiary mental health care.
2   Improving public mental health.
3   Reducing suicide.
4   Improving public safety.
5   Improving the quality of care.
6   Improving support for carers.

Of these, 1, 4 and 5 were given the most emphasis in words and actions.

Box 1.1 The National Service Framework for Mental Health standards

Standard 1 aims to ensure health and social services promote mental health and reduce the discrimination and social exclusion associated with mental health problems.
   Health and social services should:

*   promote mental health for all, working with individuals and communities;
*   combat discrimination against individuals and groups with mental health problems, and promote their social inclusion.

Standards 2 and 3 aim to deliver better primary mental health care, and to ensure consistent advice and help for people with mental health needs, including primary care services for individuals with severe mental illness.
   Any service user who contacts their primary health care team with a common mental health problem should:

*   have their mental health needs identified and assessed;
*   be offered effective treatments, including referral to specialist services for further assessment, treatment and care if they require it.

Any individual with a common mental health problem should:

*   be able to make contact round the clock with the local services necessary to meet their needs and receive adequate care;
*   be able to use NHS Direct, as it develops, for first-level advice and referral on to specialist helplines or to local services.

Standards 4 and 5 aim to ensure: that each person with severe mental illness receives the range of mental health services they need; that crises are anticipated or prevented

---

Continued…

Box 1.1 continued

where possible; prompt and effective help if a crisis does occur; and timely access to an appropriate and safe mental health place or hospital bed, including a secure bed, as close to home as possible.

All mental health service users on CPA (Care Programme Approach) should:

- receive care that optimizes engagement, anticipates or prevents a crisis, and reduces risk;
- have a copy of a written care plan that:
    - includes the action to be taken in a crisis by the service user, their carer and their care coordinator,
    - advises their GP how they should respond if the service user needs additional help,
    - is regularly reviewed by their care coordinator,
    - is able to access services 24 hours a day, 365 days a year.

Each service user who is assessed as requiring a period of care away from their home should have:

- timely access to an appropriate hospital bed or place that is:
    - in the least restrictive environment consistent with the need to protect them and the public,
    - as close to home as possible;

- a copy of a written care plan agreed on discharge that sets out the care and rehabilitation to be provided, identifies the care coordinator, and specifies the action to be taken in a crisis.

Standard 6 aims to ensure health and social services assess the needs of carers who provide regular and substantial care for those with severe mental illness, and provide care to meet their needs.

All individuals who provide regular and substantial care for a person on CPA should:

- have an assessment of their caring, physical and mental health needs, repeated on at least an annual basis;
- have their own written care plan that is given to them and implemented in discussion with them.

Standard 7 aims to ensure that health and social services play their full part in the achievement of the target set in a previous public health white paper to reduce the suicide rate by at least one fifth by 2010.

The NHS Plan

The year after the NSFMH was published the NHS Plan (Department of Health, 2000) put in place the targets and money that made parts of the NSFMH a reality – specifically improvements in forensic services and intensive community care teams. Three critical targets were the focus of much management action within mental health services:

- 50 early intervention teams to be in place by 2004
- 335 crisis resolution teams by 2004
- 220 assertive outreach teams by 2003.

Implementation of the NSFMH and NHS Plan/achievements

Supporters of mental health policy during the New Labour years tend to focus on seven key areas of achievement:

1 The reform of community care to provide a much more intensive and comprehensive service.
2 Reductions in suicide rates nationally.
3 Large investment in mental health services of perhaps £2bn in real terms and staffing increases averaging about one third.
4 Improvements in inpatient care with around 70 per cent of patients in private rooms.
5 Increased use of new drugs and therapies including psychotherapy.
6 High patient satisfaction.
7 Investment in older people's and children's services (via the two further NSFs mentioned above).

A specific analysis by NSF standard tends to show a more mixed picture. In relation to Standard 1 (Promotion and Prevention) there are very few achievements and no evidence of improved public mental health. Indeed there has been a significant deterioration of the mental health of middle-aged women as shown by epidemiological surveys. Dementia is also increasing in line with demography. Child mental health problems have remained steady at the high levels of 1990s. More recently, and subsequent to the life of the NSFMH, we are seeing more debt-related and stress problems caused by the economic environment. This poor progress is reflected by very low levels of investment in public mental health (between 2000 and 2009 only around 0.1 per cent of annual NHS mental health spend was spent on mental health promotion, the subject of Standard One). Arguably other Ministries such as Education have invested more in emotional well-being than Health.

In terms of Standards 2 and 3 (Primary Mental Health Care) there have been some ad hoc improvements, but these are hard to measure. General Practitioners (GPs) use interventions other than medication sporadically although many wish to do so. A policy of expansion of psychological therapy provision was fought for long and hard by mental health charities and professional bodies. Some initial progress has been made with extra ring-fenced funding, but in many parts of the country there is still a struggle to establish adequate and effective psychological therapy services.

The greatest achievements seem to be in relation to Standards 4 and 5 (Secondary Care), which appears to have improved in both quality and quantity and is regarded as being amongst the best in the world for a public sector mental health service. However, large resources are being spent on secure care and some inpatient care without clear outcomes. Services are still not fully user or recovery oriented although some good progress has been made.

In relation to Standard 6 (Carers) little was achieved except to introduce carers' assessments and there is little value in assessment in isolation. On Standard 7, suicide rates have been reduced and a good strategy (refreshed in 2011) was put in place, although a causal link between the two is hard to prove.

Overall, it appears that major progress was made in mental health service development during the New Labour years but with a number of key deficits:

- There were and are no plans to deal with ineffective services such as unfocused day care and counselling. Inpatient care also lacks an absolute evidence base but progress has been made to reform this.
- Secure settings and prisons seem to be used as modern asylums at huge financial and human cost.
- Services remain poorer for young adults, older people and people from ethnic minorities.
- As stated above, there is a dearth of investment in promotion and prevention.
- Services are still too medically focused and too downstream with not enough early intervention – housing and employment support services for example.
- Mental health workforce planning has created a model that is arguably still too top heavy and lacking integration, for example between psychology and other services.
- Stakeholder input into policy has been poor but input into many local services has improved.
- There is no clear hierarchy of priorities, giving the impression that policy is unachievable.

The policy challenges under the Coalition Government

This leaves us, therefore, with a number of serious challenges ahead, both in terms of establishing policies that will provide a framework for tackling these deficits, and in turning policy into everyday practice that is truly patient-centred, recovery-based and integrated, in terms of primary and secondary mental health services and support across different agencies such as housing, criminal justice and social care.

The new mental health strategy

The Coalition Government, elected in 2010, published its own new mental health strategy in January 2011 (Department of Health, 2011). This set out six key 'shared objectives', in many ways echoing the seven standards set out in the 1999 NSFMH.

The six shared objectives are:

(i)   More people will have good mental health
More people of all ages and backgrounds will have better wellbeing and good mental health. Fewer people will develop mental health problems – by starting well, developing well, working well, living well and ageing well.

(ii) More people with mental health problems will recover
More people who develop mental health problems will have a good quality of life – i.e. a greater ability to manage their own lives, stronger social relationships, a greater sense of purpose, the skills they need for living and working, improved chances in education, better employment rates and a suitable and stable place to live.

(iii) More people with mental health problems will have good physical health
Fewer people with mental health problems will die prematurely, and more people with physical ill health will have better mental health.

(iv) More people will have a positive experience of care and support
Care and support, wherever it takes place, should offer access to timely, evidence-based interventions and approaches that give people the greatest choice and control over their own lives, in the least restrictive environment, and should ensure that people's human rights are protected.

(v) Fewer people will suffer avoidable harm
People receiving care and support should have confidence that the services they use are of the highest quality and at least as safe as any other public service.

(vi) Fewer people will experience stigma and discrimination
Public understanding of mental health will improve and, as a result, negative attitudes and behaviours to people with mental health problems will decrease.

(Department of Health, 2011)

The strategy can be seen as an attempt to cement more recent policy thinking into mental health commissioning and service provision for at least the next few years. It has a welcome focus on promoting whole population mental health (which is not the same thing as simply an absence of mental disorder). It puts flesh on the policy mantra that mental health is 'everyone's business' by citing a wide range of public and private services such as education, employment and housing as essential players in improving whole population mental health, as well as enabling individuals with mental health problems to recover and lead fulfilling lives in their communities.

Importantly, the strategy is also age-inclusive, reflecting that services should be based on need, not age – a policy that was boosted by the passing of the Equality Act in 2010, which makes it illegal to provide less favourable treatment to anyone on grounds of age. This should help overcome some of the problems that people have faced getting service support at transitional times, from childhood into adulthood, and from adult services into older people's services.

Delivering policy through outcomes

There remains, of course, a significant question mark over how mental health policy, as embodied in the strategy, will be implemented. The Labour Government provided significant new funding for mental health and made targets (as set out in the NHS Plan 2000, see above) a key lever for improvements, although these were criticised by some for being arbitrary, inflexible and likely to lead to inappropriate local prioritisation. The present Coalition Government, at a time of recession, is unlikely to commit significant new sums to mental health, and has opted for delivery through outcomes as the key driver for service improvements. We therefore have a new NHS Outcomes Framework, Social Care Outcomes Framework and Public Health Outcomes Framework, all of which contain some specific outcome measures in mental health. The intention is that the proposed new NHS Commissioning Board will also create a set of outcomes, as will each local area.

It is possible, if the right recovery-based outcomes are chosen in collaboration with people who use mental health services and their carers, that an outcome-focused approach might bring significant benefits. For example, it could help to end the commissioning and provision of ineffective services, and support the wider acceptance of the social recovery model of care, which may be as much about an individual having a job and stable accommodation as about reducing clinical symptomology.

However, alongside the establishment of national outcome measures, the Government has simultaneously been promoting a policy of localism. This means that while it will be looking to local mental health services (among other public services) to deliver the outcomes it has set, it is up to local areas to decide how best to do this within its own priorities. The likely result of this is an increase in the variations in service provision between different areas, leading to continued complaints about a 'postcode lottery'.

Key areas for policy development

While mental health policy makers need to keep a wide range of issues under review, three areas might be seen as particular priorities – the mental health needs of children and older people, the quest for integrated care and the personalisation agenda.

Children and older people

If mental health policy (and funding) has primarily been directed in recent years at adults of working age, then there is growing recognition that in the coming years there needs to be a focus on developing mental health policy in respect of both children and older people.

There is an ever-growing evidence base demonstrating that the circumstances of children's early years are hugely important in terms of building emotional resilience and reducing the risk of developing mental disorders later in life, and that effective early years, family and school-based interventions are essential to minimise this risk. This is reflected in the 'starting well and developing well' elements of the first shared objective of the new mental health strategy. Over and above the simple health case for optimising our children's emotional well-being, there is a strong economic business case for investing in this area (Children and Young People's Mental Health Coalition, 2010).

At the same time, future predictions indicate that there will be a growing population of older people (post-state retirement age) in England. While we can welcome living longer, it is inevitable that many older people will move into later life with a mental health problem, or may develop a problem during their later years, alongside a range of physical health problems associated with older age. In particular, the number of people with dementia is expected to increase significantly. Mental health (and social care) policy will need to address the challenges posed by this significantly older population, not least because of the potential future costs: a King's Fund report of 2008 estimated that the annual health and social care costs of supporting people with dementia could increase in real terms from £14.8 billion in 2007 to £34.8 billion by 2026 (King's Fund, 2008). Early intervention is as important a policy for older people as it is for children and younger adults. We need to encourage more research on early intervention initiatives to learn what works best and further strengthen the evidence base.

Integrated care

Integrating a range of care and support to achieve better outcomes for people with a mental illness is hardly new. In 1949, only one year after the NHS came into being, the Chief Medical Officer reported:

an increasing interest in the factors which lead to mental illness and an interest in the less overt forms of mental illness in which environmental factors play a relatively greater part.... the part played by the parents and the home in causing the maladjustment of the child leads to attempts to improve the milieu in which the child lives... the effect of unsuitable working conditions leads to interest in vocational guidance and personnel selection, [the] effect of the domestic situation leads to interest in problems of housing, divorce, delinquency and so on.

(Ministry of Health, 1949)

For the past 60 years we have therefore understood the need to address mental health issues holistically. In that time there have been many admirable policies aimed at encouraging better joint working and integrated care within and between agencies (especially health and social care) and in parts of the country this is very successfully done. It is, however, something that has proved exceptionally hard to achieve consistently and sustainably. While one can welcome recent Government statements highlighting the need for integrated services, they can in effect be seen as an admission of this failure:

The Government is committed to integrated services that improve quality of care for patients and improve efficiency. We want to achieve this as much through cultural and behavioural change as through statutory requirements, and our proposals are intended to create a facilitative environment for the commissioning of integrated services.

(HM Government, 2011)

The policy of developing integrated services for people with mental health needs is clearly the right one, but we are going to have to get better at implementing it if we are not to be having the same discussions in 10, 20 and 30 years' time.

Personalisation

Personalisation has been defined as 'starting with the person as an individual with strengths, preferences and aspirations and putting them at the centre of the process of identifying their needs and making choices about how and when they are supported to live their lives' (Social Care Institute for Excellence, 2010). Personalisation has been a policy driver in social care provision for some years, and is being increasingly used in the context of health services. The Government's current NHS mantra of 'Nothing about us, without us' aims to place the patient as an equal partner in his or her care decisions, not just a passive recipient of care. This may be a particular challenge within mental health services, given the historic power imbalance between mental health professionals and patients.

Providing a good personalised service does not necessarily require individuals to take control of the money that is spent on their care. However, there is evidence that personal budgets for people who use mental health services for social care, housing and employment support have been proven to help keep them well, and resulted in better psychological health (Department of Health, 2008). It remains to be seen whether personal health budgets, at present being piloted, will produce the same benefits, and whether mental health professionals – trained in risk management – will support their patients in taking up budgets. Regardless of this, mental health policy should continue to be based on the principle that people who experience mental health problems have the same rights as any other citizen to be treated as an individual with personal preferences, and the presumption that, unless otherwise proven, they have the capacity to make decisions about what care they receive.

Mental health legislation

We mentioned at the start of this chapter that policy can be implemented through legislation. The Labour Government of 1997–2010 spent almost a decade trying to introduce new mental health legislation, culminating in the controversial Mental Health Act 2007 that among other things introduced Community Treatment Orders. This Act amended, but did not replace as originally intended, the Mental Health Act 1983.

We do not know what future events may grab the attention of Ministers and the media in the future to stimulate new legislation, and there has been some interest in looking at whether it would be better to create a single capacity-based piece of legislation in England (as Northern Ireland is considering) that would amalgamate current Mental Health and Mental Capacity Acts. However, it appears unlikely that there will be a major new piece of English mental health law tabled in the next 10 years. Significant shifts in mental health legislation tend to come along once a generation – the 1890 Lunacy Act was amended only by the Mental Health Treatment Act of 1930, to be followed by the 1959, 1983 and (amending) 2007 Mental Health Acts.

The wider policy picture

We also mentioned at the start of this chapter generic policies on, for example, health, welfare and housing and their potential impact on mental health. It is unrealistic and unhelpful to think of mental health policy as separate from the wider policy world established under the previous Labour Government and by and large embraced by the new Coalition Government. For example, the Government-wide drive for choice applies to mental health as much as any other part of the NHS. By the same token, the Government's strategy for public health (Department of Health, 2010) includes a commitment to build people's self-esteem, confidence and resilience right from infancy, with stronger support for early years – as suggested above, this being a key area for future mental health policy as well.

If we are serious about improving public mental health, though, a key issue for any future Government will be how to ensure that a mental health assessment is built into polices across a range of Government departments touching on all aspects of people's lives.

Conclusion

There has been widespread acceptance of the broad direction of mental health policy in England over the past 20 or 30 years, under all Governments. This has largely been a story of gradual improvements in community support for people with mental health problems following the closure of the large asylums, alongside an even more gradual shift – by no means completed – from a medical to a social model of care.

The future is likely to see a continuing evolution of the main trends that have already been set in place, such as mental health being seen as on a par with physical health (indeed, the two being inextricably linked), the recognition that people with mental health problems have rights and should be equal partners in their care, and the development of better integrated individual care pathways and care planning involving a range of support agencies. The stigma of mental illness, such a barrier to people's recovery, will hopefully lessen, although changing public attitudes and behaviour around the risk that mentally ill people pose will require a continuing policy drive based on the best evidence of what works.

In the light of the Coalition Government's NHS reforms, we will see a more diverse range of mental health service providers, with the private and voluntary sectors vying for business with more traditional statutory services. However, in the foreseeable future a great deal of mental health expenditure will continue to be targeted at relatively few patients with higher levels of support needs. At a time of severe financial constraints, there is a real risk that this will lead to many people with lower (though still significant) levels of need losing what limited support they currently get. Policies need to be developed that tackle this risk, regardless of the diversification of service providers.

Of course it is one thing to design an evidence-based mental health policy, and another ensure that that policy translates into effective practice on the ground, especially at a time of severe public service spending constraints such as we have today. Many of the service improvements we saw between 2000 and 2010 were the result of a significant amount of new money being allocated to mental health. Now that those times have passed it is perhaps incumbent on the creators of future mental health policy for England to be pragmatic about what can be achieved, without losing the vision of a future where we not only provide excellent, timely, person-centred support to anyone who experiences a mental disorder, but we reduce the number of citizens who develop such disorders in the first place.

References

Children and Young People's Mental Health Coalition (2010) *Improving Children and Young People's Mental Health: the business case*, London: Children and Young People's Mental Health Coalition.

Department of Health (1999) *National Service Framework for Mental Health*, London: Department of Health.

Department of Health (2000) *The NHS Plan: a plan for investment, a plan for reform*, London: Department of Health.

Department of Health (2008) *Evaluation of the Individual Budgets Pilot Programme: final report*, London: Department of Health.

Department of Health (2010) *Healthy Lives, Healthy People: our strategy for public health in England*, London: Department of Health.

Department of Health (2011) *No Health without Mental Health: delivering better mental health outcomes for people of all ages*, London: Department of Health.

HM Government (2011) *Government Response to the House of Commons Health Select Committee Fifth Report of Session 2010–11: commissioning*, London: HM Government.

King's Fund (2008) *Paying the Price: the cost of mental health care in England to 2026*, London: King's Fund.

Koontz, H. and Weihrich, H. (1988) *Management*, New York: McGraw-Hill.

McCulloch, A. and Parker, C. (2004) Compliance, Assertive Community Treatment and Mental Health Inquiries. Chapter in Stanley, N. and Manthorpe, J. (eds) *The Age of Inquiries*. London: Routledge.

McCulloch, A., Glover, G. and St John, T. (2003) The National Service Framework: past, present and future, *The Mental Health Review*. 8(4) 7–17.

Ministry of Health (1949)*Report of the Ministry of Health for the Year Ended 31st March 1949*, Cmd.7910, London: HMSO.

Muijen, M. and McCulloch, A. (2009) Public Policy and Mental Health. Chapter in Gelder, M. *et al.* (eds) *New Oxford Textbook of Psychiatry*. Oxford: Oxford University Press.

Sainsbury Centre for Mental Health (1999) *Policy Briefing on the National Service Framework for Mental Health*, London: The Sainsbury Centre for Mental Health.

Social Care Institute for Excellence (2010) *Personalisation – a rough guide 2008* (revised 2010), London: SCIE.

2 UK mental health policy development

A counter-argument deriving from users' experiences

Rachel E. Perkins

The many shortcomings of existing mental health services have been extensively catalogued over the years. In response, demands have generally been for 'more'. More professionals, bigger and better services. While I would not challenge the need for better services, does this really mean more professionals, bigger services? I think not.

In offering an alternative perspective on mental health policy and mental health services I write from that uncomfortable 'no (wo)man's land' between 'them' and 'us'. For thirty years I worked in mental health services. This career took me from Assistant Psychologist at Broadmoor Hospital through the ranks of Clinical Psychology to Clinical Director of rehabilitation, then general adult mental health services and on to Director of Quality Assurance and User Experience in South West London. Twenty years ago I embarked on a somewhat different psychiatric career – that of 'mental patient': a career that has put me on the receiving end of both inpatient and community mental health services. Services look very different from the other side of the fence. I felt completely at sea without map or compass: amazed at how little my professional training helped me to navigate life with mental health problems.

It was not until the early 1990s that I found a way of thinking about mental health conditions that made sense to me as both provider and recipient of mental health services. People like Judi Chamberlin, Patricia Deegan and Mary O'Hagan introduced me to ideas about recovery: an approach born not of learned professionals but of the lived experience of people who had themselves faced the challenge of living with and growing beyond a diagnosis of mental health problems (see, for example, Chamberlin, 1978; Deegan, 1988; O'Hagan, 1993). It is this approach that has guided my work over the last two decades and on which I have based the views about mental health policy. In essence I will argue that we need genuinely recovery-focused mental health policy.

What is 'recovery'?

Recovery is not about 'recovering from an illness' – it is about 'recovering a life' – rebuilding a meaningful, satisfying and contributing life. Recovery is '…the lived or real life experience of people as they accept and overcome the challenge of the disability. They experience themselves as recovering a new sense of self and of purpose within and beyond the limits of the disability' (Deegan, 1988).

Recovery is not something that services or professionals do, it is a personal journey of discovery: making sense of, and finding meaning in, what has happened; discovering your own resources, resourcefulness and possibilities; building a new sense of self, meaning and purpose in life; growing within and beyond what has happened to you; and pursuing your dreams and ambitions.

The challenge for services is to assist people in their journey. Everyone's journey is individual and uniquely personal. The writing of those with lived experience of recovery suggests that three things are critical (see Repper and Perkins, 2006; Shepherd *et al.*, 2008):

- Hope. It is not possible to rebuild your life unless you believe that a decent life is possible and you need people around who believe in your possibilities.
- Control. Taking back control over your destiny, the challenges you face and the help you receive to overcome them.
- Opportunity. The chance to do the things that you value, access those opportunities that all citizens should expect and participate in society as an equal citizen.

This experiential expertise is supported by empirical research evidence. In his extensive review of the international research literature Warner (2009) demonstrates three things to be important in recovery: optimism, empowerment and employment. Sadly, it remains the case that too often mental health services erode hope, take control over our lives and fail to assist us in pursuing our dreams and ambitions.

There are encouraging signs. Government mental health policy increasingly talks about the need to break down prejudice and discrimination, promote recovery and enable people with mental health challenges to access jobs, homes and friends (Department of Health 2009, 2011). However, the primary focus remains fixing us through treatment, prescribing what is good for us, ensuring our compliance/adherence to these prescriptions and containment under the auspices of preventing harm to ourselves or others.

If mental health policy is to be truely recovery-focused then more fundamental changes are required. Two key issues need to be addressed: the purpose of mental health services and the balance of power between services and the individuals and communities that they serve.

What is the purpose of services?

Mental health services continue to be organised around three 'C's: cure, care and containment. The overarching paradigm guiding the work of services is one of cure: the reduction/ elimination of symptoms or problems. Unless and until a person's problems can be eliminated they are 'cared for' and, should they be a threat to their own health and safety or that of others, contained. Professionals of different hues may vie for supremacy – debate whose explanatory paradigm is 'correct', whose interventions are 'best' – but the primary aim is problem removal: moving away from problems, but towards what?

Professionals think about 'the patient in our services' and start by defining a person's symptoms and problems, then prescribe interventions and the services/supports the person is deemed to 'need' in order to achieve the goal of 'cure'. Needs are defined in terms of what services have to offer, like inpatient care, assertive outreach, medication and assorted therapies, and our history becomes the history of our psychiatric becoming. Personal strengths, goals, social circumstances, activities, values, beliefs, goals etc. are considered only in so far as they inform decisions about diagnosis, treatment, support and prognosis.

Recovery-focused services start in a different place, thinking not about 'the patient in our services' but 'the person in their life'. Where we have been, what has happened, where we are now, what we have got going for us, what is important to us and what we want to do in our lives. The primary goal is to help people to move towards a future: to live the life they want to live and do the things they want to do. We do not build our futures on the basis of our deficits and dysfunctions – ambitions are realised, and dreams pursued, on the foundation of our strengths and resources. Symptoms, diagnosis, prognosis, treatment, support and services must be considered not in terms of how much they reduce problems but how far they enable (or impede) the person to do the things they want to do and live a satisfying, meaningful and valued life.

People may find a range of different treatments and therapies useful in their journey, but the removal of symptoms/problems cannot be the overarching purpose of mental health policy. Symptom removal is not a sufficient condition for rebuilding a life, neither is it a necessary condition: many have shown us that it is possible to live a meaningful, satisfying and contributing life in the presence of symptoms and ongoing challenges. 'Recovery requires reframing the treatment enterprise … the issue is what role treatment plays in recovery' (Davidson *et al.*, 2006).

Warner (2009) shows that, for the most part, there is an inverse relationship between recovery from schizophrenia and the number of learned professionals around. Not only is it the case that recovery from schizophrenia is greater, and mortality lower, in the 'developing' world, but 'One of the most robust findings about schizophrenia is that a substantial proportion … will recover completely or with good functional capacity, with or without modern medical treatment' (Warner, 2009).

Some people find treatment – whether psychological or pharmacological – helpful, but they form but a part (and probably a smaller part than most professionals would care to acknowledge) of what is often a rich tapestry of ways in which people manage the challenges they face.

> Over the years I have worked hard to become an expert in my own self-care … Over the years I have learned different ways of helping myself. Sometimes I use medications, therapy, self-help and mutual support groups, friends, my relationship with God, work, exercise, spending time in nature – all of these measures help me remain whole and healthy, even though I have a disability.
>
> (Deegan, 1993)

Recovery-focused mental health policy must have as its overarching aim supporting people to take back control, do the things they want to do and participate as equal citizens. The role of professional treatment and intervention treatment lies in supporting self-care and the pursuit of ambitions rather than 'fixing' people. A change in purpose requires a change in the means of evaluating efficacy. The question is not whether neuroleptic medication, psychological therapy or assertive outreach alleviates symptoms but whether these enable someone to take back control and pursue their ambitions in life. We need a whole new evidence base.

Changing the balance of power

Mental health services maintain clear demarcations between 'them' and 'us': professionals and patients. There is one set of experts – the learned professionals – who it is assumed have access to a body of knowledge that cannot be understood by non-experts. Therefore the task of professionals is to tell people what they should do and get them to comply with these prescriptions.

Because of their special knowledge, reality in mental health services is defined by professionals in terms of the theories on which their profession is based (see Perkins and Moodley, 1993). Professionals do not always agree. Arguments ensue about whether 'reality' is defined in organic, psychological, systemic or social terms, or alternatively 'fusion' theories

– like a 'bio-psychosocial' approach – may be adopted. However, the principle remains the same: professionals define the patients reality in terms that their profession has invented, then try to persuade the patient of the veracity of our explanation – 'a correct attitude to a morbid change in oneself' (Lewis, 1934) – and deem them to lack insight if they disagree (David, 1990). Professionals then prescribe how it might be put right and then ensure compliance – for the person's own good, of course! 'Given the established efficacy of neuroleptic drugs in psychotic disorders, and the devastating consequences of relapse, non-compliance is one of the major preventable causes of psychiatric morbidity and a research priority in the NHS' (Kemp *et al.*, 1996).

Attempts to increase compliance have been many and varied, from mental health legislation allowing forced medication, through suggestions that welfare benefits be contingent on treatment compliance (Thompson, 1996) to the development of 'compliance therapy' (Kemp *et al.*, 1996, 1998).

Ideas about recovery start from a different place. Each person is the expert in their own recovery and has a right to define their own reality. In recovery-focused services there are two sets of expertise: 'experts by profession' whose expertise derives from empirical research evidence and 'experts by lived experience' whose expertise is founded on personal narratives and experience. Mental health professionals should be, as Winston Churchill said of scientists, 'on tap' and not 'on top' (Churchill, 1964). Instead of prescribing what is good for a person, professionals need to put their empirically based knowledge at the disposal of those whom they serve: make available their expertise, interventions and supports for us to use if/when we find them helpful in our recovery journey and looking after ourselves along the way.

We must move beyond ideas about 'user involvement'. For professionals, 'involvement' typically means involving 'them' in 'our' services and treatment/support decisions. In recovery-focused services the question is reversed: do they want to involve 'us' (professionals/services) in 'their' lives. Recovery-focused services would bring together the expertise of lived experience and professional expertise on equal terms in a process of genuine co-production to create a range of options that people want to utilise in their recovery journeys. At the heart of such co-production lies a fundamental shift in the balance of power at all levels: from the design and development of policy, through the development and delivery of treatment and services, to shared decision making at the level of the individual.

> Shared decision making diverges radically from compliance because it assumes two experts – the client and the practitioner – must share respective information and determine collaboratively optimum treatment.... It helps to bridge the empirical evidence base, which is established on population averages, with the unique concerns, values and life context of the individual client. From the vantage point of the individual healthcare client, the efficacy of a particular medication is not certain ... the question of how the medication will affect the individual becomes an open experiment for two co-experimenters – the client and the practitioner.
>
> (Deegan and Drake, 2006)

The development of 'personal health budgets' that allow people to purchase the support, treatment and services they find helpful have the potential to really change the balance of power and make a reality of co-production (see Alakeson, 2011).

In creating services based on self-management and self-direction, recovery-focused mental health policy must help people to use their own resources and resourcefulness. This might involve:

- 'Coaching' rather than 'therapeutic' relationships. Therapeutic relationships necessarily involve an expert 'therapist' and a 'patient/client' and should be restricted to technical therapy sessions. A coaching relationship is one that helps a person to arrive at their own decisions about what is important to them and recognise their own strengths and resources, and use these to achieve their goals. The coach is not 'more expert' than the person they are coaching; their role is to enable the person to realise their own potential – Rafael Nadal has a coach, but he is without doubt not a better tennis player than Rafael himself!
- An educational approach:

> reinforcing and developing people's strengths rather than adding to the attention placed on what is 'wrong' with them … [helping people to] discover who they are, learn skills and tools that promote recovery, what they can be, and the unique contributions they have to offer.
>
> (Ashcraft and Anthony, 2005)

How much of what we currently do as 'therapy' or 'groups' could be better done in the form of seminars, workshops and courses? Courses co-produced and co-delivered where experts by experience, people who are close to them and professionals could learn together? These might incude developing the skills of both professionals and those whom they serve to participate in the co-production/shared decision making (see Deegan *et al.*, 2008; The Health Foundation, 2008).

- A different approach to providing information: helping people to do their own research, and providing opportunities for them to gain intelligence from their peers.
- Providing opportunities for people to develop their own Recovery Plans (see Copeland, 2000; Perkins and Rinaldi, 2007)
- A different kind of workforce: no longer 'them' and 'us'.

People who have travelled a similar journey are often the best travelling companions. If you need to have heart surgery, then you would be best advised to consult a qualified heart surgeon, but if you have to live with a damaged heart then someone who is facing similar challenges – maybe someone who is a few steps farther down the road than you – is probably more useful to you. Most heart surgeons have never themselves faced the challenges of those on whom they operate. Similarly, if you want psychotherapy, then you would be best advised to find a qualified psychotherapist, but they are unlikely to be expert in rebuilding life with a mental health condition.

Peer support helps people to feel less alone, fosters hope and images of possibility and support from someone who better understands what you are going through because they have been through similar things themself. It allows people to share experiences, understanding, ideas about dealing with challenges, and is of mutual benefit by enabling people to use their experience to help others facing similar challenges (see, for example, Bassett *et al.*, 2010; Repper and Carter, 2010). There are many ways of gaining peer support (naturally occurring peer support, informal arrangements, self-help groups) and changing the workforce to include formalised or intentional peer support, by training and employing peer support workers. If the expertise of lived experience is important in recovery then it must be available within mental health services (Ashcraft and Anthony, 2005). Peer support workers are not just another set of professionals. Peer support involves a different kind of relationship: mutual support provided by people with similar life experiences as they move through difficult situations (Repper and Carter, 2010).

Much, if not most, of what mental health services do is *not* technical treatment – so why do we need professionals to do it? Might 'experts through lived experience' be better placed? Are there not risks in using professionals to provide support in areas in which they are not expert – living with and rebuilding life with a diagnosis of mental illness? Not only do we deprive people of the expertise of lived experience, we also risk deskilling and disempowering those whom we serve, not to mention wasting scarce resources (see Shepherd *et al.*, 2008).

> As services become more truly focused on service users' needs and accept the value of 'lived experience' ... we expect to see a greatly expanded role for 'peer professionals' in the mental health service workforce of the future. We recommend that organisations should consider a radical transformation of the workforce, aiming for perhaps 50% of care delivery by appropriately trained and supported 'peer professionals'.
>
> (Sainsbury Centre for Mental Health, 2010)

Changing the balance of power: what about compulsory detention and treatment?

Any consideration of the balance of power in mental health policy would be incomplete without addressing the powers of compulsion afforded by the state in mental health legislation to those who provide mental health services. 'Power ... is what the system is all about.... The existence and widespread use of involuntary commitment affects all aspects of mental health care ... Most clients never face commitment but they know the power is there' (Chamberlin, 1978).

The 1983 Mental Health Act allows people to be detained in hospital and treated against their will on the grounds of their own safety or for the protection of others. It is not really possible to change the balance of power in services – really enable people to take control over their own lives and foster genuine co-production and shared decision making – if, at the bottom line, the professional can force the patient to do what they think is best.

Mental health legislation is intrinsically discriminatory. It affords powers to compulsorily detain and treat people deemed to have 'mental disorders' in a manner that would be inconceivable among those with physical health conditions (see, for example, Dawson and Szmukler 2006; Szmukler *et al.*, 2010). In England and Wales compulsory treatment of people defined as having 'physical' conditions is governed by the 2005 Mental Capacity Act while those defined as having 'mental' conditions are subject to the additional powers of the 1983 Mental Health Act. If a person with a physical health condition is able to understand the nature of treatment, why it is being proposed and the consequences of accepting it or not then they cannot be forced to accept treatment even if refusal would be damaging to their health. They can make a decision in light of the things that are important to them. Even if the treatment may save or prolong their life, if they consider the costs to outweigh the benefits they have a right to refuse it. Not so for people deemed to have 'mental disorders' (the definition of which is very broad). Even if a person has 'capacity' as defined in the 2005 Mental Capacity Act, they can be detained and forcibly treated if their 'mental disorder' is deemed by professional experts to be of a nature and degree that makes treatment 'appropriate' and 'necessary' for the person's health and safety or for the protection of others. So if I am deemed to have cancer I can decide what treatment I have; if I am deemed to have bipolar disorder I am denied that right. So much for the maxim that can often be heard on the lips of practitioners: 'mental illness is an illness like any other' (see Sayce, 2000)!

Compulsory powers extend beyond a paternalistic concern about what is good for the person – to consideration of risk to others. Most citizens cannot be deprived of their liberty because someone thinks they might commit an offence: even if they, for example, drink and have a short temper they are 'innocent until proved guilty' under the law. But if you have a 'mental disorder' you can be deprived of your liberty if someone thinks you might be a risk. Remember, people who are considered to have a serious mental disorder are responsible for only a small fraction of the violence in our society and violence is no more predictable in those with a mental disorder than in those without (see Fazel and Grann, 2006, 2009; Szmukler *et al.*, 2010).

The existence of mental health legislation denies people deemed to have 'mental disorders' their rights. The UK has ratified the 2006 United Nations Convention on the Rights of Persons with Disabilities, which explicitly includes people with longer term mental health problems within the rubric of disability. This convention states that there must be respect for inherent human dignity and individual autonomy including the freedom to make one's own choices (article 3), people must enjoy legal capacity on an equal basis with others in all aspects of life (article 12) and that the existence of disability shall in no case justify a deprivation of liberty (article 14). As indicated by the Annual Report of the High Commissioner for Human Rights (Office of the High Commissioner for Human Rights, 2009) the 1983 Mental Health Act does not meet these requirements.

Mental health legislation also actively reinforces the destructive myths that result in discrimination and exclusion: that people with mental health conditions have lost the ability to 'act rationally' (and so are unpredictable and dangerous and must be detained for the good of others) and/or have lost the ability of 'sound reasoning' (and therefore their expressed views, wishes and preferences can be disregarded – for their own good, of course).

It is particularly alarming that, at the same time as we have seen ideas about recovery and the need to break down prejudice and discrimination appearing in mental health policy (Department of Health, 2009, 2011), the number of people forcibly detained and treated has increased and the powers of compulsion have been extended. Care Quality Commission (2010) data show that the number of detentions in hospital under the Mental Health Act increased from 23,982 in 1989/90 to 41,828 in 1999/2000 and 45,755 in 2009/10. At the same time, the 2007 Mental Health Act extended the powers of compulsion to include Community Treatment Orders (CTOs) compelling people to receive treatment in the community and allowing for recall to hospital if they failed to comply. The rhetoric ran that it would allow for earlier discharge and reduce hospital admissions if people could be compelled to receive treatment in the community, therefore the number of people detained in hospital would decrease. Initial estimates were that there would be around 400–600 CTOs per year (see Lawton-Smith, 2010). The reality has proved very different. CTOs were introduced in November 2008. In the first full year of their operation the number of people compulsorily detained in hospital increased from 43,999 in 2008/9 to 45,755 in 2009/10 and in 2009/10 there were an additional 4017 CTOs: a staggering increase of 5773 people in a single year being subject to compulsory powers.

Recovery-focused mental health policy requires that we rethink our approach to mental health legislation, possibly along the lines of that proposed by Szmukler *et al.* (2010). They have proposed the abolition of specific mental health legislation and its replacement with a single capacity-based law covering treatment without consent of all conditions – 'physical' and 'mental' – in all health care settings.

> ... one that requires us to assess the ability of a person to understand, recall, use and weigh relevant treatment information, and to communicate a treatment decision ... a legal regime that ... relies squarely on the incapacity of the person to make necessary treatment decisions, in association with a 'best interests' test, as the key justification for intervention in their life.
>
> (Szmukler *et al.*, 2010)

But we also need to consider the relationship between discriminatory mental health legislation and the position of people deemed 'mentally ill' in society. In his book *Long Walk to Freedom* Nelson Mandela (1995) described a situation where his fellow prisoners on Robben Island were campaigning for the better treatment of Blacks in prison. He remarked that the position of Blacks in prison was unlikely to improve until the position of Blacks in society changed. Maybe similar wisdom might apply to 'mental patients'.

Changing the individual or changing the world?

Recovery-focused mental health policy requires a shift from a primary focus on problem/symptom removal to helping people to live the lives they want to lead, do the things they want to do and participate as equal citizens. Therefore it is necessary to consider not only ways of changing the person so they 'fit in' (by treating symptoms and remedying skills deficits), but changing the world so it can accommodate the person. Mental health conditions do not occur in a vacuum; they exist in a social context: one in which people defined as 'mentally ill' are among the most excluded (Social Exclusion Unit, 2004).

In the broader disability world, people were told by professionals that the problems lay within them – in their lack of mobility, hearing, etc. However, disabled people came to realise that their impairments were a given, not a problem: that the real problems lay in barriers in the environment – in people's attitudes and the lack of equipment, adjustments and support that they needed to do the things they wanted to do. Therefore, although for many treatment remains important, a 'medical' or 'clinical' model of disability was replaced by a 'social model' and an approach based on rights not 'cure'. It is such an approach that underpins the United Nations Declaration on the Rights of Disabled People, and the 1995 UK Disability Discrimination Act and, for the most part, the 2010 Equality Act. The premise that the real barriers to building/rebuilding a life and participating as an equal citizen lie not within the individual but in society can be seen in development of ideas about recovery among people with lived experience of mental health conditions, and some have drawn parallels with counterparts in the disability movement (see, for example, Deegan, 1988, 1992; Chamberlin, 1993, 1995; Sayce, 2000).

> If we think about it, having a psychiatric disability is, for many of us, simply a given. The real problems exist in the form of barriers in the environment that prevent us from living, working and learning in environments of our choice. [The task is] to confront, challenge and change those barriers and to make environments accessible ... If we remember that environments are not just physical places but also social and interpersonal environments, then it is clear that those of us with psychiatric disabilities face many environmental barriers that impede and thwart our efforts to live independently and gain control over our lives and the resources that affect our lives.
>
> (Deegan, 1992)

Having access to those opportunities that all citizens should expect as well as access to, and control over, the support and adjustments that you need to do the things you want to do are central. The challenge is therefore one of creating communities that can accommodate all of us, but the enormity of the task should not be underestimated.

> We must begin to turn toward the people we now isolate – the troubled (and troubling) relatives and friends we both love and fear. It will not be easy. The mental hospital system developed precisely because it is a job that we would rather leave to others.
>
> (Chamberlin, 1978)

Mental health services: from centre stage to the margins

Developments in mental health policy increasingly recognise that mental health is not the preserve of mental health services but permeates all of our society. Yet we have a long way to go in creating communities that genuinely include and value all of us. We may have broken down the old asylums, but we continue to see 'mental health problems' as the province of 'experts' and to marginalise those who experience them.

As Mary O'Hagan (2007) has described, paradoxically, mental health professionals and services (whether they be statutory or voluntary) can, albeit unwittingly, serve to perpetuate marginalisation and exclusion in a kind of vicious cycle. Those of us with mental health problems have come to believe that experts hold the key to our difficulties. Our nearest and dearest have believed we are unsafe in their untrained hands – they should leave it to the experts. So we all become less and less used to finding our own solutions and embracing distress as a part of ordinary life.

> The biggest challenge that we face is not creating better access to bigger and better professional services, it is maximising the life chances of people with mental health conditions. The real challenge is how to do things differently and use resources differently: recognise the limitations of traditional expertise, the value of the expertise of lived experience …
>
> (Perkins, 2010)

Mental health professionals have a role, but it is a smaller, supporting role, making available technical support and help if and when it is useful to those who need it. It must become as absurd for someone's primary identity to be that of 'mental health service user' as it would be for someone to define themself as a 'general practice service user' (Perkins, 2010). Like general practitioners, mental health professionals should be there in the background providing easy access to a range of treatments when needed to assist people to thrive in those roles that are important to them: as partners, parents, workers, footballers …

Mental health policy should focus on creating (or re-creating) communities that can accommodate all of us: helping both individuals and the communities we serve to discover their own resources and resourcefulness. 'People with mental health problems, as well as communities, need to start believing they hold most of the solutions to human problems, instead of professionals and services' (O'Hagan, 2007).

This cannot be a professional endeavour. If professionals are educating communities about people with mental health conditions then we will simply reinforce beliefs that professionals hold all the answers. The challenge we face is to hand over control to individuals and communities, by 'fostering service-user leadership in recovery and in services, integrating with other sectors, and engaging in community development and social inclusion work' (O'Hagan, 2007).

Perhaps the most useful approach would be to integrate mental health policy with the broader disability arena and the social model and rights-based approach on which it is founded. Focus attention on those rights to which we are entitled within the United Nations Declaration on the Rights of Persons with Disabilities – the rights to independent living on which broader disability policy is predicated.

> All disabled people having the same choice, control and freedom as any other citizen – at home, at work and as members of the community. This does not necessarily mean disabled people 'doing everything for themselves' but it does mean that any practical assistance people need should be based on their own choices and aspirations.
>
> (Office for Disability Issues, 2008)

A rights-based approach based on a social model of disability would change the focus of policy from treatment to recovery and inclusion and, in conjunction with the control afforded by personal budgets, change power relationships by placing professionals 'on tap' rather than 'on top'.

References

Alakeson, V. (2011) *Active Patient. The case for self-direction in healthcare*, University of Birmingham/The Centre for Welfare Reform Joint Policy Paper, 5 January

Ashcraft, L. and Anthony, W.A. (2005) A story of transformation. An agency fully embraces recovery, *Behavioral Healthcare Tomorrow*, 14, 12–21

Bassett, T., Faulkner, A., Repper, J. and Stanou, S. (2010) *Lived Experience Leading the Way. Peer support in mental health*, London: Together

Care Quality Commission (2010) *Monitoring the Use of the Mental Health Act in 2009/10*, London: Care Quality Commission

Chamberlin, J. (1978) *On Our Own*, New York: Hawthorn

Chamberlin, J. (1993) Psychiatric disabilities and the ADA. An advocates perspective, in Gostin, L.O. and Beyer, H.A. (Eds) *Implementing the Americans with Disabilities Act*, Baltimore, MD: Brookes

Chamberlin, J. (1995) Psychiatric survivors: Are we part of the disability movement?, *Disability Rag and Resource*, March/April, 4–7

Churchill, W. L. S. quoted in Churchill. R.S. (1964) *Twenty-one Years*, London: Weidenfeld & Nicolson

Copeland, M. E. (2000) *Guide to Developing a WRAP – Wellness Recovery Action Plan*, www.mentalhealthrecovery.com

David, A. (1990) Insight and psychosis, *British Journal of Psychiatry*, 156, 798–808

Davidson, L., O'Connell, and M. Tondora, J. (2006) The top ten concerns about recovery encountered in mental health system transformation, *Psychiatric Services,* 57, pp. 640-645

Dawson, J. and Szmukler, G. (2006) Fusion of mental health and incapacity legislation, *British Journal of Psychiatry*, 188, 504–509

Deegan, P. (1988) Recovery: The lived experience of rehabilitation, *Psychosocial Rehabilitation Journal*, 11, 11–19

Deegan, P. (1992) The independent living movement and people with psychiatric disabilities: Taking back control over our lives, *Psychosocial Rehabilitation Journal*, 15, 3–10

Deegan, P. (1993) Recovering our sense of value after being labelled mentally ill, *Journal of Psychosocial Nursing and Mental Health Services*, 31, 7–11

Deegan, P. and Drake, R. (2006) Shared decision making and medication management in the recovery process, *Psychiatric Services*, 57, 1636–1639

Deegan, P., Rapp, C., Holter, M. and Reifer, M. (2008) A program to support shared decision making in an outpatient psychiatric medication clinic, *Psychiatric Services*, 59, 603–605

Department of Health (2009) *New Horizons. A Shared Vision for Mental Health*, London: HM Government

Department of Health (2011) *No Health without Mental Health: A Cross-Government Mental Health Outcomes Strategy for People of All Ages*, London: HM Government

Fazel, S. and Grann, M. (2006) The population impact of severe mental illness on violent crime, *American Journal of Psychiatry*, 163, 1397–1403

Fazel, S., Gulati, G., Linsell, L., Geddes, J.R. and Grann, M. (2009) Schizophrenia and violence: Systematic review and meta-analysis, *PLoS Medicine*, 1000120, http://www.plosmedicine.org/article/info%3Adoi%2F10.1371%2Fjournal.pmed.1000120

Kemp, R., Hayward, P., Applewhaite, G., Everitt, B. and David, A. (1996) Compliance therapy in psychotic patients: Randomised controlled trial, *British Medical Journal*, 312, 315–319

Kemp, R., Kirov, G., Everitt, B., Hayward, P. and David, A. (1998) Randomised controlled trial of compliance therapy: 18 month follow-up, *British Journal of Psychiatry*, 172, 413–419

Lawton-Smith, S. (2010) *Supervised Community Treatment*, Mental Health Alliance, Briefing Paper 2, www.mentalhealthalliance.org.uk/resources/SCT_briefing_paper.pdf

Lewis, A. (1934) The psychopathology of insight, *British Journal of Medical Psychology*, 14, 332–348

Mandela, N. (1995) *Long Walk to Freedom*, London: Abacus

Office for Disability Issues (2008) *Independent Living. Cross Givernment Strategy About Independent Living for Disabled People*, London: HM Government

Office of the High Commissioner for Human Rights (2009) Annual Report of the High Commissioner for Human Rights to the General Assembly, A/HRC/10/49, presented 26 January

O'Hagan, M. (1993) *Stopovers on My Way Home from Mars*, London: Survivors Speak Out

O'Hagan, M. (2007) Parting Thoughts, *Mental Notes* (Mental Health Commission, Wellington, New Zealand), 18, 4–5

Perkins, R. (2010) Professionals: From centre stage to the wings, in Sainsbury Centre for Mental Health, *Looking Ahead. The Next 25 years in Mental Health*, London: Sainsbury Centre for Mental Health

Perkins, R. and Moodley, P. (1993) The arrogance of insight?, *Psychiatric Bulletin*, 17, 233–234

Perkins, R. and Rinaldi, R. (2007) *Taking Back Control. A Guide to Planning Your Own Recovery*, London: South West London & St George's Mental Health NHS Trust

Repper, J. and Carter, T. (2010) *Using Personal Experience to Support Others with Similar Difficulties. A review of the literature on peer support in mental health services*, London: Together

Repper, J. and Perkins, R. (2006) *Social Inclusion and Recovery: A Model for Mental Health Practice*, Edinburgh: Baillière Tindall

Sainsbury Centre for Mental Health (2010) *Implementing Recovery. A framework for organisational change*, London: Sainsbury Centre for Mental Health

Sayce, L. (2000) *From Psychiatric Patient to Citizen*, London: MacMillan

Shepherd, G., Boardman, J. and Sade, M. (2008) *Making Recovery a Reality*, London: Sainsbury Centre for Mental Health

Social Exclusion Unit (2004) *Mental Health and Social Exclusion,* London: Office of the Deputy Prime Minister

Szmukler G., Daw R. and Dawson J. (2010) A model law fusing incapacity and mental health legislation, *Journal of Mental Health Law Special Issue*, 20, 1–140

The Health Foundation (2008) *Co-creating Health Briefing*, www.health.org.uk/publications/co-creating-health-briefing-paper

Thompson, C. (1996) *Letter to the Committee from the Royal College of Psychiatrists (ICB 20)*, House of Commons Social Security Committee, Session 1996–1997

Warner, R. (2009) Recovery from Schizophrenia and the Recovery Model, *Current Opinion in Psychiatry*, July 2009, 22, 4, 374–380

3 Collaborative partnerships with service users

Models that work

Alan Simpson

The secret of the linen cupboard

Those of us who trained in the UK as mental health nurses in the 1980s or before will have spent the majority of our student years studying and working in a Victorian-era mental hospital. Before the development of community-focused care, these massive asylums, often built out in the countryside away from mainstream society, housed thousands of 'mental patients' in scores of impersonal wards at the ends of miles of polished corridors. Those living in these managed communities wandered between the dance hall and the church, from arts and crafts to industrial therapy, through the acres of cricket pitches and bowling greens to the hospital farm.

Hidden within such sprawling facilities and often well-meaning beneficence lay a grim reality of power imbalance and abuse, and loss of personal freedoms, choice and individuality. For the young mental health nursing student, the impersonal warehousing of people experiencing mental distress (alongside shocking histories of those admitted for being pregnant or gay) was probably symbolised most astutely when the charge nurse or sister sent you off to sort out the linen cupboard. This tedious duty, usually performed during long evening shifts or even longer weekends, involved sorting through the mounds of trousers, skirts, shirts, blouses, belts, socks, ties, braces, pants and jumpers in an attempt to create sets of clothing that might best approximate the height and girth of particular patients on the 30-bed ward. For while it may seem astonishing now, as recently as the mid-1980s mental health patients rarely had their own clothes; they were kitted out in whatever combination of garments the frustrated student could find and then squeeze the poor, confused patient into. Alternatively, belts were yanked in as tight as possible to ensure the billowing trousers stayed put during the journey over to occupational therapy and back.

Now, after almost 30 years and many policy changes and service developments, that keen but woefully underprepared student has made a number of transitions and career changes and whilst continuing to agitate for further improvements in mental health service provision, also recognises the immense changes that have taken place. The distant asylums have been replaced by smaller psychiatric units that in turn saw the development of local community-focused care provided by multidisciplinary teams. The language of asylums, patients and chronicity has become one of recovery and service users – perhaps even citizens and rights.

These changes have not come about by accident. They are the result of a complex merging of various economic, social and political, and medical developments (Murphy, 1991). Not least within those forces was the power of the emancipatory movements that swept across Western society from the 1950s onwards, including civil rights, feminism, gay rights and the disability rights movement. Out of and alongside these emerged anti-asylum, anti-psychiatry campaigners and a growing if splintered service user movement (Rogers and Pilgrim, 1991) campaigning for, variously, the end to institutionalisation, the end of psychiatry and the abuse of powers within psychiatry, and for the improvement of mental health services (Wallcraft and Bryant, 2003; Campbell, 2005).

As a result, mental health policies in most Western countries now require that service users are actively involved in making decisions about their treatment and care. Service users are now participants in the recruitment and selection of mental health nursing students and staff; and take part in the education and training of psychiatrists, psychologists, nurses and social workers. Mental health service providers increasingly employ service users in a range of posts across their organisations while others chair and attend NHS Trust committees and make sure that user-led service audits and improvements are acted on. Mental health researchers collaborate with service users in the design and execution of research studies, while other user researchers lead their own funded studies. There has been a quiet revolution that has brought partnership with service users into the mainstream of mental health services, education and research.

In this chapter I will explore this move towards greater partnership working and collaboration between mental health staff and service users. I will provide illustrations of effective partnership working in clinical practice, in service development and delivery and in mental health education. Then, I will consider where this journey might next take us – towards personalisation and co-production of health, positive outcomes and citizenship – and some of the challenges we are likely to face along the way.

Identifying the drivers

Over the last two decades, there has been a consistent drive to include service users and carers, patients and public in the commissioning, design, delivery and evaluation of health and social care services (Department of Health, 1999a, 1999b, 2000, 2005a).

The drivers are several. There is the political impetus aimed at making health and social care services more responsive to the needs of the public, often in order to nullify the perceived power of the professions. Consumer choice and influence has also been fuelled by a less deferential populace, progressively more informed through access to the internet and other sources of information. In particular, patients with long-term conditions often exhibit extensive knowledge and understanding of their ailments, care and treatments, which has led to recognition of these 'expert patients' as valuable partners in the health care journey (Department of Health, 2001). And there is a moral recognition that as citizens the public is entitled to have a voice in all aspects of the health service (Telford *et al.*, 2002).

But the most significant driver is quality improvement and a belief that the involvement of users and carers leads to deeper clinical understanding and improvement in relations between health care professionals and patients and a consequent increase in the quality of care and treatment provided (Wykurz and Kelly, 2002). Through valuing and listening to 'experts through experience', staff can provide the interventions perceived to be most appropriate and effective in the manner that is most acceptable to those receiving the service.

Studies evaluating patient involvement in planning and developing health care services have reported positive changes in service delivery and staff attitudes (Crawford *et al.*, 2002, 2003). And a small number of projects involving users in the delivery and evaluation of mental health services also found improved patient experiences (Simpson and House, 2002). However, there is also evidence that even when user involvement is actively pursued, beyond any immediate gains for those service users directly involved, the outcomes may be more complex and uncertain than is often suggested (Fudge *et al.*, 2008).

The direction of travel

Murray-Neill (2011) has outlined a suggested direction of travel that those of us involved in mental health care have been following. Starting out in segregated, institutional care in the old asylums, the 'lunatics, cripples and idiots' were subjected to broadly medically based attempts at cure in an environment where 'doctor knows best'. The move towards community-focused care and support saw the emergence of 'clients and service users' as health and social care was delivered by multidisciplinary 'professionals' in teams. Now we are arguably moving into an era characterised by individualised, personalised support within a socially based approach where citizens have equal rights and opportunities. Cure or care is superseded by recovery, independent living and self-directed services where the individual works in partnership or co-production with professional staff, when and where they find that beneficial.

Central to this new focus is the adoption of the recovery approach, covered in detail elsewhere in this book, which is increasingly influencing and informing mainstream mental health policy and practice. Recovery does not necessarily mean 'clinical recovery', which is usually defined in terms of symptoms and cure, but is more about individualised or 'social recovery' – building a life beyond illness without necessarily achieving the elimination of the symptoms of illness (Watkins, 2007). Recovery is about individualised approaches and helping people in mental distress find meaning and purpose in their lives and experiences and to develop a satisfying and fulfilling life, as defined by each person. Recovery is often described as a journey, with its inevitable ups and downs, setbacks and leaps forward, and people often describe themselves as being *in recovery* rather than recovered.

The recovery approach emerged from the service user movement and directly from service user experiences across the world (Slade, 2009). People that had experienced mental distress or illness and who had used mental health services often spoke of being given a 'life sentence' and of being advised that they would have this illness for the rest of their lives; that they would probably have to take medication for ever; and were often advised to forget ideas of completing education, of meaningful employment, even fulfilling relationships. Yet within the user movement were people who had found meaning from their experiences, who found purpose and achieved goals and found fulfilment in returning to education, obtaining and succeeding in jobs and having successful friendships, relationships and families – often despite the lack of support from health services.

Recovery advocates speak of providing hope and encouraging others to identify their strengths and interests. People in distress are encouraged and supported to take more responsibility and control over their lives and for their recovery, to develop personal recovery plans with personalised strategies for managing symptoms, setting personal goals and developing social support systems (Gingerich and Mueser, 2005).

In England, a joint position paper was published in 2007 as the result of a collaboration between the Care Services Improvement Partnership (CSIP), Royal College of Psychiatrists (RCPsych) and Social Care Institute for Excellence (SCIE). This important report recommended that the key principles and values of the recovery approach should inform mental health practice in all areas of care and underpin service structures and individual practice. It was based on the core belief that 'adopting recovery as a guiding purpose for mental health services favours hope and creativity over disillusionment and defeat' (ibid, pvi). Similar position statements have been published by policy makers in New Zealand, the USA and Ireland.

More recently in England the coalition government's new legislative framework for health, *Liberating the NHS* (Department of Health, 2010), has a stated intention to 'put patients at the heart of the NHS, through ... greater choice and control' and has a clear focus on the service user experience and shared decision making. Furthermore, its new mental health policy,

'*No health without Mental Health*' (HMG/DH, 2011), contains guiding values and principles that include supporting people to reach their potential; to take more responsibility and control over their health and care; and to promote personalisation. It also includes talk of fairness and the need to ensure equality, justice and human rights.

Just how far these fine words will extend to the interests of people with mental illness remains to be seen and there are many who fear these policies are more about removing state protection and finances for society's more vulnerable members, than they are about promoting recovery and citizenship for all. Alongside this promotion of the recovery agenda, England has witnessed a staggering growth in the use of Community Treatment Orders (CTOs), which require patients to comply with treatment or face recall to hospital, far in excess of the figures expected (Rugkasa and Burns, 2009). It seems that the direction of travel is perhaps not one-way.

Nonetheless, the extent of the distance travelled on the recovery journey is evident in a position statement published by consultant psychiatrists at two leading NHS Trusts in London in which they state that:

> The principles and values of Recovery ideas have been formulated by, and for, service users to describe their own experiences. It is service users that 'do Recovery'. Professionals (and mental health services) can influence Recovery and Recovery journeys in that they can impede them, but they can also facilitate them. It is this idea of the facilitation of Recovery that must be central to the role of professionals.
>
> (South London and Maudsley NHS Foundation Trust and
> South West London and St George's Mental Health NHS Trust, 2010, p5)

They outline how this might shape the way that psychiatrists adapt the way they work and how partnership working with service users will be central to that new approach:

> ...as psychiatrists we need to rethink how we work alongside, in partnership with, people who use our services to enable them to get on with their life from the point when they first access services.
>   ...the challenge for us is to look beyond clinical recovery and to measure effectiveness of treatments and interventions in terms of the impact of these on the goals and outcomes that matter to the individual ... and their family.
>   ...shared decision making in mental health has the potential to improve mental health care as it impacts on quality of life, autonomy, choice and health outcomes.
>
> (ibid, p3)

Similar sentiments for genuine partnerships and collaboration with service users are now standard across the mental health professions (Department of Health, 2006a). How far the intentions will be translated into real-world practice may depend on the support and encouragement provided for clinicians to disentangle and make sense of the often conflicting demands they face when working in an inherently and understandably risk-averse mental health service with all the imbalances of power and entitlements that brings. However, much good practice is emerging and there is considerable hope for the future.

Partnership in practice: from CPA to WRAP and beyond

Across mental health services, case management frequently provides the underpinning framework for the delivery of services where interventions and support from a range of multidisciplinary staff and various organisations can be coordinated to ensure consistency of approach and effective communications between staff and with the service user and their family.

In Britain, the Care Programme Approach (CPA), a form of case management, was introduced in mental health services in England and Scotland in the early 1990s and Wales in 2003. Implementation of the CPA has been variable in all three nations and consequently has been subject to various reforms (Department of Health, 2008; Welsh Assembly Government, 2011).

At its heart, the aim of the CPA is to ensure care is effective, efficient and communicated clearly through a single written care plan and regular reviews, with meaningful involvement of service users, their families and carers. It aims to ensure care is coordinated with regular communication between multidisciplinary staff and health and social care agencies. It is designed to reduce risk and help services meet the multiple, complex health and social care needs of service users and their carers. Additionally, great emphasis is now placed on the principles underpinning these processes, and *partnerships* between users and professionals are described as key to care which is personalised, safe and oriented towards recovery (ARW, 2008; Department of Health, 2008).

However, there is strong evidence that the implementation of the CPA remains problematic and in particular there are serious questions concerning the continued failure to consistently and meaningfully involve service users in the care planning and review processes.

In England, the most recent national survey of over 17,000 community mental health service users across 66 mental health NHS Trusts reported the experiences of the 43 per cent that had their care coordinated under the CPA (CQC, 2010). Of those, most (84 per cent) knew who their care coordinator was and around two thirds (62 per cent) said their care was coordinated well. However, over a quarter (30 per cent) said that they had not been given or offered a copy of their care plan and of those with care plans almost a half (47 per cent) did not fully understand them. A similar proportion did not really think their views were taken into account during care planning with similar numbers uncertain that goals were clear or addressed by services. Limitations were also identified in the inclusion of crisis and contingency plans and the usefulness of care review meetings.

These findings contrast strongly with policy makers' aspirations where 'care planning' is intended to be a collaborative, recovery-oriented process encompassing consideration of individual and family needs, safety, roles and relationships and the optimisation of health and well-being (ARW, 2008; Department of Health, 2008).

There are various attempts to increase the level of partnership working under the CPA and to make the process more individualised and recovery-focused. One that appears to be proving popular is the introduction of 'first person' care plans, making CPA more recovery-focused, where the service user is encouraged to develop their own care plan written in the first person. Questions or prompts are used to guide the user to provide the information they think important and want staff to consider. These might include:

- 'This is how I best describe myself at the moment.'
- 'These are my experiences that have led me to have contact with the community mental health team.'
- 'This is where I see myself in one year's time.'
- 'These are my strengths, aspirations and hopes.'
- 'These are the areas where I need the most support and this is what the team can do to support and aid my recovery and moving on.'

Here is an example where a nursing home resident has identified their need to walk regularly:

After I eat breakfast and get dressed, I want to walk with staff. I will accompany you anywhere. I like to help while we are together. I can fold linen and put things away with you. I do not like to nap. If weather permits, please walk outside with me. I like to keep walking in the evening until I go to bed. I sit when I am tired, so don't fuss over asking me to sit.

Such processes are clearly quite different to a more traditional, profession-led approach and documentation, in that they foreground the user's voice and priorities over those of medical or nursing models and service agendas. Similarly, the increased use of advanced directives and statements and relapse prevention plans aim to promote partnership working with the service user in order to increase the potential for services to be user-focused and responsive to the individual.

Consultations conducted with service users in East London found that their concerns around the CPA could be grouped succinctly under four headings:

- Communication: 'Help me understand what is happening and why.'
- Involvement: 'I want to be involved in decisions about my care.'
- Individuation: 'Recognise my individual circumstances and strengths.'
- Preparation: 'Make sure my care review meetings are well organised with the right people there and someone who knows me chairing.'

In relation to care reviews, many local service providers are also training and employing service users to audit clinical practice and recommend developments designed to ensure good practice. In Newham, East London, this has been underway for several years and has led to the production of user-led standards for conducting CPA care review meetings (ELFT, 2008). The good practice recommendations include the following:

- Care coordinator informs service user and carer about purpose of review and the aims and choices available.
- Care coordinator offers to meet service user before meeting to prepare and support.
- Care coordinator will inform key individuals at least two weeks prior to meeting.
- Professionals unable to attend should send a report concerning progress and any issues to discuss.
- Users should be encouraged to invite a family member, advocate or friend to attend the meeting.
- CPA reviews should not start later than 15 minutes after allocated start time.
- Users and carers will be notified of any delays and staff should aim to be present from the start.
- Introductions of all present should highlight role in user's care, not job title alone.
- Mobile phones should be switched off.
- Jargon should be avoided and language should be easily understandable.
- Permission should be requested for any student to be present for training purposes.
- The care coordinator should ensure everyone has an opportunity to express their views.
- The care coordinator should meet with the user after the CPA review to ensure the content was understood and to discuss any issues arising from the meeting.
- Users (and carers and others agreed with the user) should receive a typed copy of the care plan within two weeks.

However, perhaps the reality is that after 20 years of often frustrated attempts to encourage staff to work in partnership within this framework, it is time to embrace a more recovery-focused approach. Emerging from the USA, self-management programmes for people with chronic health problems play an important part in patient-centred care. These programmes have been shown to produce positive changes in health outcomes, attitudes and behaviours through providing information and skills aimed at managing symptoms, maintaining health and well-being and enhancing quality of life (see summary in Cook *et al.*, 2011). Similar programmes have been developed in mental health, most prominently Wellness Recovery Action Planning (WRAP).

WRAP is usually taught or delivered by service users in stable recovery over 8–12 week sessions. Participants create an individualised plan to achieve and maintain recovery by learning to utilise wellness maintenance strategies, identify and manage symptoms and crisis triggers, and to cope with crises when they occur. Peer modelling and support is central to the approach, with peer facilitators drawing on the experiences of themselves and their students to illustrate key concepts of self-management and recovery (Copeland, 1997).

WRAP and similar self-management programmes are proving to be popular amongst service users and there is a now an extensive programme in the USA, which is rapidly expanding throughout many Western and Oceanic countries, although research into the effectiveness of WRAP has been far less extensive (Cook *et al.*, 2009). However, the results of a recently published randomised controlled trial of 519 adults with severe mental illness on an 8-week WRAP intervention or a waiting-list control condition with usual care has produced impressive results. After six months, compared with those people receiving usual care, service users who had received WRAP showed significant alleviation of symptoms of mental illness, significantly greater improvement in hopefulness and enhanced quality of life (Cook *et al.*, 2011). The results indicate that peer-delivered self-management training may be effective in delivering recovery-focused interventions.

The success of such approaches perhaps suggests a challenge for mental health professionals in that the content of WRAP draws on user accounts and experiences and is delivered by peer facilitators. It suggests that service user peers may be more able to connect with, enthuse and empower their fellow peers than perhaps more distant practitioners. Or perhaps there are clues in the work of peer providers that can inform clinicians on ways to 'up their game' in terms of developing effective partnerships.

Cook *et al.* (2011) suggest the process of illness self-management, such as the WRAP programme, has its conceptual foundation in the psychological theory of self-determination (Ryan and Deci, 2000). In this framework, health behaviour change occurs and continues through autonomous motivation where the person feels a sense of volition, self-initiation and endorsement of their behaviour. Such motivation is more likely to occur in supportive environments where those providing the support understand the person's perspective, acknowledge his or her feelings, offer choices and provide information (Williams *et al.*, 2007). Additionally, perceived confidence is important as those who feel more competent in a particular health-related behaviour are more likely to carry it out (Williams *et al.*, 2006).

The social support provided by peer facilitators may enhance these critical components of health behaviour change not least because the peer provider aims to provide an understanding, accepting, environment while simultaneously demonstrating and modelling the very competencies required to enhance recovery.

Service users are increasingly volunteering or being trained and employed to provide mental health services to their peers, and the peer specialist roles are being developed in inpatient and community services in the USA, Australia, Scotland and now in England (Clay, 2005; Bluebird, 2008; Maclean *et al.*, 2009: Ley *et al.*, 2010). Reviews of the research evidence suggest peer support is well received by service users and can be highly effective (Davidson *et al.*, 2006;

Repper and Carter, 2011). In light of these developments, traditionally qualified mental health staff may need to think more about how they will work in partnership with peer supporters, peer WRAP trainers and peer advocates as well as the service users themselves. These new roles are both exciting and challenging and issues around communication and boundaries, roles and responsibilities, integrated versus complementary services, career development and progression for peer specialists, will all have to be considered and negotiated.

Personalisation and partnership

Personalisation and the trend towards 'co-production' has emerged as a means to increase consumer choice, autonomy and access to individually tailored services provided by public, private and third-party or voluntary sector agencies (Department of Health, 2005b, 2006b, 2009). As will be seen, personalisation also has major implications for partnership working.

At the heart of the personalisation agenda is the desire to encourage health and social care service providers to rethink their whole approach to supporting people with mental health problems. It is predicated on the idea that in the future people and their families will take much more control over their own support and treatment options. Linked to that will be new levels of partnership and collaboration between citizens and professionals (Duffy, 2010, p3). Building on the recovery approach, Duffy (2010) suggests the shift towards personalisation means:

- Tailoring support and services to fit the specific needs of the individual.
- Respecting the important relationships the person has with families and friends.
- Supporting people to take more control over their lives and their supports.
- Enabling people to define the outcomes that are important to them.
- Improving the responsiveness and flexibility of services and supports.
- Increasing the involvement of local communities.

Personalisation is also about encouraging service providers to work more closely with communities and local organisations to develop more flexible, responsive services and reduce the causes of mental ill health. But central to personalisation is the idea of self-directed support and co-production.

In line with core concepts of recovery is the idea that people with mental health problems can improve their journey towards recovery and better manage their mental health problems when they play a bigger role in designing and controlling their own support. Through providing information about options available and increasing direct involvement and choice over accessing supports and services, people can take more responsibility and greater control over their recovery, their treatment and support and their own well-being.

Echoing the work on self-management programmes such as WRAP, self-directed support encourages the individual to identify their needs, problems or goals and then, before thinking about professional support, identify the personal, family and community strengths, abilities, supports, networks and resources that may be called upon. Then a personal plan of support is developed that may or may not involve professional support. Where appropriate and desired, the person may request or purchase professional support as required, such as when they wish to benefit from professional knowledge and expertise about a particular condition, treatment or intervention. Such a model offers a major rethink to the way services may be provided in the future and has massive implications for the way that professionals provide support and are organised and employed. But there are considerable opportunities for 'service users' – or perhaps it is now more appropriate to say 'citizens' – to pick, choose and buy-in the particular professional supports and interventions he or she requires and for professional mental health staff to work as co-producers of support and care alongside the individual and family, friends, peers and various supports.

One aspect of the personalisation agenda that has received a lot of attention is that of direct payments and personal budgets. Direct payments are cash payments given to service users in place of community care services they have been assessed as needing and are intended to give users greater choice in their care. The payment must be sufficient to enable the service user to purchase services to meet their needs and must be spent on services that they need. Personal budgets are an allocation of funding given to users after an assessment that should be sufficient to meet their assessed needs. Users can either take their personal budget as a direct payment or, while still choosing how their care needs are met and by whom, leave local authorities with the responsibility to commission the services. Or they can have some combination of the two. As a result, they provide a potentially good option for people who do not want to take on the responsibilities of a direct payment (Mithran, 2011).

Research commissioned by the Social Care Institute for Excellence (Newbronner *et al.*, 2011) into people's experiences of using self-directed support and personal budgets in pilot areas, concluded that while individual budgets could enhance people's sense of control and satisfaction with services, there was substantial variation in the benefits and experiences of older people and people with mental health problems. Importantly though, people with mental health problems reported a significantly higher quality of life and improved psychological well-being as a result of using individual budgets. However, some people found there were difficulties in organising personal budgets and accessing support, consistent with earlier research evidence on the barriers to the take-up of direct payments.

Newbronner *et al.* (2011) conclude that as local authorities gear up to make personal budgets available to more and more people who use services, they need to find ways to keep the personal budget process 'personal'. They acknowledge that with high workloads and resource constraints this is easy to say and very difficult to do but stress the

> very central place of the relationship between personal budget holders and their social care practitioner or care coordinator. This human factor cannot be underestimated, and so giving staff support, training and time to work with personal budget holders properly is crucial.
>
> (Newbronner *et al.*, 2011, p66)

The report concluded that a successful personal budget process requires a series of effective partnerships to be established between individuals and agencies and that this process inevitably takes time.

This conclusion reflects Duffy's (2010) stance that self-directed support should not mean leaving people to do everything on their own. Different people need different degrees of control and support and many people with mental health problems have complex needs that require interaction and engagement with a vast array of services and supports, including health, social care, housing, benefits, employment and education, substance misuse services and the criminal justice system. Care management systems, like the CPA mentioned earlier, have been designed to help manage these complexities by providing care managers or coordinators to work in partnership with service users to help navigate the systems. But the personalisation approach aims to take these practices to a new level of partnership with much closer, more individualised support provided.

Duffy's (2010) personalisation model draws on the CPA to suggest that a care manager works in partnership with the person to provide professional coordination and expertise across both health and social care, while drawing on a range of professional and non-professional support from family, friends and others within the community. The care manager or coordinator needs to ensure that:

- The person's needs are assessed and they are accessing everything they are entitled to, whether through traditional services or through personal and/or direct payments.
- The person's plans make sense, are safe and likely to be effective.
- The plans are regularly reviewed in partnership with the individual to ensure that progress is being made against their personalised, recovery-focused goals.

Underpinning this approach is an appreciation that informal and formal support can also be provided by family, friends and peers and greater use of community resources and networks, such as user-led facilities, voluntary groups, churches, mosques and faith-based groups, employers and educational facilities.

Many professional mental health staff will already be employing such personalised approaches to partnership working but for others this approach may be more challenging. So it is crucial that pre-registration education and continuing professional development for mental health staff provides a focus on recovery, personalisation and partnership working.

Partnership in educating and training mental health staff

For many people, the key to changing the attitudes, values and approaches employed by mental health professionals lies in the education of mental health students, whether doctors, nurses, psychologists or other health and social care staff, and the training or continuing professional development of qualified staff. There has been much progress in how professionals are educated and prepared for practice, for example all health and social care staff educational bodies now require service users to be involved in the design and delivery of professional education and development (QAA, 2005).

One of the drivers for increased patient or service user involvement in medical, health and social care education is the increasing acknowledgement of the 'patient voice' in health care. This reflects the wider involvement of service users and carers and the 'personalisation' of care in public services discussed above. This shift towards a partnership and personalised care agenda emphasises the role of clinicians not only as practitioners but also as partners in care (London Deanery, 2011). It follows then that this shift needs to be reflected in the content and delivery of education and training.

As an example, to strengthen pre-registration mental health nurse education, the Chief Nursing Officer for England's review of mental health nursing recommended that users and carers should be routinely involved in four key areas of the educational process: recruitment, curriculum planning, teaching and assessment (Department of Health, 2006b). Suggestions and some evidence for the creative, supportive and effective involvement of users and carers in nursing education have been published by Mental Health Nurse Academics UK (Simpson, 2006).

By ensuring that user and carer perspectives are threaded throughout the educational process, it is anticipated that staff will be more attuned to work within and help develop a user-focused service. Classroom involvement of service users in the education of pre-registration mental health students has been associated with reduced use of professional 'jargon', greater empathy with users' distressing experiences, less use of defensive 'distancing' and an increased tendency to adopt an individualised approach to assessment and intervention (Wood and Wilson-Barnett,

1999). Greater awareness and understanding of the patient experience and stated intentions to take that learning into practice has also been reported by students interacting online with service users during enquiry-based learning exercises (Simpson *et al.*, 2008). Studies of user participation in postgraduate nurse education have also reported positive changes in attitudes towards service users, greater understanding of their perspectives and developments in clinical practice (Happell and Roper, 2003; Khoo *et al.*, 2004). And Stickley *et al.* (2010) have also explored how service users can participate in the assessment of students in clinical practice.

However, a comprehensive literature review of user and carer involvement in the education and training of health care staff reported that whilst overall it was a positive process, well received by the service users and carers, students and teachers involved, the impact in relation to ensuing health care behaviour had rarely been evaluated (Repper and Breeze, 2004).

Furthermore, Collier and Stickley (2011) suggest that whilst there may be good examples of user involvement and collaborative working in some programmes or universities (McKeown *et al.*, 2010), overall the picture is patchy and uneven with isolated examples of good practice, and it remains subject to major philosophical and organisational challenges. They argue that there is little evidence of truly collaborative models becoming mainstream in nurse (or other health care) education to really create the shift to establish genuine partnership working in mental health care.

As a result, they conclude that not only can educators not claim to know what effect greater partnership in education is having on the education of students, beyond their reported perceptions, views and opinions, but they are not confident that their own well-established collaborative project will have a lasting influence on the practice of nurses of the future. 'It is not that we doubt the efficacy of the work that we have accomplished; it is rather that we acknowledge the strong social forces at play that maintain the *status quo*' (Collier and Stickley, 2011, p10).

The combined counterforce of professional protectionism, organisational inflexibility and the continuing fear, prejudice and stigmatisation experienced by people with mental illness may yet outweigh the undoubted positivity and hope of those pursuing a journey or recovery, personalisation and partnership. But essentially, as an optimist, I take heart that although the journey may at times seem troubled and slow, we have come a long way in just the few years since I worked as a student nurse picking through bundles of clothing in that linen cupboard.

References

ARW Training & Consultancy and Practice Based Evidence (2008) *Making the CPA work for you.* London: Department of Health.

Bluebird, G. (2008) *Paving new ground: Peers working in in-patient settings.* Alexandria, VA: National Technical Assistance Centre.

Campbell, P. (2005) From Little Acorns – The mental health service user movement. In Bell, A. and Lindley, P. (eds) *Beyond the water towers: The unfinished revolution in mental health services 1985–2005.* London: Sainsbury Centre for Mental Health. pp73–82.

Care Services Improvement Partnership (CSIP)/Royal College of Psychiatrists (RCPsych)/Social Care Institute for Excellence (SCIE) (2007) *A common purpose: Recovery in future mental health services. London: Social Care Institute for Excellence.*

Clay, S. (2005) *On our own, together: Peer programs for people with mental Illness.* Nashville, TN: Vanderbilt University Press.

Collier, R. and Stickley, T. (2011) From service user involvement to collaboration in mental health nurse education: developing a practical philosophy for change. *The Journal of Mental Health Training, Education and Practice*, 5, 4, 4–11.

Cook, J.A., Copeland, ME., Hamilton, M., *et al.* (2009) Initial outcomes on a mental illness self-management program based on wellness recovery action planning. *Psychiatric Services*, 60, 246–249.

Cook, J.A., Copeland, M.E., Jonikas, J.A., Hamilton, M.M., Razzano, L.A., Grey, D.D., Floyd, C.B., Hudons, W.B., Macfarlane, R.T., Carter, T.M. and Boyd, S. (2011) Results of a randomized controlled trial of mental illness self-management using wellness recovery action planning. *Schizophrenia Bulletin Advance Access*, doi:10.1093/schbul/sbr012.

Copeland, M.E. (1997) *Wellness recovery action plan*. Dummerston, VT: Peach Press.

CQC (2010) *Community mental health services survey 2010*. London: Care quality Commission. http://www.cqc.org.uk/aboutcqc/howwedoit/involvingpeoplewhouseservices/patientsurveys/communitymentalhealthservices.cfm. Accessed 21 July 2011.

Crawford, M.J., Rutter, D., Manley, C. *et al.* (2002) Systematic review of involving patients in the planning and development of health care. *British Medical Journal*, 325, 7375, 1263.

Crawford, M.J., Aldridge, T., Bhui, K. *et al.* (2003) User involvement in the planning and delivery of mental health services: a cross-sectional survey of service users and providers. *Acta Psychiatrica Scandinavica*, 107, 6, 410–414.

Davidson, L., Chinman, M., Sells, D. and Rowe, M. (2006) Peer support among adults with serious mental illness: a report from the field. *Schizophrenia Bulletin*, 32, 3, 443–450.

Department of Health (1999a) *National Service Framework for Mental Health: Modern standards and service models*. London: HMSO.

Department of Health (1999b) *Patient and public involvement in the new NHS*. London: Department of Health.

Department of Health (2000) *The NHS Plan*. London: Department of Health.

Department of Health (2001) *The expert patient*. London: HMSO.

Department of Health (2005a) *Creating a patient-led NHS: Delivering the NHS improvement plan*. London: HMSO.

Department of Health (2005b) *Our health, our care, our say*. London: Department of Health.

Department of Health (2006a) *Our health, our care, our say: Making it happen*. London: Department of Health.

Department of Health (2006b) *From values to action: The Chief Nursing Officer's review of mental health nursing*. London: Department of Health.

Department of Health (2008) *Refocusing the care programme approach: Policy and positive practice guidance*. London: Department of Health.

Department of Health (2009) *Primary care and community services: Personal health budgets: first steps*. London: Department of Health.

Department of Health (2010) *Liberating the NHS: Legislative framework and next steps*. London: Department of Health.

Duffy, S. (2010) *Personalisation in mental health centre for welfare reform*. Yorkshire and Humberside Improvement Partnership, Care Pathways and Packages Project. Association of Directors of Adult Social Services. http://www.centreforwelfarereform.org/library/by-date/personalisation-in-mental-health.html. Accessed July 2011.

ELFT (2008) *Newham Locality Community Services: Standards for CPA meetings. Service user information leaflet*. London: East London Foundation NHS Trust.

Fudge, N., Wolfe, C.D.A. and McKevitt, C. (2008) Assessing the promise of user involvement in health service development: ethnographic study. *British Medical Journal*, 336, 313. http://www.bmj.com/content/336/7639/313.full. Accessed 22 July 2011.

Gingerich, S. and Mueser, K. (2005) Illness management and recovery. In Drake, R., Merrens, M. and Lyne, D. (eds) *Evidence-based mental health practice: A textbook*. New York: WW Norton. pp. 395–424.

Happell, B. and Roper, C. (2003) The role of a mental health consumer in the education of postgraduate psychiatric nursing students: the student's evaluation. *Journal of Psychiatric and Mental Health Nursing*, 10, 3, 343–350.

HMG/DH (2011) *No health without mental health: A cross-government mental health outcomes strategy for people of all ages*. London: Department of Health.

Khoo, R., McVicar, A. and Brandon, D. (2004) Service user involvement in postgraduate mental health education: does it benefit practice? *Journal of Mental Health*, 13, 5, 481–492.

Ley, A., Roberts, R. and Willis, D. (2010) How to support peer support: evaluating the first steps in a healthcare community. *Journal of Public Mental Health*, 9, 1, 16–25.

London Deanery (2011) *Involving patients in clinical teaching.* http://www.faculty.londondeanery.ac.uk/e-learning/involving-patients-in-clinical-teaching. Accessed 27 July 2011.

McKeown, M., Malihi-Shoja, L. and Downe, S. (2010) Beyond the campus: universities, community engagement and social enterprise. In M. McKeown, L. Malihi-Shoja and S. Downe (eds) *Service User and Carer Involvement in Education for Health and Social Care*. Oxford: Wiley-Blackwell.

McLean, J., Biggs, H., Whitehead, I., Pratt, R. and Maxwell, M. (2009) *Evaluation of the delivering for mental health peer support worker pilot scheme.* Edinburgh: The Scottish Government.

Mithran, S. (2011) *Expert guide to direct payments, personal budgets and individual budgets.* http://www.communitycare.co.uk/Articles/19/08/2011/102669/direct-payments-personal-budgets-and-individual-budgets.htm Accessed 12/12/2011.

Murphy, E. (1991) *After the asylums: Community care for people with mental illness.* London: Faber and Faber.

Murray-Neill, R. (2011) *Personalisation: A journey of discovery.* Presentation to East London NHS Foundation Trust, London.

Newbronner, L., Chamberlain, R., Bosanquet, K., Bartlett, C., Sass, B. and Glendinning, C. (2011) *Keeping personal budgets personal: Learning from the experiences of older people, people with mental health problems and their carers.* London: Social Care Institute for Excellence.

QAA (2005) *Partnership quality assurance framework for healthcare education in England.* London: Social Care Institute for Excellence.

Repper, J. and Breeze, J. (2004) *A review of the literature on user and carer involvement in the training and education of health professionals.* Sheffield: Sheffield University. http://www.shef.ac.uk/content/1/c6/03/21/77/Finalreport.pdf. Accessed 27 July 2011.

Repper, J. and Carter, T. (2011) A review of the literature on peer support in mental health services. *Journal of Mental Health*, 20, 4, 392–411.

Rogers, A. and Pilgrim, D. (1991) 'Pulling down churches': accounting for the British Mental Health Users' Movement. *Sociology of Health & Illness*, 13, 2, 129–148.

Rugkasa, J. and Burns, T. (2009) Community treatment orders. *Psychiatry*, 8, 12, 493–495.

Ryan, R.M. and Deci, E.L. (2000) Self-determination theory and the facilitation of intrinsic motivation, social development and well-being. *American Psychologist*, 55, 68–78.

Simpson, A. (2006) Involving service users and carers in the education of mental health nurses. *Mental Health Practice*, 10, 4, 20–24.

Simpson, A., Reynolds, L., Light, I. and Attenborough, J. (2008) Talking with the experts: evaluation of an online discussion forum with mental health service users and student nurses. *Nurse Education Today*, 28, 5, 633–640.

Simpson, E.L. and House, A.O. (2002) Involving users in the delivery and evaluation of mental health services: a systematic review. *British Medical Journal*, 325, 7375, 1265.

Slade, M. (2009) *Personal recovery and mental illness: A guide for mental health professionals.* Cambridge: Cambridge University Press.

South London and Maudsley NHS Foundation Trust and South West London and St George's Mental Health NHS Trust (2010) *Recovery is for all. Hope, agency and opportunity in psychiatry. A position statement by consultant psychiatrists.* London: SLAM/SWLSTG.

Stickley, T., Stacey, G., Pollock, K., Smith, A., Betinis, J. and Fairbank, S. (2010) The practice assessment of student nurses by people who use mental health services. *Nurse Education Today*, 30, 1, 20–25.

Telford, R., Beverley, C.A., Cooper, C.L. & Boote, J.D. (2002) Consumer involvement in health research: fact or fiction? *British Journal of Clinical Governance*, 7 (2), 92–103.

Wallcraft, J. and Bryant, M. (2003) *The mental health service user movement in England.* London: Sainsbury Centre for Mental Health.

Watkins, P. (2007) *Recovery: A guide for mental health practitioners.* London: Churchill Livingstone Elsevier.

Welsh Assembly Government (2011) *Implementing the Mental Health (Wales) Measure 2010: Guidance for local health boards and local authorities*. Cardiff: Welsh Assembly Government.

Williams, G.C., McGregor, H.A., Sharp, D. *et al.* (2006) Testing a self-determination theory intervention for motivating tobacco cessation: supporting autonomy and competence in a clinical trial. *Health Psychology*, 25, 91–101.

Williams, G.C., Lynch, M.F., Glasgow, R.E. (2007) Computer-assisted intervention improves patient-centered diabetes care by increasing autonomy support. *Health Psychology*, 26, 728–734.

Wood, J. and Wilson-Barnett, J. (1999) The influence of user involvement on the learning of mental health nursing students. *NT Research*, 4, 4, 257–270.

Wykurz, G. and Kelly, D. (2002) Learning in practice – developing the role of patients as teachers: literature review. *British Medical Journal*, 325, 7368, 818–821.

4 The care pathway approach

A contemporary, inclusive and outcome-focused rationale for service provision

Sylvia Tang

According to NHS guidelines, clinical care pathways are 'both a tool and a concept that embed guidelines, protocols and locally agreed, evidence-based, patient-centred, best practice, into everyday use for the individual patient. In addition, and uniquely to Integrated Care Pathways (ICPs), they record deviations from planned care in the form of variances' (National Health Service, 2007).

Mental health services have been leading the way in using a pathways-based approach as a means of achieving a move away from hospital-based care. This started with the closure of the institutions and then gathered momentum in the late 1990s with the National Service Framework for Mental Health. However, in the last two years a new approach to care pathways development has been driven through the Yorkshire-based work on care clusters for mental health payment by results, and then the subsequent national pilots and proposed adoption of the cluster-based model for progression of currency development.

Another driver for modernization has been the adoption of service line management, which has been fundamental to Monitor's expectation of a business model for foundation trusts. Monitor is the independent regulator of NHS foundation trusts, which authorises and regulates these trusts and supports their development, ensuring they are well-governed and financially robust. While acute trusts have based their business lines on hospital-based specialties such as surgery or emergency medicine, mental health trusts have adopted a care pathways approach. This uses the clusters for payment by results to define the service lines (business units), which then drive the care pathways approach, through which an outcomes-based delivery leads the configuration and delivery of mental health services.

'Relatively little is known internationally at present about how to create clinical care pathways in a manner that best supports their implementation and routine use in the long term, so further information needs to be gathered' (NHS London, Mental Health Clinical Care Pathway Group, Final Report, Graham Thornicroft and David Monk, January 2008). The report goes on to suggest that any approach should:

- Adopt a wider social model of mental healthcare, including criminal justice, social services and housing contributions to clinical care pathways
- Incorporate a whole person focus of care
- Present clear and easy to understand options that empower consumers
- Provide clear expectations of what should happen at each stage of the care journey.

South London and Maudsley NHS Foundation Trust (2009) suggest that guiding principles for the development of Clinical Academic Groups (CAGs) should include:

- Improving the quality of services and increasing user satisfaction.
- Providing more specialist services and more focused interventions.
- Integrating physical, psychological and social approaches.
- Enhancing multidisciplinary approaches.
- Empowering teams to innovate.
- Promoting partnerships with stakeholders.

In addition to these guiding principles for care pathways development we should add: the strength of the evidence base, including National Institute for Clinical Excellence (NICE) guidelines, any professional standards of good practice and local agreement with commissioners, GPs and other key partners. The transparency of the care pathways and offering appropriate choice for service users wherever this is possible will bring closer engagement and empowerment of service users and introduce appropriate personalization to care plans within a care pathways model. A care pathways model dictates a protocol-based approach and counters personalized individual care planning, albeit that this is informed by highly trained clinical staff. The argument that care pathways improve the standards of care of all professionals and set a standard of commissioning for services and delivery of care for providers that is evidence based and transparent is a robust one.

Psychiatry has often been accused of being the least scientific of medical specialties but the same cannot be said for the research carried out into service model evaluation post the Mental Health National Service Framework (NSF). The relentless focus on the community perspective, with alternatives to hospital admission wherever feasible and the measurement of outcomes and user satisfaction of different models is impressive. The application of these findings has made an exciting and significant contribution to commissioning and provision in the modernization of services that has followed the NSF. The commitment to major programmes of service evaluation of the models proposed by policy makers, along with assessments of the local populations needs by commissioners, followed by the application of the best evidence and findings to service delivery, represents a radical and welcome shift.

The care pathways approach in mental health could arguably deliver even more significant bed reductions and alternatives to admission if a vertical integration model was adopted, bringing specialist mental health trusts and acute services together, for example tackling the numbers of inappropriate admissions to emergency departments, often leading to a hospital admission for the confused or demented elderly population. Health care providers of acute services have largely ignored the lessons from mental health, which in just over a decade has moved to over 90 per cent of care now being delivered in community-based settings in the statutory sector and more than this in the voluntary sector.

The approach to care pathways delivery driven by Monitor's service line management definitions, which defines each business unit as having a discrete set of resources to manage a patient's needs, uses the patient journey as the basis for the care pathway. This requires a sensitive consideration to the integration of service provision, which is key to a patient journey and therefore a successful care pathway. This of course is a challenge in the payment by results model. Other complications are the localization of social care provision and the Any Willing Provider model for health provision. The integration of the whole pathway therefore requires close collaboration amongst partners in all sectors including social care, private sector, voluntary sector and NHS secondary and primary care. One approach that has been considered is the commissioning of whole care pathways with one lead provider responsible for outcomes delivery, with the subcontracting by that lead provider with other providers for elements of the care pathway. The interface issues immediately present a risk in the delivery of the integrated and seamless care and clear definition of the outcomes for each part of the pathway and clear management of any interface issues is crucial.

In order for this to be achieved triage needs to be skilled, with assessments being delegated to the appropriate services and individuals with the skills to do this, without duplicating assessments unnecessarily. Referrers commonly complain about the complex systems in mental health trusts with various names for teams, which do not necessarily describe their function, and the mix of geographical, GP aligned, specialist and tiered teams, which serve to confuse and lead to 'bouncing around' of the referrer who often has only a few minutes to refer. We have all experienced the response that it is the wrong team and to call the other team (often a name or acronym you cannot catch) and then finding the number given is wrong or when helpfully put through, the phone cutting off or ringing dead. We should aim for simple systems of referral that learn from the best skills in customer service. The referral points and numbers should be sustainable despite a change of services, teams, care pathways or even the providers behind them.

This has led to the popularity of single points of entry though critics argue that such a mechanism is designed to keep referrals out. If this is true it will be mitigated by the payment by results (and activity) future for mental health, where clearly it would be a disincentive to refuse income. Meanwhile a service model designed with an outward focus, which builds strong relationships with referrers, and with a threshold for assessment and advice that is lower than that for ongoing service provision, has a number of clear advantages over a more restrictive model. Teams who provide that single entry point are designed to skillfully triage referrals, delegating quickly to treatment services where appropriate, for example substance misuse, crisis home treatment teams, early intervention for psychosis service, memory clinics or psychological services. Everyone wants any member of their family to have ready access to a senior expert assessment, formulation, advice and ongoing care where this is what is needed, and all undertaken swiftly and by a single team. This has been well documented since the early 2000s when community mental health services were reviewed by Tom Burns. Assessment teams require highly experienced clinical and social care staff. This is strongly supported by a joint publication from the Royal College of Psychiatrists, London School of Economics and the NHS Confederation (2009), 'Mental health in times of economic crisis'.

When designing new services it is useful to underpin any national developments with local planning and evidence, for example surveys of local GPs and other referrers. Piloting (or early adopting) of potential new models with evaluation of effectiveness and further satisfaction surveys are helpful prior to reconfiguration plans and implementation. Our experience locally in the Trust was that there were many different views on what a good assessment model would be, although most accepted the principle of improvement needed in standardising response to referrers, with variable views on whether improvements were required. Different models were piloted in different areas and though GP feedback was not conclusive due to small numbers, GP leads consistently wanted to see a universal model and response across the patch, with direct relationships with consultants to be maintained as much possible. Of course the balance for localised and personal service, within the constraints of standard and equitable service, is a challenge. However, it is clear that GPs and other stakeholders have suggested that a responsive single point of access to mental health services for new service users would be helpful in reducing 'bouncing' of referrals around the system. There is a need to standardise responses to referrals to jointly deal with health related and social care related issues and ensure a uniform threshold and quality. The threshold for assessment and advice should be lower than that for providing an ongoing service.

The pilots of different assessment models have shown comprehensive skilled assessments mean fewer people have ongoing assessments due to uncertain needs. The innovators also highlight which models are sustainable and what the workforce for the model should be. A clear understanding of the evidence base for effective treatments will lead to fewer people receiving interventions that do not improve outcomes. Sessions by clinicians with expert knowledge will meet the need for specialist assessments and this will allow for specialist expertise to be strengthened, e.g. for Asperger's or adult attention deficit hyperactivity disorder (ADHD).

Ongoing pathways were informed using the needs-based clustering tool that underpins payment by results in mental health for working age adults and older people. Service line planning groups similar services together so, for example, those with similar interventions and approaches like the services that use a recovery approach and treat longer term psychosis, or those with an assertive approach requiring intensive treatments for psychosis like early intervention services and assertive outreach services (see Figure 4.1).

Each cluster could form the basis of a care pathway with NICE guidelines informing the interventions for the care pathway and timeline. The challenge for specialist services is to coordinate effectively with general services such as community mental health teams (CMHTs), or to expand their services to provide for care coordination, attention to physical health, care management, social care and a pathways approach. The tradition of specialist services has been for inclusion and exclusion criteria, without consideration to engagement or motivational work if the service user is pre-contemplative for psychotherapeutic intervention or not ready as self-managing with substance or alcohol and in a defensive position, or has an unsettled social situation. Whilst this is understandable where the interventions have no benefit unless the service user is ready for the intervention, there is little structure to facilitate the resolution of social issues, provide support or to offer motivational therapy and provide a holistic patient journey. The other parts of the pathway tend to be picked up by general services such as CMHTs, which become the back-stop for all services. The danger of this approach is that there is a loss of focus on the evidence base for each individual diagnostic pathway and the risk that care coordination and support become the proxy for therapeutic interventions.

The care pathway approach should coordinate sequencing of support and engagement, social interventions, motivational work and general well-being work leading to the specialist treatment phase. Following specialist treatment the next phase would be follow-up, support and recovery approaches for educational, employment and social reintegration. Whilst some of the models for psychosis and rehabilitation have used this approach for some years this is a less commonly considered approach for non-psychotic illnesses. Some of the NSF models for psychosis do not focus on care pathways through to the point of discharge from specialist services, so risk creating a dependency model due to services being commissioned for a capacity defined by number of service users, rather than one focused on service user defined outcomes.

In the service line model in our Trust we have grouped the clusters in care pathways. Each one is led by clinical and managerial leads who are responsible for delivering the care pathways for the clusters in the service line, including defining the interventions, the clinical audit plans – including NICE guidelines – the competencies required to deliver the care pathways and planning and putting in place the workforce.

Each care pathway needs to have identified measurable outcomes, including appropriate clinical outcomes, service user experience satisfaction and performance data, including the requirements for regulators such as the Care Quality Commission, and the leads must be accountable for the productivity of the care pathway, adopting innovative approaches to deliver improvements wherever these are warranted, in line with their business plan. They rely on an information system that can capture the data and report in meaningful form about their service

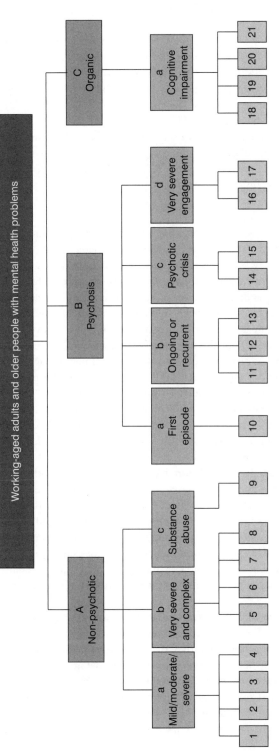

Figure 4.1 Yorkshire clusters decision tree. Reproduced with kind permission of the Department of Health.

1 – Common Mental Health Problems (Low Severity)
2 – Common Mental Health Problems (Low Severity With Greater Need)
3 – Non–Psychotic (Moderate Severity)
4 – Non–Psychotic (Severe)
5 – Non–Psychotic Disorders (Very Severe)
6 – Non–Psychotic Disorder of Over-Valued Ideas
7 – Enduring Non–Psychotic Disorders (High Disability)
8 – Non–Psychotic Chaotic and Challenging Disorders
9 – Blank Cluster
10 – First Episode Psychosis
11 – Ongoing or Recurrent Psychosis (Low Symptoms)

12 – Ongoing or Recurrent Psychosis (High Disability)
13 – Ongoing or Recurrent Psychosis (High Symptoms and Disability)
14 – Psychotic Crisis
15 – Severe Psychotic Depression
16 – Dual Diagnosis
17 – Psychosis and Affective Disorder – Difficult to Engage
18 – Cognitive Impairment (Low Need)
19 – Cognitive Impairment or Dementia Complicated (Moderate Need)
20 – Cognitive Impairment or Dementia Complicated (High Need)
21 – Cognitive Impairment or Dementia (High Physical or Engagement)

Further clusters for Child and Adolescent Mental Health Service (CAMHS) and for Forensic will follow as they are developed.

line's activity and cost performance. This of course can be a challenge, particularly when the interfacing of different systems required to capture health, as well as social care costing flows, is absent or embryonic.

In our Trust, reorganisation into care pathways highlighted that not all services had the capacity to provide for social care, self-assessment for personalized care or medical interventions. These gaps could fuel the criticism from GPs that mental health trusts provide a 'psychosis only' service and, to remedy this, resources need to be reallocated from CMHTs to provide these functions in care pathways for non-psychotic disorders. The resource requirements need to be calculated, by carrying out an assessment of current CMHT caseloads.

Another major consideration in reorganising services along care pathways is the complexity of the integration of social care. While it might seem tempting to develop services that are divided both by functionalised needs and local authority requirements, it could lead to a rapid increase in the numbers of teams and pathways. I would strongly endorse an approach that attempts to engage social care partners and commissioners in a collaboration to deliver cross-borough or joint and fully integrated services.

The resources per borough/authority can then be clearly defined but managed in a joint, integrated pathway, avoiding the need to develop borough-specific services. This leads to a reduction in the postcode lottery, but may be increasingly difficult to deliver, dependent on approaches adopted in future commissioning arrangements. Commissioning must focus on whole services and pathways to achieve the desired outcomes, rather than micro-management of the operational processes or quality detail. Using clearly agreed and meaningful outcomes, rather than process measures, will direct the attention of both commissioners and providers to delivering the best and most cost-effective, high quality outcomes-based service for individuals.

The other consideration is for age-defined services versus needs-defined services. The focus on needs is generally accepted but as they are less clearly defined than age this can lead to increased interface issues and time wasted on boundary disputes. A collaborative 'can do' attitude is needed and this needs to be modelled by senior managers to whom these issues should be rapidly escalated. Again much of this may be mitigated by the Payment by Results (PbR) implementation. Currently there is a sense that resources do not follow service users and therefore boundary disputes are fuelled by a sense of pressure and being 'put upon' without 'reward'. Our experience has been that adopting a collaborative attitude leads to smoother care for the service user and less wasted energy and time in negotiation or even conflict. The issues arise where a qualitative term such as physical frailty or functional impairment is used, which is not clearly defined. The sourcing of 'easy to use' tools, which are not implemented rigidly, can helpfully inform such discussions to reach a decision. Alternatively, if a clinical team have a view that the needs of a service user could be best met in another pathway, for example in a case of pre-senile dementia or physical frailty but no dementia, then there should be an acceptance of that referral. If the integrity of the referrer is respected it leads to a smoother transition and better morale.

Our local experience was that this was well illustrated when rehabilitation services stopped reassessing the functional impairment of service users for transfer to rehabilitation services and subsequently refusing people on the grounds that they did not have rehabilitation needs. Instead they accepted referrals and approached the service user in order to engage them, with an automatic assumption that they would be taken on. This reduced the subjective impression that there was some sort of hurdle or test to be passed in order to be accepted for services. The same could be applied to assertive outreach team (AOT) services where service users feel rejected, or that they have failed a test when not accepted, despite their clinical teams having felt this was indicated.

The care pathway model should allow teams to remove the need for duplication. In current models it is not uncommon for service users to have intensive treatment and support from a rehabilitation or inreach/outreach and require full care coordination from another team. Streamlining of these processes is essential in delivering a care pathways approach.

There are potential exceptions to the care pathway encompassing the whole patient journey for one set of needs. The model of service should not set up services that require referral between care pathways, unless the service users need change. Examples of where this might happen might be the development of a whole new set of needs due to the emergence of a psychotic illness or cognitive illness. The exception might be the 'acute care pathway' model for mental health, based on alternatives to inpatient care, establishing whether there are 'least restrictive' alternatives appropriately based on risk and clinical need, delivered with gate-keeping of beds. The principle of always taking the least restrictive alternative follows the ethos of the Mental Health Act 1983. Most mental health trusts would boast that this part of the care pathway would be managing the minority of the total caseload at any one time. For most trusts, between 90 and 97 per cent of the services would be outside the hospital at any one time. The resources required to deliver hospital services and alternatives might require these provisions to be seen as a separate care pathway within other care pathways. It is unlikely that it is cost-effective to deliver the acute care pathway in each care pathway separately.

The acute care pathway is broadly defined as all services that are currently in place to manage what was traditionally (within the last 15 years) hospital care. The alternatives include home treatment crisis resolution services that gate-keep all admissions to acute beds and crisis beds for short-term, non-hospital-based stays. These often do not require medical or nursing intervention but provide a safe space for review, 'timeout', assessment of alternatives, respite for carers, re-establishment of medication, medical review and assessment of risk.

The recent model of linking daytime interventions at recovery centres, which are focused day hospitals providing short-term interventions, has provided a flexible alternative of around 12 weeks of daytime intervention, linked with either a few weeks of home visits and supervision of medication, or a short one to four week stay in crisis beds without needing to access hospital-based care. This is a model established in Camden, which has been supported by commissioners and service users alike and has received wider endorsement, for example from the Care Quality Commission.

An earlier model of crisis bed provision that has shown improved satisfaction for over a decade, compared to hospital admission, is the women's crisis house in Islington (Killaspy *et al.*, 2000). The evidence base for crisis resolution teams that followed from the Mental Health NSF found that informal admissions were prevented and there was increased satisfaction from service users with alternatives to hospital (Johnson *et al.,* 2010; McCrone *et al.*, 2009).

More recent early data by Osborn *et al.* (unpublished) examined one year of admissions to six crisis beds at a mental health recovery centre in Camden, and found they had a turnover higher than that of an acute ward and length of stays of one week on average where, previously, over 70 per cent of users had been admitted to an inpatient ward in a hospital for a longer time and half of this group had previously been detained. These initial findings appear to indicate that the recovery centre with short-term crisis beds provides an alternative to hospital admission, with a consequent reduction in acute bed utilization. The data for acute bed usage may be confounded by other improvements in the pathway, such as approaches to gate-keeping and in the use of assessment wards in the acute setting that have been introduced at the same time. The crisis beds are linked to a daytime recovery centre and crisis teams, which are all co-located in one environment that has been specifically designed to meet their needs.

Assessment wards, which are entirely focused on assessment and diagnosis to provide a deliberately short intervention, with daily ward input from the consultant, working together with crisis teams committed to alternatives to hospitals and patients' early discharge when safe, appear to be having an impact on our length of stay. The intensive model has resulted in an increase in trimmed average length of stay (ALOS) of 10 days. However, ALOS locally has two peaks, one at less than 10 days and one at over 65 days. This would suggest there are broadly two groups in the population using inpatient beds. While crisis interventions, crisis houses and the use of a recovery centre might have an impact on the '10 day peak', they appear not to impact on the '65 day peak'. Further development planned in the rehabilitation pathway, driven by robust service line management and full adoption of the care pathway approach could have some effects on this group of service users but this is as yet untested.

The most advanced care pathway has been that of acute care, due to the essential need to maximize productivity and innovation, driven by the high cost of hospital service, coupled with a commitment to improve the service user experience. Having the right multidisciplinary teams of skilled practitioners in place and 'lined up' is the first stage of a successful care pathway. Process mapping with full involvement of all staff stakeholders from each component of the care pathway has served to reduce the blockages and improve interface issues. Having clear accountability for clinical and operational managerial leadership has ironed out any disincentives between services. Close working with housing services and accommodation teams who are part of the pathway has helped to promote a clearer flow through service for service users, by releasing tenancies earlier in supported housing projects when it becomes clear that someone is not able to safely return within a reasonable period (one year). This has markedly reduced delayed transfers of care (people remaining in hospital unnecessarily, waiting for suitable supported housing).

Clear identification of the treatment goals for the acute ward, in order to achieve rapid access back to home treatment, and also swiftly addressing social factors that may impact on timely discharge have been the other successes that have helped us to achieve improved outcomes and supported our ability to reduce overall bed numbers. The assessment ward has also introduced rapid dispensing of medication in order that service users ready for discharge, or for a trial of home treatment, do not need to wait for hours in hospital for medication to be ready before they can leave, a change that service users understandably appreciate.

The other dilemma facing those who commission and provide mental health services is to recognize that the best approach to delivering assertive outreach, through specialist teams, means accepting the evidence of the REACT trial led by Dr Helen Killaspy (Killaspy *et al.*, 2006) and hence changing the standard model of delivery. Based on Dr Killaspy's follow-up study on AOT (Killaspy *et al.*, 2009) there would be a possible rationale for incorporating the AOT functions with high-need CMHT clients into a care pathway. Research trials on AOT show CMHTs are as successful in achieving health outcomes; however, the AOT model has higher satisfaction with service users. We consider satisfaction a very important measure and it is also a core component of the National Outcomes Framework for mental health. We also have high numbers of people in the clusters relating to AOT services, greater than the capacity for these services. We know from our work locally that features of the service that are valued by service uses are effective team-working, extended hours, the ability to supervise medication and to increase and reduce input as required. We have been examining the use of the functional assertive community treatment (FACT) model from The Netherlands, which would allow these positive and flexible features of the AOT service to be retained but with an increased total caseload. This model also prioritises attention on recovery (daytime activities, meaningful relationships, physical activity) rather than the traditional focus on engagement and active treatment – though naturally these elements are important. Clearly more evidence will emerge as the model is tested further in England.

The application of the growing evidence base and a constant striving to improve outcomes should be fundamental to planned changes to service models. Care coordination, whilst a successful model in delivering integrated care, is not an intervention but a method of coordinating the interventions required. Care coordination in some areas has sometimes become a substitute for the therapeutic interventions. It can also deskill professional staff. The integrated community mental health team model is an excellent model for delivering services to those with ongoing psychotic illnesses but the same model is not evidenced for other disorders.

For non-psychotic disorders there are very clear guidelines for interventions that are proven to work. It is not possible to be expert in treating a condition unless one sees people with the condition frequently. It is important to develop specialist services in order to have experts in diagnosis and treatment of those conditions, particularly for non-psychotic conditions. This supports the need locally for trauma services, personality disorder services, improving access to psychological treatment (IAPT) and others. Unfocused interventions can lead to longer, chaotic use of various services without improvement.

Careful mapping of the medical, therapeutic and social care interventions required in the care pathway will inform the workforce requirements, and the clinical and social care outcomes, as well as process measures, such as safeguarding alerts, lengths of stay and the activity flows related to population need, all essential elements for truly effective pathway management. This will lead to a clear business plan for each care pathway or groups of care pathways. The demonstration of the productivity and innovation in the acute care pathway I have described are possible in all care pathways. The reorganization and implementation of these will take careful planning and time. The care pathways may look different in different trusts or areas of the country subject to population needs, commissioning patterns and configurations of organizations but this is the freedom that the NSF did not allow. The NSF brought real achievements of new income and new models outside hospitals but this new generation of pathways development, thinking about patient journeys and patient identified goals, outcomes and satisfaction, is bringing innovative thinking and creativity back into mental health services. The cultural shift to journeys through services rather than dependence on them can help us all focus on true recovery approaches and to change the culture to one of co-production rather than paternalism and dependence.

References and further reading

Department of Health (1999) *National Service Framework for mental health*, London, December.

Department of Health (2002) *Community mental health teams – mental health policy implementation guide*, London, June.

Department of Health (2010) *Transforming community services*, London, November

Johnson, S., Nolan, F., Pilling, S., Sandor, A., Hoult, J., Mckenzie, N., White, I.R., Thompson, M. and Bebbington, P. (2005a) Randomised controlled trial of acute mental health care by a crisis resolution team: the north Islington crisis study. *BMJ (Clinical Research Ed.)* 331(7517):599–602.

Johnson, S., Nolan, F., Hoult, J., White, I.R., Bebbington, P., Sandor, A., Mckenzie, N., Patel, S.N. and Pilling, S. (2005b) Outcomes of crises before and after introduction of a crisis resolution team. *Br J Psychiatry* 187:68–75.

Johnson, S., Wood, S., Paul, M., Osborn, D.P., Wearn, E., Lloyd-Evans, B. *et al.* (2010) *Inpatient mental health staff morale: a national investigation*. Final report. London, NIHR Service Delivery and Organisation programme.

Killaspy, H., Dalton, J., McNicholas, S. *et al.* (2000) Drayton Park, an alternative to hospital admission for women in acute mental health crisis. *Psychiatric Bulletin* 24:101–104.

Killaspy, H.T., Bebbington, P. E., Blizard, R., Johnson, S., Nolan, F., Pilling, S. and King, M. (2006)The REACT study: randomised evaluation of assertive community treatment in North London. *BMJ (Clinical Research Ed.)* 332(7545):815–820.

Killaspy, H., Kingett, S., Bebbington, P.E., Blizard, R., Johnson, S., Nolan, F. and Pilling, S.K.M. (2009) Three year outcomes of participants in the REACT (Randomised Evaluation of Assertive Community Treatment in North London) study. *Br J Psychiatry* 195:82–83.

McCrone, P., Johnson, S., Nolan, F., Pilling, S., Sandor, A., Hoult, J., McKenzie, N., White, I.R. and Bebbington, P. (2009)Impact of a crisis resolution team on service costs in the UK. *The Psychiatrist* 33: 17–19.

National Health Service. Protocols and Care Pathways Library (2007) http://www.library.nhs.uk/pathways/ London, National Health Service.

NHS London, Mental Health Clinical Care Pathway Group (2008) *Final Report,* Graham Thornicroft and David Monk, http://healthcareforlondon.steel-ltd.com/about-the-mental-health-project/, January.

NICE (2011) Advice from NICE aims to improve commissioning of services for people with common mental health disorders, http://www.nice.org.uk/newsroom/pressreleases/CommonMentalHealthDisordersCommissioningGuide.jsp

Pathways and Packages Project (2009) Clustering booklet, http://www.cppconsortium.nhs.uk/docs.php (July–December).

Royal College of Psychiatrists, London School of Economics and the NHS Confederation (2009) *Mental health in times of economic crisis.* London, November.

South London and Maudsley NHS Foundation Trust (2009) *Framework for CAG care pathway development,* November .

Part II
Characteristics of new mental health services

5 Home treatment for mental health crises

Presenting the evidence and potential for improvement

Fiona Nolan

Introduction

This chapter will describe the background to crisis resolution teams in mental health, the body of evidence available to support their continued use, their core characteristics and the potential for development and improvements to this type of care. Definitions of home treatment have been inconsistent, as has the nomenclature of the services, which are known varyingly as 'crisis resolution teams', 'crisis teams', 'home treatment' teams and 'crisis assessment and treatment' teams. For ease and consistency, the services will be referred to in this chapter as crisis resolution teams (CRTs).

Background

Home treatment for acute mental health problems is not a new concept. It has been delivered in various different guises throughout the past 200 years, with documented initiatives to provide this type of care since the 1800s. Home treatment for people in mental health crises has reached its current level of acceptance within the past 40 years in England, following the process of deinstitutionalisation and closure of the large asylums that began in the 1950s and has culminated with the current model of multi-professional teams embedded within the NHS. Early proponents of this type of care were found in Belgium (Gheel, 1800s), Holland (Amsterdam, 1930) and the USA (Kentucky and Colorado, 1960s), while within the UK centres were set up in Scotland (Dingleton, 1960s), Sussex (Worthing, 1950s) and North London (Barnet, 1970s).

Prior to deinstitutionalisation the advocates of home treatment such as Dr Arie Querido in Amsterdam, and the Mental After Care Association in London (MACA, founded 1879) aimed to avoid institutional care thus relieving some of the stigma associated with mental illness. They also worked to address the social problems associated with mental illness, such as poverty and poor living conditions. After the 1950s there were more chronic patients living in the community in the UK than at any time in the preceding 200 years, many of them institutionalised and needing some form of care. This period witnessed the widespread introduction of psychotropic drugs, which enabled psychiatric beds to be used in a similar way to medical beds, with a focus on medication. The interest in home treatment stemmed from social necessity, changes in the treatment of mental illness, and ongoing endeavours to incorporate a more humane and less stigmatising model into mainstream service provision.

The development of this form of home treatment has two primary strands: therapeutic radicalism and fiscal conservatism. The first has been led by individuals who were motivated to provide what they saw as an improvement in the then traditional treatment of the mentally ill, for example Lasalle (Belgium), Querido (Amsterdam), Polak (Denver) and Hoult (Sydney). The second strand has been directed by economic and political forces, relocating health care provision from the institution and into the community. Both strands were interlinked up to the 1980s (and beyond), with the redeployment of care from hospital to the community gaining momentum as inpatient beds in large institutions were closed.

The model of home treatment that emerged from early work in the 1960s and 1970s incorporated a crisis theory (Caplan, 1964) stipulating that the patient and care workers should use a crisis as an opportunity to make meaningful and positive changes in behaviour. The therapeutic value of gainful activity was also given importance in this work, which emphasised teaching or facilitating the patient to live in the community. Descriptions of the core components of crisis teams were developed in government papers (Department of Health, 2002) following their introduction into national policy in 2000. The strength of these formulations of crisis team care was in the organisational components, which have provided service managers with clear guidance on setting up teams, and provided a measure of fidelity in subsequent work (Glover, Arts and Babu, 2006). Describing the content of care delivered by the teams presented more challenges, the most comprehensive attempt being made by Johnson and Needle (2008), incorporating the views of experts in the field. The CRT model is thus an underspecified model, lacking fidelity measures or evidence on which interventions work. The most effective ingredients of CRTs are not known, nor in what combinations can these ingredients be best used.

Crisis theory originated from the work of Gerald Caplan, who identified three types of crisis: developmental, or 'rites of passage' crises, occurring at critical moments in normal life; situational crises, relating to traumatic events, such as death of a loved one; and complex crises, which are not those routinely encountered in everyday life. Crises associated with severe mental illness are described as complex crises. There has been some scepticism among the developers of home treatment as to the applicability of crisis theory to the population served by mental health services, particularly as the theory has not been subject to evaluation.

However, Rosen (1997) has described crisis theory as congruent with the principles of crisis intervention, which provides 'rapid service, intense work in the short term, and a practical here-and-now therapeutic focus'.

Crisis theory, in identifying the crisis as an opportunity for change and development, provides a framework of optimism in which to build on and enhance the resources of the individual who is undergoing difficulties. In this respect it has a similar platform to the recovery approach, which has been developed in recent years and now features prominently in psychiatric discourse.

In 2005 the National Institute for Mental Health in England (NIMHE) endorsed the recovery model as a principle to guide mental health service provision and public education. The core elements of recovery have been identified by Repper and Perkins (2006) as finding hope, having supportive relationships, being empowered to make decisions and included in society, developing coping strategies, and finding a meaning in life. It is important to note, however, that the effectiveness of these principles and how best to apply them in the treatment of mental health problems has not been evaluated.

There is considerable overlap between recovery principles and Caplan's crisis theory, which draws on the strengths of the person undergoing a mental health crisis in learning new skills during the period of crisis, in order to develop more effective ways of coping. While the recovery model has been adopted in rehabilitation services, little work has been done to incorporate the principles into treatment of mental health crises. The work of Stein and

Test in the Training in Community Living Programme (1980), continued by Muijen *et al.* in the Daily Living Programme (1992) adopted principles of social inclusion, engagement and gainful employment, which were implemented as soon as possible after the crisis presented, and continued once the crisis had resolved. While the relevance of crisis theory to this work has not been highlighted, it is apparent in the use of the period immediately following the crisis as an opportunity to engage the person undergoing the crisis and facilitate their use of more effective coping strategies.

Organisational characteristics and core components of CRTs

The first step in the development of a new policy on crisis services in the UK was the stipulation in the National Service Framework for Mental Health (Department of Health, 1999) that 24-hour access to emergency assessment must be available, and that local services should be able to offer home treatment as an alternative to hospital admission. The National Service Framework did not specify a particular model of service organisation as the mandatory method of delivering these types of care. However, when its standards were operationalised in the NHS Plan (Department of Health, 2000), the CRT model was selected as the vehicle for delivering emergency assessment and home treatment. The NHS Plan required that 335 CRTs should be established by 2004, each treating 20 to 30 people at a time. The *Mental Health Policy Implementation Guide* (Department of Health, 2001a) contains more detailed guidance on their staffing and operation. Uptake of the teams was swift, and the National Mapping Service provided by the University of Durham reported that 267 were operating by March 2005 (Glover, Arts and Babu, 2006).

Key organisational features are described in the *Policy Implementation Guide* (PIG) (Department of Health, 2001a) by Brimblecombe (2001) and also in the Sainsbury Centre for Mental Health publication on Crisis Resolution (2001). These features are also identified by Health (2005). Having adequate funding to allow a low patient staff ratio, a 24-hour service and the opportunity to engage in handover discussions during the day are seen as essential. The team approach, with a sharing of responsibility for patients across the team, necessitates time for handing over information and discussion. The multidisciplinary aspect, with psychiatrists performing home visits and working alongside team members, is also seen as important. The gate-keeping role is acknowledged, but the PIG does not stipulate how CRTs should be integrated into the wider acute care system, nor does it identify CRTs as actively participating in inpatient reviews, or facilitating early discharge from hospital. This organisational aspect has been discussed by Nolan and Tang (2008) who compared three different ways in which CRTs can function within the acute care system based on case studies of teams in England. Whilst the guidance advocates CRT working with existing community care services to promote effective liaison and handover of treatment at the end of the crisis, the authors describe ways of working effectively with acute care services in managing the crisis. Targeting a population of patients suffering from symptoms severe enough to warrant admission to hospital and offering a brief period of home treatment are also seen as important characteristics of the service.

A debate around one essential organisational characteristic of CRTs has yet to be resolved. This is whether the teams should be separate from other services, and function as 'stand-alone' teams, or whether they should be part of existing CMHTs. Of the ten experts interviewed by Johnson and Needle (2008), only three were strongly of the opinion that CRTs should be separate teams, believing that the strength of the CRT focus on treating acutely ill people in the community would be weakened if team members worked alongside, or shared duties with, clinicians who had a broader remit.

Box 5.1 Core interventions for CRTs

- Comprehensive initial assessment, including risk, symptoms, social circumstances and relationships, substance use and physical health status.
- Engagement – intensive attempts to establish a therapeutic relationship and negotiate a treatment plan which is acceptable to patients.
- Symptom management, including starting or adjusting medication.
- Medication administered to patients in the community and their adherence encouraged and supervised, twice daily if needed.
- Practical help – support with resolving pressing financial, housing or childcare problems, getting home into a habitable state, obtaining food.
- Opportunities to talk through current problems with staff, brief interventions aimed at increasing problem-solving abilities and daily living skills.
- Education about mental health problems for patients and carers.
- Identification and discussion of potential triggers to the crisis, including difficulties in family and other important relationships.
- Relapse prevention work and planning for management of future crises.
- Discharge planning beginning at an early stage, so that continuing care services are available as soon as the crisis has resolved.

The core interventions that should be delivered by CRTs are discussed in Johnson *et al.* (2008, Chapter 6). The expert consensus derived from the interviews described above was that all the interventions delivered in a hospital setting should be provided, as a minimum standard, by these teams within the home. The interventions are listed in Box 5.1. Most have their roots in the early studies and models of CRTs, such as offering practical help, working with families and carers, and administering medication in the home. Establishing a therapeutic relationship with patients on their own terms was seen as important, and was also identified as a high priority for patients by Killaspy *et al.* (2009) in a qualitative study of the content of care delivered by assertive outreach teams.

Working with the patient to make a thorough assessment of their situation, identify possible triggers and enable future relapses to be avoided or managed more easily are seen as central to CRT interventions. Use of brief interventions, suitable for the short period of engagement with CRTs, is encouraged. However, throughout the literature, there have been no descriptions of formalised approaches to delivering these interventions. In this respect, CRT interventions are somewhat nebulous. It appears that the principle of their delivery is addressed, but not the practice. The role of psychologists in delivering brief interventions has been discussed by Hoult and Nolan (2008). Their survey of a small number of psychologists working in CRTs in England indicated that these interventions are delivered in some teams. No evidence is currently available as to which interventions work, who can deliver them effectively and which patients are likely to benefit.

Evidence for home treatment

There have been ten clinical trials to date to investigate the effectiveness of home treatment in a mental health crisis. Five of these trials were conducted in North America: Pasamanick *et al.* (1964), Langsley *et al.* (1971), Polak and Kirby (1976), Fenton *et al.* (1979) and Stein and Test

(1980). One was conducted in India (Pai and Kapur, 1983), one in Australia (Hoult *et al.*, 1983) and three in London (Merson *et al.* (1992), Marks *et al.* (1994) and Johnson *et al.* (2005b)). In addition, seven quasi-experimental studies have been carried out, using designs of either geographical comparisons of control and experimental sites with matched pairs, or 'before and after' implementation comparisons. Five of these studies were conducted in the UK (Grad and Sainsbury (1966), Dean *et al.* (1993), Minghella *et al.* (1998), Johnson *et al.* (2005a) and Tyrer *et al.* (2010)). One was conducted in Australia (Hugo *et al.*, 2002) and one in North America (Guo *et al.*, 2002). Other uncontrolled studies have been carried out to provide evidence on the types of patients that CRTs can treat most effectively (Tufnell *et al.* (1985), Bracken and Cohen (2000); on patient and carer satisfaction with treatment (Fulford and Farhall, 2001); on the content of care delivered by the teams (Boomsa *et al.*, 1999), and the effect of working in CRTs on levels of staff burnout (Nelson *et al.*, 2009)). The impact of the introduction of CRTs on admission rates and hospital stays has also been investigated (Dean and Gadd (1990), Brimblecombe *et al.* (2003) and Cotton *et al.* (2007)).

The evidence from the controlled trials, quasi-experimental studies and other uncontrolled studies had been overwhelmingly supportive of their positive effect on bed use, patient satisfaction and carer experiences.

The impact on bed use has been investigated throughout each study, providing substantial evidence for the continued implementation of this type of service due to the financial benefits to society. The impact on carers has been evaluated in the trials, but numbers have been low and measures of satisfaction variable in quality, limiting the robustness of the findings. Evaluations of patient satisfaction were incorporated only in the later studies, and investigated most thoroughly and identified as primary outcomes in Johnson *et al.* (2005a, 2005b). These studies used an established measurement, the Client Satisfaction Questionnaire (Atkisson and Zwick, 1982; Atkisson and Greenfield, 1999) in addition to further questions investigating specific aspects of treatment. The results from both studies were significantly in favour of CRT treatment. Further investigations linked to these studies were of carer satisfaction with treatment and the views of GPs. Numbers of carer participants were low, although still higher than in any previous study (33 in the control and 54 in the treatment group) and indicated that carer satisfaction with treatment was higher in the experimental group for treatment by community services and for treatment overall. Perceived carer stress was not increased when the client was treated by a crisis team. No other trial has investigated the views of associated or referring professionals, and data linked to the Johnson *et al.* (2005b) study demonstrated no significant difference in GP satisfaction between groups (Nolan, 2011).

The CRT model has been implemented widely, but the form of service delivery should be guided by evidence. The evidence is robust enough to underpin this widespread and continued implementation in the UK given the findings of these studies, particularly in terms of cost-effectiveness. However, further research is necessary in eight principle areas. These are:

- Patients' experiences of home treatment, using measures with established psychometric properties that cover a range of needs. Qualitative evaluations conducted alongside larger scale studies, with comparison of results from both methods, would further illuminate this complex area.
- Carers' views and experiences of home treatment, within large-scale studies with adequate power.
- Staff experiences of working in crisis teams, compared to other mental health services, using both quantitative tools to measure job satisfaction, stress and burnout, and qualitative interviews to complement these.

- Obtaining the views of staff in linked services such as CMHTs and inpatient wards would be valuable. Longitudinal evaluations of staff turnover and sickness in crisis teams compared to other acute care and community services should be conducted where the teams are well developed and these data are available.
- The content of care delivered by crisis teams compared to other mental health services. The processes used within crisis teams have not been identified, and the results of comparison of clinical and social outcomes between CRTs and other services are equivocal.
- The safety of home treatment: The impact of crisis teams on deaths or suicides has not been evaluated due to the necessity of large sample sizes in order to have adequate power on which to base findings. Adverse events of violence, self-harm, self-neglect and being a victim of exploitation of violence due to vulnerability have not been adequately explored. Deaths associated with home treatment could be evaluated using routinely collected data from Trusts nationally.
- Comparison between stand-alone crisis teams and crisis services provided within generic CMHTs: No study has investigated home treatment delivered by augmented standard care services. A provision of CMHTs managing crises by increasing contacts over a short period, and having extended hours, including evening and weekends, with 24-hour on call, needs to be compared with stand-alone service. Indications from a qualitative study (Nolan, 2011) linked to Johnson *et al.* (2005b) were that continuity of care is appreciated by patients, and established relationships with CMHT workers are difficult to replicate with brief interventions from unknown staff (Nolan, 2011). It would be beneficial for patients to talk to workers with whom they have established relationships, and would lessen the incidence of mistrust identified by many of the qualitative sample. Variations in ways of providing acute care services (Nolan and Tang, 2008) in which crisis team and ward staff are part of a cohesive acute care service, and are readily accessed by CMHT staff, may also impact on outcomes. Differences in length of hospital admissions are unlikely to be as great as within comparisons between standard care and crisis teams, so larger numbers would be needed in any evaluations. Length of community crisis treatment could, however, be investigated within a smaller sample. The efficacy of specific interventions should also be tested within different means of service delivery.
- Developing measure of fidelity to a model of CRTs is necessary. In order to do this, critical ingredients for the model need to be established and tested for their effectiveness. Fidelity scales are intended to measure how far a service adheres to a model based on best evidence about the most effective practice (Mowbray *et al.*, 2003). Once a fidelity scale for CRTs has been established, further research can be conducted to test whether the model adherence does indeed result in better outcomes, so that fidelity scale development and outcome measurement may be an iterative process as such evidence accumulates.

Implications for service planning and clinical practice

The findings from the studies of CRTs indicate that while this type of service appears to have tangible benefits, there is also room for improvement in the ways in which the teams address individual needs. In addition to the organisational characteristics and core interventions described by Johnson *et al.* (2008), a model for CRTs should emphasise the areas in which practice might be improved. These improvements can potentially be achieved in terms of changes to clinical practice within teams and to the planning of services within provider organisations.

Clinical practice within teams should focus on developing strong therapeutic relationships with patients, using non-coercive means. These may include assisting with practical problems, especially in the initial stages of treatment. Staff should base all interactions on an empathetic approach, and exhibit kindness, patience and tolerance. The often highly pressured nature of CRT work, with high caseloads and quick turnover, can easily inhibit the expression of these qualities. Instilling an ethos within teams of exhibiting kindness and working collaboratively with patients is therefore a challenge, but may be achieved through supportive leadership and role modelling. Adequate time should be allocated for visits. This could potentially be achieved by having a standard duration for each visit, with flexibility in implementation. Information on this standard time period should be routinely given to patients, so that they have realistic expectations. This would also assist staff in planning their visits, and in determining caseload sizes. Workload allocation should take gender into account; where possible, female patients should not be visited by male staff alone. When team staffing makes this unavoidable, patients should be given a choice of whether to have a visit or not. Visits by two male staff have been identified by both male and female patients as intimidating (Nolan, 2011), and should also be avoided. Consideration should be given to an appropriate gender mix when appointing staff, and when planning the team work rota.

Working with families and social systems should be prioritised. Identifying people who form part of the patients' social system should be the initial stage of this work, followed by discussion with them about the content of the intervention they would like the team to have with their friends or relatives.

Patients should have quick access to prescribing from CRTs. This can be facilitated by the presence of non-medical prescribers in each team, which would supplement the work of medical prescribers. In addition, use of Patient Group Directions (PGDs) or group protocols (Medicines and Healthcare Products Regulatory Agency, 2010) within teams would enable nursing staff to prescribe from a limited formulary, and provide patients with quick access to medication, until a review by a prescriber can occur. Improved continuity of care between community services and CRTs is needed. CRTs should encourage joint visits to patients with care coordinators or key workers from community services as part of standard practice. Liaison between services without the knowledge of the patient is not enough. Visible working between services is required to engender trust between the patient and CRT staff. Continuity of care within CRTs can be facilitated by restricting the numbers of staff involved in each treatment period, while maintaining a team approach.

Being employed appears to be linked with increased satisfaction (Nolan, 2011). CRTs could thus improve outcomes in this area by providing support and advice on employment and activities, and developing links with local vocational services.

Monitoring of practice within teams is necessary to ensure that standards are upheld. Use of regular supervision sessions, provided by staff within the team, or by outside facilitators for whole team supervision, can provide forums in which staff can reflect on their practice and look for possible improvements. Use of senior staff employed with a remit to improve practice, such as nurse consultants or practice development staff, should also be considered for CRTs. Such staff have been traditionally employed in inpatient services, but would be potentially of benefit within the CRT setting.

Ongoing use of patient evaluation measures within teams would promote staff awareness of their performance from the patients' perspective. Feedback from these evaluations should be incorporated into CRT practice, through regular (e.g. monthly) analysis of results and team discussions.

Service planning within organisations should aim to ensure that CRTs are part of a cohesive acute care service. This would involve greater integration of CRTs, acute inpatient wards and acute care day hospital services. This model is described by Nolan and Tang (2008), and has been in operation in Norfolk and Waveney NHS Foundation trust since 2004, where it has demonstrated positive impacts on patient satisfaction and bed use. The model potentiates more effective liaison between services through staff working in each service on a rotational basis, providing cover between services when necessary, and the use of service-wide recording documents for assessment and care planning. Streamlining the process of referral, assessment and joint working between CMHT and acute care services can impact on continuity of care.

Provider organisations in the UK should also ensure that CRTs are part of each Trust Acute Care Forum (National Institute for Mental Health in England, 2009), which have the remit of improving practice in services through use of local initiatives.

A thorough evaluation of the interventions provided by CRTs, and their adherence to a model of fidelity, once established, is needed. A suitably skilled workforce is also required to deliver these interventions, and organisations need to ensure that appropriate training is provided.

Conclusion

CRTs have been part of mainstream service provision in the UK since 2001 and have demonstrated significant fiscal benefits, along with increased levels of satisfaction in those they treat. Thus, there is a strong argument for their continued provision, particularly during periods of economic constraint. There is scope for improvement to their clinical practice, evidenced by recent studies in England, in addition to developing of a model of fidelity to provide a marker for teams. Priorities in implementing this improved service are increased work with families and carers, a flexible approach, tighter liaison with other acute care services and provision of an appropriately skilled workforce.

References

Atkisson, C. C. and Zwick, R. (1982) 'The client satisfaction questionnaire: psychometric properties and correlations with service utilization and psychotherapy outcome', *Evaluation & Program Planning*, vol. 5, no. 3, pp. 233–237.

Attkisson, C. C. and Greenfield, T. K. (1999) 'The UCSF client satisfaction scales: I. the client satisfaction questionnaire-8'. In M. E. Maruish (ed.) *The Use of Psychological Tests for Treatment Planning and Outcomes Assessment*, Mahwah, NJ: Lawrence Erlbaum Associates.

Boomsa, J., Dassen, T., Dingemans, C. and van de Heuvel, W. (1999) 'Nursing interventions in crisis-orientated and long-term psychiatric care', *Scandinavian Journal of Caring Sciences*, vol. 13, pp. 41–48.

Bracken, P. and Cohen, B. (2000) 'Home treatment in Bradford', *Psychiatric Bulletin*, vol. 23, pp. 349–352.

Brimblecombe, N. (2001) 'Developing intensive home treatment services: problems and issues'. In N. Brimblecombe (ed.) *Acute Mental Health Care in the Community: Intensive Home Treatment*, London: Whurr, pp. 187–210.

Brimblecombe, N., O'Sullivan, G., and Parkinson, B. (2003) 'Home treatment as an alternative to inpatient admission: characteristics of those treated and factors predicting hospitalization', *Journal of Psychiatric and Mental Health Nursing*, 10, 683–687.

Caplan, G. (1964) *Principles of Preventive Psychiatry*, New York: Basic Books.

Cotton, M. A., Johnson, S., Bindman, J., Sandor, A., White, I., Thornicroft, G., Nolan, F., Pilling, S., Hoult, J., McKenzie, N. and Bebbington, P. (2007) 'An investigation of factors associated with psychiatric hospital admission despite the presence of crisis resolution teams', *BMC Psychiatry*, vol. 7, no. 1, p. 52.

Dean, C. and Gadd, E. M. (1990) 'Home treatment for acute psychiatric illness', *BMJ*, vol. 301, no. 6759, pp. 1021–1023.

Dean, C., Phillips, J., Gadd, E. M., Joseph, M. and England, S. (1993) 'Comparison of community based service with hospital based service for people with acute, severe psychiatric illness', *BMJ*, vol. 307, no. 6902, pp. 473–476.

Department of Health (1999) *A National Service Framework for Mental Health: Modern Standards and Service Models*, London: Department of Health.

Department of Health (2000) *The NHS Plan*, London: The Stationery Office.

Department of Health (2001a) 'Crisis resolution/home treatment teams'. In *The Mental Health Policy Implementation Guide*, London: Department of Health.

Department of Health (2002) *Acute Adult In-patient Care: Policy Implementation Guide*, London: Department of Health.

Fenton, F. R., Tessier, L. and Struening, E. L. (1979) 'A comparative trial of home and hospital psychiatric care. One year follow-up', *Archives of General Psychiatry*, vol. 36, pp. 1073–1079.

Fulford, M. and Farhall, J. (2001) 'Hospital versus home care for the acutely mentally ill? Preferences of caregivers who have experienced both forms of service', *Australian & New Zealand Journal of Psychiatry*, vol. 35, no. 5, pp. 619–625.

Glover, G., Arts, G. and Babu, K. S. (2006) 'Crisis resolution/home treatment teams and psychiatric admission rates in England', *British Journal of Psychiatry*, vol. 189, pp. 441–445.

Grad, J. and Sainsbury, P. (1966) 'Evaluating the community psychiatric service in Chichester: results', *Milbank Memorial Fund Quarterly*, vol. 44, no. 1, p. Suppl-78.

Guo, S., Biegel, D. E., Johnsen, J. A. and Dyches, H. (2002) 'Assessing the impact of community-based mobile crisis services on preventing hospitalization', *Psychiatric Services*, vol. 52, no. 2, pp. 223–228.

Heath, D. (ed.) (2005) *Home Treatment for Acute Mental Disorders: An Alternative to Hospitalization*, London: Routledge.

Hoult, J., Reynolds, I., Charbonneau-Powis, M., Weekes, P. and Briggs, J. (1983) 'Psychiatric hospital versus community treatment: the results of a randomised trial', *Australian & New Zealand Journal of Psychiatry*, vol. 17, no. 2, pp. 160–167.

Hoult, J. and Nolan, F. (2008) 'Symptom management'. In S. Johnson, J. Needle, J. Bindman and G. Thornicroft (eds), *Crisis Resolution and Home Treatment in Mental Health*, London: Cambridge University Press.

Hugo, M., Smout, M. and Bannister, J. (2002) 'A comparison in hospitalization rates between a community-based mobile emergency service and a hospital-based emergency service', *Australian and New Zealand Journal of Psychiatry*, vol. 36, no. 4, pp. 504–508.

Johnson, S. and Needle, J. (2008) 'Crisis resolution teams: rationale and core model'. In S. Johnson, J. Needle, J. Bindman and G. Thornicroft (eds), *Crisis Resolution and Home Treatment in Mental Health*, London: Cambridge University Press.

Johnson, S., Needle, J., Bindman, J. and Thornicroft, G. Eds (2008) *Crisis Resolution and Home Treatment in Mental Health*, Cambridge: Cambridge University Press.

Johnson, S., Nolan, F., Hoult, J., Pilling, S., White, I., Bebbington, P., Sandor, A., McKenzie, N. and Patel, S. (2005a) 'The outcomes of psychiatric crises before and after introduction of a crisis resolution team', *The British Journal of Psychiatry*, vol. 187, pp. 68–75.

Johnson, S., Nolan, F., Pilling, S., Sandor, A., Hoult, J., McKenzie, N., White, I. R., Thompson, M. and Bebbington, P. (2005b) 'Randomised controlled trial of acute mental health care by a crisis resolution team: the north Islington crisis study', *British Medical Journal*, vol. 331, p. 599–602.

Killaspy, H., Johnson, S., Pierce, B., Bebbington, P., Pilling, S., Nolan, F. and King, M. (2009) 'Successful engagement: a mixed methods study of the approaches of assertive community treatment and community mental health teams in the REACT trial', *Social Psychiatry and Psychiatric Epidemiology*, vol. 44, no. 7, pp. 532–540.

Langsley, D. G., Machotka, P. and Flomenhaft, K. (1971) 'Avoiding mental hospital admission: a follow-up study', *American Journal of Psychiatry*, vol. 127, no. 10, pp. 1391–1394.

Marks, I., Connolly, J., Muijen, M., Audini, B., McNamee, G. and Lawrence, R. (1994) 'Home-based versus hospital-based care for people with serious mental illness', *British Journal of Psychiatry*, vol. 165, pp. 179–194.

Merson, S., Tyrer, P., Onyett, S., Lack, S., Birkett, P., Lynch, S. and Johnson, T. (1992) 'Early intervention in psychiatric emergencies: a controlled clinical trial', *Lancet*, vol. 339, no. 8805, pp. 1311–1314.

Medicines and Healthcare Products Regulatory Agency (MHRA), Department of Health (2010) *Patient Group Directions in the NHS*. London: Department of Health.

Minghella, E., Ford, R., Freeman, T., Hoult, J., McGlynn, P. and O'Halloran, P. (1998) *Open All Hours: 24-hour Response for People with Mental Health Emergencies*, London: Sainsbury Centre for Mental Health.

Mowbray, C.T., Holter M.C., Teague G.B. and Bybee D. (2003) 'Fidelity criteria: development, measurement, and validation', *American Journal of Evaluation*, vol. 24, no. 3, pp. 315–340.

Muijen, M., Marks, I. M., Connolly, J., and Audini, B. (1992) 'The Daily Living Programme: Preliminary comparison of community versus hospital-based treatment for the seriously mentally ill facing emergency admission', *British Journal of Psychiatry*, 160, 379–384.

Nelson, T., Johnson, S. and Bebbington, P. (2009) 'Satisfaction and burnout among staff of crisis resolution, assertive outreach and community mental health team', *Social Psychiatry and Psychiatric Epidemiology*, vol. 44, no. 7, pp. 541–549.

National Institute for Mental Health in England (NIMHE) (2009) *The Capable Acute Care Forum*. London.

Nolan, F. (2011) 'An evaluation of the crisis resolution team model of mental health care', unpublished thesis, University College London.

Nolan, F. and Tang, S (2008) 'Early discharge and joint working between crisis teams and hospital services'. In S. Johnson, J. Needle, J. Bindman and G. Thornicroft (eds) *Crisis Resolution and Home Treatment in Mental Health*, London: Cambridge University Press.

Pai, S. and Kapur R. L. (1983) 'Evaluation of home care treatment for schizophrenic patients', *Acta Psychiatrica Scandinavica*, vol. 67, pp. 80–88.

Pasamanick, B., Scarpitti, F. R. and Dinitz, S. (1967) *Schizophrenics in the Community: An Experimental Study in the Prevention of Hospitalization*, New York: Century-Crofts.

Pasamanick, B., Scarpitti, F. R., Lefton, M., Dinitz, S., Wernet. J. J., & McPheeters, H. (1964) 'Home versus hospital care for schizophrenics', *Journal of the American Medical Association (JAMA)*, vol. 187, pp. 177–181.

Polak, P. R. and Kirby, M. W. (1976) 'A model to replace psychiatric hospitals', *Journal of Nervous & Mental Disease*, vol. 162, no. 1, pp. 13–22.

Querido, A. (1954) 'Experiment in public health', *Bulletin of the World Federation for Mental Health*, vol. 6, pp. 203–216.

Repper, J. and Perkins, R. (2006) *Social Inclusion and Recovery: A Model for Mental Health Practice*, Edinburgh: Baillière Tindall.

Rosen, A (1997) 'Crisis management in the community'. *Medical Journal of Australia*, 1997; 167: 633–638.

Sainsbury Centre for Mental Health (2001). *Mental Health Topics: Crisis Resolution*. London: Sainsbury Centre for Mental Health.

Stein, L. I. and Test, M. A. (1980) 'Alternative to mental hospital treatment. I. Conceptual model, treatment program, and clinical evaluation', *Archives of General Psychiatry*, vol. 37, pp. 392–397.

Tyrer, P., Gordon, F., Nourmand, S., Lawrence, M., Curran, C., Southgate, D., Oruganti, B., Tyler, M., Tottle, S., North, B., Kulinskaya, E., Kaleekal, J.T. and Morgan, J. (2010) 'Controlled comparison of two crisis resolution and home treatment teams', *The Psychiatrist*, vol. 34, no. 2, pp. 50–54.

6　Contemporary rehabilitation

Helen Killaspy

Rehabilitation remodelled

Until the latter half of the 20th century, most people with mental health problems in the UK received care in large, Victorian asylums, usually located on the periphery of major towns and cities. At their peak in the 19th century, asylums operated as self-contained institutions, with little focus on rehabilitation. Individuals were admitted voluntarily or committed, sometimes for life, and 'rehabilitation' mainly comprised work in the laundry, kitchen or gardens or in industrial therapy units where factory style production lines operated.

The development of modern rehabilitation services is inextricably linked to the closure of the asylums. De-institutionalisation gathered apace from the 1950s onwards, fuelled by the development of phenothiazine medications (the first antipsychotic drugs), an increasing awareness of the negative effects of institutionalisation (see for example, Goffman, 1968; Wing and Brown, 1970), the ever increasing asylum population size and the untenable costs of upkeep of the institutions. These factors gradually led to a shift in socio-political attitudes away from the benevolent Victorian concept of 'asylum', towards the socially inclusive concept of 'care in the community' (Department of Health and Social Security, 1981).

Many rehabilitation practitioners were proactive protagonists of de-institutionalisation and rehabilitation began to focus on supporting individuals to gain skills and confidence to make a successful move to the community. That ethos is apparent in the following definition of rehabilitation given by John Wing (1980): 'The process of minimising psychiatric impairments, social disadvantages and adverse personal reactions so that the disabled person is helped to use his or her talents and to acquire confidence and self-esteem through experiencing success in social roles.'

As the process of de-institutionalisation progressed, rehabilitation practitioners became increasingly involved in the 'resettlement' process. Individuals with more complex problems and higher levels of need were often moved to small, community-based residential facilities. Some were purpose-built and many were converted from large (often Victorian) houses. Those with the most complex needs were the last to leave the asylum and often placed in innovative 'wards in the community' or 'houses in the hospital grounds'. All these facilities offered communal living to a relatively small number of residents. The Team for the Assessment of Psychiatric Services (TAPS) carried out a comprehensive longitudinal study to investigate the outcomes for individuals of de-institutionalisation. Overall, the results were very positive. Five years after leaving the asylum, the majority, even those with the most complex problems, had increased their social networks, gained independent living skills, improved their quality of life and not required readmission to hospital (Leff and Trieman, 2000; Trieman and Leff, 2002).

The development of community mental health services

As community mental health care further evolved, multidisciplinary community mental health teams (CMHTs) became established, staffed by psychiatrists, nurses, psychologists, occupational therapists and social workers. Community mental health and social care provision became an increasingly complex system to navigate and case management was developed to address this by assigning individual staff to coordinate an individual's treatment and care. In the UK, this system is organised through the statutory framework of the Care Programme Approach (Department of Health, 1990, 1999a).

In 1999, the National Service Framework for Mental Health (Department of Health, 1999b) detailed the implementation across England of three new models of community mental health services alongside CMHTs: early intervention services (for people experiencing their first episode of psychosis); crisis resolution and home treatment services (providing home-based, short-term care for people in acute mental distress); and assertive outreach services (longer term, intensive case management for people who have difficulties engaging with CMHTs and are high users of inpatient care). Patient satisfaction with all three services has been shown to be greater than standard CMHT care, and early intervention and crisis resolution services have also been shown to be clinically cost-effective (Craig *et al.*, 2004; Johnson *et al.*, 2005). However, assertive outreach teams have not shown clinical advantage over CMHTs in the UK (Killaspy *et al.*, 2006, 2009a; Glover *et al.*, 2006), perhaps because of inadequate implementation of the model, particularly in operating an extended hours service and the sharing of clinical responsibility between staff, or because CMHTs already offer some of the key elements of assertive outreach such as home visiting and having full clinical responsibility for all clients (Killaspy, 2010a).

Rehabilitation of service users

Despite the investment in specialist community mental health services, there remains a group of patients who do not recover adequately to be discharged home following an acute psychiatric admission. This is the group who are referred to contemporary mental health rehabilitation services. Most have a diagnosis of schizophrenia (Killaspy *et al.*, 2008) though at any time, only around 1 per cent of people with schizophrenia are in receipt of inpatient rehabilitation (Holloway, 2005). Delayed recovery is usually due to complexities in the person's presentation that are related to long-term psychosis, pre-existing or co-morbid problems. Multiple problems can, of course, compound the situation. These include: treatment resistance (i.e. non-response to adequate trials of medication), which occurs in one fifth to one third of people with a diagnosis of schizophrenia (National Institute for Health and Clinical Excellence, 2010); cognitive impairments, especially those affecting frontal lobe function (planning and organisational skills); negative symptoms (apathy, amotivation, blunting of affect and poverty of thought); co-morbid depression, anxiety, substance misuse, brain injuries; pre-morbid learning disabilities, developmental disorders and personality disorders; and challenging behaviours produced by these problems (Wykes & Dunn, 1992; Green, 1996; Meltzer, 1997; Holloway, 2005; Killaspy *et al.*, 2008). People referred to contemporary mental health rehabilitation services have usually been unwell for many years and been recurrently admitted. Though they are relatively few in number, they have such complex needs that they require lengthy, expensive admissions; they are a 'low volume, high need' group. In 2009–10, 51 per cent of the total direct costs of adult mental health and social care were related to services for people with longer term mental health problems and of these, around half (25 per cent of the total £6bn budget) was spent on designated rehabilitation services and specialist mental health supported accommodation (Mental Health Strategies, 2010).

Serious mental health problems, especially schizophrenia and related disorders, are associated with a number of problems that interact and exacerbate social exclusion. These include: poor social and functional skills; poor educational attainment and unemployment; poverty; poor housing and homelessness; social isolation (poor social networks and being single); stigma and discrimination; exploitation and victimisation. Since rehabilitation services focus on individuals with the most complex needs and greatest levels of functional impairment, they work with one of the most socially excluded groups in society (Social Exclusion Unit, 2004). Nevertheless, positive outcomes have been demonstrated in longer term studies. Harding *et al.* (1987) showed that half to two thirds of patients who had received rehabilitation were significantly improved or recovered 32 years later. The markers of recovery were impressive, i.e. not requiring medication to control symptoms; working; having good relationships with family and friends; showing no overt behaviours indicative of ever having had a psychiatric problem. Similarly, a large international multicentre study found that amongst people diagnosed with schizophrenia, global outcomes were favourable in over half 15 and 25 years after diagnosis (Harrison *et al.*, 2001). These results suggest that therapeutic optimism in the longer term is appropriate. As contemporary mental health services have become increasingly focused on shorter term outcomes, holding therapeutic optimism and a long-term view are key features of the culture of rehabilitation services.

Ethos of contemporary rehabilitation services

In 2005 a national survey of rehabilitation services was undertaken and key clinicians were asked their views on what they felt the term 'rehabilitation' meant. From their responses a contemporary definition was collated:

> A whole systems approach to recovery from mental illness that maximizes an individual's quality of life and social inclusion by encouraging their skills, promoting independence and autonomy in order to give them hope for the future and leads to successful community living through appropriate support.
>
> (Killaspy *et al.*, 2005)

This definition encompasses therapeutic optimism in terms of holding hope when other services and the service user themselves may feel stuck and demoralised. It also emphasises the need for a whole care pathway to support service users as they recover. Rehabilitation services operate across the whole spectrum of care, not just in inpatient or community settings and work in partnership with other statutory and non-statutory services to support and enable service users over a number of years to maximise their independence in all aspects of their life. The range of services required includes housing, welfare benefits, education and employment, and liaison with primary health care to promote fitness and manage physical health problems.

Collaborative partnerships are also of paramount importance between service users and staff and rehabilitation services were early adopters of the 'Recovery' approach, a key feature of which is collaborative partnership working with service users. Although a full description of the concept and origins of what is meant by 'Recovery' is beyond the scope of this chapter, its ethos can be summarised in the most widely quoted definition:

> A deeply personal, unique process of changing one's attitudes, values, feelings, goals, skills and roles. It is a way of living a satisfying, hopeful and contributing life even with limitations caused by the illness. Recovery involves the development of a new meaning and purpose in one's life as one grows beyond the catastrophic effects of mental illness.
>
> (Anthony, 1993)

Though a relatively recent 'movement', Recovery is not a new concept. William Tuke, a successful Quaker businessman and philanthropist, is credited with the establishment of a clinical philosophy known as 'moral treatment' in the early 19th century. Appalled by the conditions in the York asylum at the time, he raised funds to found a private asylum (The Retreat) with a philosophy based on kindness, compassion, collaboration and hope (Tuke, 1855). These qualities remain key to a service's Recovery orientation, which also encompasses a focus on collaborative working with service users rather than paternalism, choice rather than coercion, enablement rather than being 'looked after', and shared holding of responsibility, including around issues related to risk. All modern mental health services are strongly encouraged to adopt a Recovery orientation (Shepherd *et al.*, 2008, 2010; Sainsbury Centre, 2009).

In the US, Liberman and Kopelowicz (2002) have suggested a number of 'markers of Recovery' including working, studying and participating in leisure activities in mainstream settings; good family relationships; living independently; having control of one's self-care, medication and money; having a rewarding social life; taking part in the local community; voting; and satisfaction with life. Many of these clearly also reflect a more 'socially included' life. It therefore follows that a Recovery orientated service will also be one that promotes service users' social inclusion.

This focus on social functioning is of central importance in rehabilitation. Even with optimum medication, complete resolution of 'positive' psychotic symptoms is not always possible. However, it is the 'negative' symptoms and impairments of cognitive functioning that are often more problematic in terms of a person's social and everyday functioning, but it is often these that are the most difficult to treat. Few medications specifically target 'negative' symptoms and the person may have become increasingly deskilled through the course of their illness and admission/s. Anyone who has experienced a period of physical illness can probably relate to the loss of confidence in one's own abilities engendered by having to accept help from others whilst debilitated. Given the severity and complexity of problems that rehabilitation service users experience, it is not surprising that the process of 'reskilling' can take many years. Some service users will have become unwell prior to adulthood and may never have gained independent living skills. Key to this process is the identification of the person's existing strengths that can be built on, as well as a full understanding of the person's particular difficulties. This 'strengths' approach embodies a therapeutic positivity, facilitating the service user to gain confidence through encouragement and positive reinforcement of their existing interests and skills (however insignificant they may appear).

Interventions and skills

The specific treatments and interventions delivered by inpatient and community rehabilitation services will vary according to service users' particular needs, but they follow evidence-based guidance (e.g. those detailed in the NICE guidelines for the treatment of schizophrenia) and include medications for treatment-resistant psychosis and affective disorders, physical health promotion, psychological interventions such as cognitive behavioural therapy and family interventions, occupational therapy and supported employment. Although occupational therapy is currently lacking in terms of an evidence base, it is known that many people with schizophrenia spend many hours a day doing absolutely nothing (Curson *et al.*, 1992). Occupational therapy is key in motivating service users to engage in activities (Cook and Birrell, 2007). The implementation of specific interventions in rehabilitation settings is described in detail in *Enabling Recovery: The Principles and Practice of Rehabilitation Psychiatry* (Roberts *et al.*, 2006). The rehabilitation team therefore has to have an appropriate skill mix to assess service users' needs and deliver support and interventions that are tailored to each individual. Incremental steps are required for progress to be made, and it has been noted that rehabilitation staff need to be of a temperament that is low in 'expressed emotion' (Shepherd, 2006). In other words, the ideal rehabilitation practitioner is a person who is calm, patient, therapeutically optimistic and encourages a person to build on their strengths rather than criticising them for their deficits.

An average inpatient rehabilitation unit in England has 14 beds and is staffed by a multidisciplinary team comprising a full-time rehabilitation psychiatrist, a full-time occupational therapist, a part-time clinical psychologist and a full complement of nursing and support workers (Killaspy *et al.*, 2005). Increasingly, services employ non-registered staff to facilitate service users' access to community activities and some services employ ex-service users (not necessarily of the same service) as staff members, for example in support worker or peer supporter roles. All staff are likely to be involved in the delivery of lower intensity psychological interventions such as motivational interviewing, relapse prevention and insight orientated work, and treatment and care plans should, wherever possible, be drawn up collaboratively with service users and, where possible, family and carers.

As service users recover, they are encouraged and supported to expand their repertoire of activities on the unit and in the community, including, ultimately, engagement in education and work. Rehabilitation practitioners, especially occupational therapists, are often key in building bridges with educational establishments and employment agencies to facilitate this. At the same time, support to gradually (re)gain competence in managing activities of daily living (self-care, laundry, cleaning, budgeting, shopping and cooking) continues as service users move on from inpatient to community settings. Nurses, support workers and occupational therapists are all involved in facilitating service users with these skills.

The rehabilitation care pathway

A range of hospital and community-based units are required to support service users in their rehabilitation and recovery. Both shorter term (length of stay less than one year) and longer term units are required to serve a locality (local authority area or borough). The Faculty of Rehabilitation and Social Psychiatry of the Royal College of Psychiatrists has published *A Template for Rehabilitation Services* (Wolfson *et al.*, 2009) that describes in detail the types of inpatient and community-based services required in a whole system rehabilitation care pathway. At a locality level these generally include high dependency inpatient rehabilitation units (usually locked units that take detained patients, often with challenging behaviours), 'open' rehabilitation units (usually community based, that take non-detained patients and focus on developing everyday living skills in a domestic environment) and longer term complex care units (either hospital or community based, for patients with high levels of disability). At a regional level, secure rehabilitation units provide for those who have a history of offending as well as complex mental health needs, and specialist units provide for those with complex mental health needs co-occurring with other special needs such as organic brain damage or Autism Spectrum Disorder.

As individuals recover, they are able to move on to less supported settings. The higher intensity inpatient and community rehabilitation services described above are, ideally, supported in this process by the provision of a full range of supported accommodation in each locality (MacPherson *et al.*, 2004). In England, around a third of working age adults with severe mental health problems reside in supported accommodation provided by health and social services, voluntary organisations, housing associations and other independent providers.

These include nursing and residential care homes, group homes, hostels, blocks of individual or shared tenancies with staff on site, and independent tenancies with 'floating' or outreach support from staff. In 2006 around 12,500 people with mental health problems in England were in a nursing or residential care home (National Statistics, 2006) and around 40,000 were receiving floating outreach (Department of Communities and Local Government, 2006). Not all this group will necessarily have come through a rehabilitation care pathway, but the mixed economy of supported accommodation provides a flexible range of supported facilities for service users that they can move through according to their needs. Most staff in supported accommodation services do not have mental health professional qualifications. They provide day-to-day support to service users to assist them in managing their tenancy and activities of daily living and accessing community activities (education, leisure, work). More specialist mental health supervision and interventions are provided by local mental health services. In some areas, community rehabilitation teams provide care coordination to service users in supported accommodation and in others this is provided by generic CMHTs.

Disinvestment in rehabilitation services and the use of out of area placements

The investment in specialist community mental health services facilitated by the National Service Framework for Mental Health (Department of Health, 1999b) was associated with an overly optimistic expectation on the part of some commissioners and managers of services that rehabilitation services would no longer be required. The absence of rehabilitation services from the National Service Framework for Mental Health did little to challenge this assumption (Department of Health, 1999b). There followed a period of disinvestment, with patchy closures of rehabilitation units across England and rebadging of around one third of community rehabilitation teams as assertive outreach services (Mountain *et al.*, 2009). However, even with intensive community services such as assertive outreach teams, the 'low volume, high need' group continued to require longer term inpatient care. In turn, this led to a rise in the use of 'out of area' placements where patients were transferred to inpatient or community-based nursing/residential care provided by the independent sector, often geographically displaced from their area of origin.

Many out of area placements provide good quality care and some focus on very specialist care, where the small number of service users in a locality does not support a case for investment in local provision. However, concerns have been raised about the distance that many people are placed from their local community, family and friends, the lack of 'rehabilitation' provided, with practices that may deskill individuals rather than encouraging their autonomy (for example providing meals rather than supporting self-catering), difficulties in accessing specialist input from mental health services local to the placement, and delays in accessing appropriately supported accommodation in the area of origin when the individual is ready to move (Ryan *et al.*, 2004). The phenomenon of out of area placements has been referred to as a 'virtual asylum' (Poole *et al.*, 2002) and a similar process of 'reinstitutionalisation' has also been reported elsewhere in Europe (Priebe *et al.*, 2005). A survey by the Faculty of Rehabilitation and Social Psychiatry of the Royal College of Psychiatrists of all primary care trusts (PCTs) and local authorities (LAs) in England found that of the 30,000 mental health placements made in 2008–9, 21 per cent were made out of area. This figure was clearly much higher than could be explained by the need for specialist regional placements for individuals with especially complex needs. The cost of an out of area placement was on average 67 per cent greater than local placements and the estimated total annual cost was estimated at £330m (Killaspy and Meier, 2010b).

Some areas have implemented review systems to identify people placed out of area who can be 'repatriated' to appropriately supported accommodation in their area of origin, with the associated financial flows being reinvested into local rehabilitation services and supported housing (Killaspy *et al.*, 2009b). These kinds of initiatives rely on successful collaboration between commissioners and service providers in the NHS, voluntary and independent sectors. Local reinvestment in provision for service users with longer term and more complex needs not only provides appropriate resources to facilitate the ongoing rehabilitation of those returning from out of area placements, it also builds local competence in working with this group, thus reducing future reliance on out of area placements.

The current economic downturn has focused more attention on the potential efficiencies of a well managed system for the review and repatriation of out of area placements. In 2010 the Department of Health commissioned a work stream on this topic as part of its 'Quality Innovation, Productivity and Prevention' initiative, the product of which is a web-based toolkit for mental health commissioners and providers published by Royal College of Psychiatrists (2011). This attention on the issue is certainly welcome but it is vital that repatriation is accompanied by local investment in rehabilitation and supported housing services for the process to work, otherwise any short-term financial gains will quickly be lost as those with more complex needs once again become stuck in acute admission wards.

Quality and effectiveness of rehabilitation services

In England, the Care Quality Commission is the regulatory body for care provided by the NHS, local authorities, private companies and voluntary organisations. Most countries have similar systems for the registration and review of the quality of health and social care facilities. However, until recently there were no specific tools for the assessment of the quality of mental health rehabilitation units, though standards were set and reviewed. The DEMoBinc study addressed this gap (Development of a European measure of best practice for people with longer term mental health problems in institutional care).

This three-year project was funded by the European Commission and involved ten European countries at different stages of de-institutionalisation, with the aim of building a quality assessment toolkit specifically for longer term mental health units (average length of stay over six months). The product was a web-based toolkit that is completed by the unit manager, the Quality Indicator for Rehabilitative Care (QuIRC). It is available as an online application (www.quirc.eu) and takes about an hour to complete. It assesses seven domains of care (Living Environment; Therapeutic Environment; Treatments and Interventions; Self-Management and Autonomy; Social Interface; Human Rights; and Recovery Based Practice). These domains were identified for inclusion in the toolkit through triangulation of the results from: i) a review of care standards in each country; ii) a systematic literature review of the components of care (and their effectiveness) in mental health units (Taylor *et al.*, 2009); and iii) an international Delphi exercise with four stakeholder groups (service users, carers, professionals, advocates) (Turton *et al.*, 2010). The content of the QuIRC was agreed by an international panel of experts in the field. The toolkit has excellent inter-rater reliability (Killaspy *et al.*, 2011a) and the ratings (provided from the answers provided by the unit manager) have been shown to reflect service users' ratings of their experiences of care and the unit's promotion of their autonomy (Killaspy *et al.*, 2011b). The QuIRC produces a report for each unit that compares the domain scores to the average scores for similar units in the same country. It also details the areas that could be focused on to improve quality in each domain.

The QuIRC has been incorporated into the UK's peer accreditation system for inpatient rehabilitation units (AIMS-Rehab) coordinated by the Royal College of Psychiatrists' Centre for Quality Improvement, and similar initiatives are underway in other countries. It will therefore be possible in the future to compare the quality of units in different economic and socio-political contexts. The QuIRC data is also useful for research purposes, local audit, regional, national and international benchmarking.

Contemporary mental health rehabilitation is a complex intervention and, in the UK, there have been no studies investigating its effectiveness. In order to address this, the National Institute of Health Research has funded a five-year programme of research in this area (the Rehabilitation Effectiveness for Activities for Life study; www.ucl.ac.uk/REAL-Study). The programme includes a detailed national survey of mental health rehabilitation services in England, a randomised controlled trial to investigate the efficacy of an intensive staff training intervention (derived from occupational therapy and organisational psychology theory) that aims to facilitate service users' activities, and a naturalistic cohort study to investigate service users' outcomes over time. The findings will allow a better understanding of the current provision and components of these services and help to identify which interventions and aspects of rehabilitation are most beneficial for service users.

References

Anthony, W.A. (1993) Recovery from mental illness: the guiding vision of the mental health service system in the 1990s, *Psychosocial Rehabilitation Journal*, 16: 11–23.

Cook, S. and Birrell, M. (2007) Defining and occupational therapy intervention for people with psychosis, *British Journal of Occupational Therapy*, 70(3): 96–106.

Craig, T., Garety, P., Power, P. *et al.* (2004) The Lambeth Early Onset (LEO) Team: randomised controlled trial of the effectiveness of specialised care for early psychosis, *British Medical Journal*, 329: 1067.

Curson, D.A., Pantelis, C., Ward, J. et al. (1992) Institutionalism and schizophrenia 30 years on. Clinical poverty and the social environment in three British mental hospitals in 1960 compared with a fourth in 1990, *British Journal of Psychiatry*, 160: 230–241.

Department of Communities and Local Government. (2006) *Research into the Effectiveness of Floating Support Services for the Supporting People Programme. Final Report.* London: Communities and Local Government.

Department of Health. (1990) *The Care Programme Approach for People with a Mental Illness Referred to the Specialist Psychiatric Services.* London: HMSO.

Department of Health. (1999a) *Modernising the Care Programme Approach: Effective Co-ordination of Mental Health Services.* London: HMSO.

Department of Health. (1999b) *National Service Framework for Mental Health: Modern Standards and Service Models.* London: HMSO.

Department of Health and Social Security. (1981) *Care in the Community.* London: HMSO.

Goffman, E. (1968) *Asylums: Essays on the Social Situation of Mental Patients and Other Inmates.* New York: Doubleday; London: Penguin.

Glover, G., Arts, G. and Babu, K.S. (2006) Crisis resolution/home treatment teams and psychiatric admission rates in England, *British Journal of Psychiatry*, 189: 441–445.

Green, M.F. (1996) What are the functional consequences of neurocognitive deficits in schizophrenia? *American Journal of Psychiatry*, 153: 321–330.

Harding, C., Brooks, G., Asolaga, T. and Breier, A. (1987) The Vermont longitudinal study of persons with severe mental illness, 1. Methodological study sample and overall status 32 years later, *American Journal of Psychiatry*, 14: 718–726.

Harrison, G., Hopper, K., Craig, T. *et al.* (2001) Recovery from psychotic illness: a 15 and 25 year international follow up study, *British Journal of Psychiatry*, 178, 506–517.

Holloway, F. (2005) *The Forgotten Need for Rehabilitation in Contemporary Mental Health Services. A Position Statement from the Executive Committee of the Faculty of Rehabilitation and Social Psychiatry*. London: Royal College of Psychiatrists.

Johnson, S., Nolan, F., Pilling, S. *et al.* (2005) Randomised controlled trial of acute mental health care by a crisis resolution team: the north Islington crisis study, *British Medical Journal*, 331: 599.

Killaspy, H., Harden, C., Holloway, F. and King, M. (2005) What do mental health rehabilitation services do and what are they for? A national survey in England, *Journal of Mental Health*, 14; 157–165.

Killaspy, H., Bebbington, P., Blizard, R. *et al.* (2006) The REACT study: randomised evaluation of assertive community treatment in north London, *British Medical Journal*, 332: 815–820.

Killaspy, H., Rambarran, D. and Bledin, K. (2008) Mental health needs of clients of rehabilitation services: a survey in one Trust, *Journal of Mental Health*, 17: 207–218.

Killaspy, H., Kingett, S., Bebbington, P., Blizard, R., Johnson, S., Nolan, F., Pilling, S. and King, M. (2009a) Randomised evaluation of assertive community treatment: 3 year outcomes, *British Journal of Psychiatry*, 195: 81–82.

Killaspy, H., Rambarran, D., Harden, C., McClinton, K., Caren, G. and Fearon, D. (2009b) A comparison of service users placed out of their local area and local rehabilitation service users, *Journal of Mental Health*, 18: 111–120.

Killaspy, H. (2010a) Assertive community psychiatry – worth the investment? *Irish Psychiatrist*, 11(3): 136–138.

Killaspy, H. and Meier, R. (2010b) A fair deal for mental health rehabilitation services, *The Psychiatrist*, 34: 265–267.

Killaspy, H., White, S., Wright, C. *et al.* (2011a) The development of the Quality Indicator for Rehabilitative Care (QuIRC): a measure of best practice for facilities for people with longer term mental health problems, *BMC Psychiatry*, 11: 35

Killaspy, H., White, S., Wright, C. *et al.* (2011b) Association between service user experiences and staff rated quality of care in European facilities for people with longer term mental health problems, *British Journal of Psychiatry*, submitted.

Leff, J. and Trieman, N. (2000) Long stay patients discharged from psychiatric hospitals. Social and clinical outcomes after five years in the community. TAPS Project 46, *British Journal of Psychiatry*, 176: 217–223.

Liberman, R.P. and Kopelwicz, A. (2002) Recovery from schizophrenia: a challenge for the 21st century, *International Review of Psychiatry*, 14: 245–255

Macpherson, R., Shepherd, G. and Edwards, T. (2004) Supported accommodation for people with severe mental illness: a review, *Advances in Psychiatric Treatment*, 10: 180–188

Meltzer, H. (1997) Treatment-resistant schizophrenia – the role of clozapine, *Current Medical Resident Opinion*, 14: 1–20

Mental Health Strategies. (2010) *The 2009/10 National Survey of Investment in Mental Health Services*, London: Department of Health.

Mountain, D., Killaspy, H. and Holloway, F. (2009) Mental health rehabilitation services in the UK in 2007, *Psychiatric Bulletin*, 33: 215–218.

National Institute for Health and Clinical Excellence. (2009) *Core Interventions on the Treatment and Management of Schizophrenia in Adults in Primary and Secondary Care* (Update edition). London: NICE.

National Statistics. (2006) *Community Care Statistics 2006. Supported Residents (Adults), England*. London: The Information Centre, part of the Government Statistical Service.

Poole, R., Ryan, T. and Pearsall, A. (2002) The NHS, the private sector, and the virtual asylum, *British Medical Journal*, 325: 349–350.

Priebe, S., Badesconyi, A., Fioritti, A. *et al.* (2005) Reinstitutionalisation in mental health care: comparison of data on service provision from six European countries, *British Medical Journal*, 330: 123–126.

Roberts, G., Davenport, S., Holloway, F. and Tattan, T. (eds) (2006) *Enabling Recovery: The Principles and Practice of Rehabilitation Psychiatry*. London: Gaskell.

Royal College of Psychiatrists. (2011) In Sight and in Mind: a toolkit to reduce the use of out of area mental health services. Royal College of Psychiatrists, http://www.rcpsych.ac.uk/pdf/insightandinmind.pdf

Ryan, T., Pearsall, A., Hatfield, B. *et al.* (2004) Long term care for serious mental illness outside the NHS: a study of out of area placements, *Journal of Mental Health*, 13: 425–429.

Sainsbury Centre for Mental Health. (2009) *Implementing Recovery: A New Framework for Organisational Change.* Position paper. London: Sainsbury Centre for Mental Health.

Shepherd, G., Boardman, J. and Slade, M. (2008) *Making Recovery a Reality.* London: Sainsbury Centre for Mental Health.

Shepherd, G., Boardman, J. and Burns, M. (2010) *Implementing Recovery: A Methodology for Organisational Change.* London: Sainsbury Centre for Mental Health.

Social Exclusion Unit. (2004) *Mental Health and Social Exclusion.* London: Social Exclusion Unit.

Taylor, T., Killaspy, H., Wright, C. *et al.* (2009) A systematic review of the international published literature relating to quality of institutional care for people with longer term mental health problems, *BMC Psychiatry*, 9: 55

Turton, P., Wright, C., White, S. *et al.* (2010) Promoting recovery in long term mental health institutional care: an international Delphi study, *Psychiatric Services*, 61(3): 293–299.

Trieman, N. and Leff, J. (2002) Long-term outcome of long-stay psychiatric inpatients considered unsuitable to live in the community: TAPS Project 44, *British Journal of Psychiatry*, 181: 428–432.

Tuke, D.H. (1855) William Tuke, the Founder of the York Retreat, *Journal of Psychological Medicine and Mental Pathology*, 8: 507–512.

Wing, J.K. and Brown, G.W. (1970) *Institutionalism and Schizophrenia: A Comparative Study of Three Mental Hospitals 1960–1968.* Cambridge: Cambridge University Press.

Wing, J.K. (1980) Innovations in social psychiatry, *Psychological Medicine*, 10: 219–230.

Wolfson, P., Holloway, F. and Killaspy, H. (eds) (2009) *Enabling Recovery for People with Complex Mental Health Needs: A Template for Rehabilitation Services.* London: Royal College of Psychiatrists.

Wykes, T. and Dunn, G. (1992) Cognitive deficit and the prediction of rehabilitation success in a chronic psychiatric group, *Psychological Medicine,* 22(2): 389–398.

7   Recovery

A journey of discovery for individuals and services

Julie Repper and Rachel E. Perkins

> All I knew were the stereotypes I had seen on television or in the movies. To me, mental illness meant Dr Jekyll and Mr Hyde, psychopathic serial killers, loony bins, morons, schizos, fruit-cakes, nuts, straightjackets and raving lunatics. They were all I knew about mental illness, and what terrified me was that professionals were saying I was one of them.
>
> (Deegan, 1993)

To be diagnosed with mental health problems is a devastating and life-changing event. Not only do you have to cope with strange, and sometimes frightening, experiences. Maybe the ordinary everyday things that you usually take in your stride become impossibly difficult. People start treating you differently. It is easy to lose confidence in yourself. You feel alone and very frightened. Frightened about what is happening to you. Frightened about the prospect of using mental health services. Frightened you will lose everything you value in life, like your friends, your work, your home, your college place, your position in the community. Frightened that you won't be able to achieve your ambitions, do all the things you had planned to do in life – like raise a family, travel, get a good job.

> At a young age we had both experienced a catastrophic shattering of our world, hopes and dreams ... He was an athlete and had dreamed of becoming a professional in the sports world. I was a high school athlete and had applied to become a gym teacher. Just days earlier we knew ourselves as young people with exciting futures, and everything collapsed around us. As teenagers we were told we would be 'sick' or 'disabled' for the rest of our lives.
>
> (Deegan, 1988)

To be diagnosed with a mental health condition is a form of bereavement. Too often a diagnosis is associated with multiple losses: loss of a sense of self, meaning and purpose in life, loss of valued social roles, loss of power and control, loss of hopes and dreams. These losses often leave you feeling alienated and disconnected from yourself, from your friends and family and from the communities in which you live (Spaniol and Koehler, 1994).

> For some of us, an episode of mental distress will disrupt our lives so we are pushed out of the society in which we were fully participating. For others, the early onset of distress will mean social exclusion throughout our adult lives, with no prospect of training for a job or hope of a future in meaningful employment. Loneliness and loss of self-worth lead us to believe we are useless, and so we live with this sense of hopelessness, or far too often choose to end our lives.
>
> (Social Exclusion Unit, 2004)

Recovery – a personal journey of discovery

'You have the wondrously terrifying task of becoming who you are called to be.... Your life and dreams may have been shattered – but from such ruins you can build a new life full of value and purpose' (Deegan, 1993).

Like anyone who experiences a major bereavement that knocks the bottom out of your world, people diagnosed with a mental health condition face the challenge of recovering a meaningful, satisfying and valued life. This is a personal journey of discovering and building a new sense of who you are, what is important to you and where you want to go in life. This can be very frightening – there are no rules or formulae. Everyone must find their own way. However, in this journey of discovery, three things repeatedly emerge as important. Hope – believing in your own possibilities. Control – taking back control over your life and destiny. Opportunity and participation – the chance to do the things that matter to you and be a valued member of your community.

Rekindling hope

'Hope lies at the heart of the individual's ability and willingness to take on the challenge of rebuilding and recovery. Acceptance of what has happened can be too terrifying in the absence of hope' (Repper and Perkins, 2003).

Deegan (1996) draws a distinction between optimism and hope. She characterises optimism as being like a cheerleader – there for a brief period and then gone. Hope is about believing in yourself and being willing to 'hang on in there': persevere and pick yourself up again when you are knocked down. Hope does not arrive like a bolt of lightning – it begins as a small and fragile flame that can be fanned or snuffed out (Repper and Perkins, 2003).

As with any bereavement, a diagnosis of mental health problems is often accompanied by a tsunami of emotions. Feelings of shame, terror, hopelessness, despair, isolation, anger and denial: 'it's not true', 'this cannot be happening to me', 'it's all a terrible mistake'. These are ordinary human responses to bereavement and loss, but in someone with a diagnosis of mental health problems they are too often seen as 'symptoms' or part of their 'disorder'.

Denial is seen as 'lack of insight'

> We didn't believe our doctors ... we adamantly denied and raged against their bleak prophecies for our lives. We felt it was just all a mistake, a bad dream ... in a week or two things would be back to normal again ... Our denial was an important stage in our recovery. It was a normal reaction to an overwhelming situation. It was our way of surviving those first awful months.
>
> (Deegan, 1988)

Hopelessness and despair are viewed as 'negative symptoms' or 'depression'. 'We both gave up. Giving up was a solution for us. It numbed the pain of our despair. All of us who have experienced catastrophic illness and disability know the experience' (Deegan, 1988).

Anger, resentment and blame directed at staff, family members and peers is interpreted as the aggression inherent in the person's disorder.

> Anger follows in the footsteps of despair. Anger at the illness which has so devastated us. Anger at the helping system that may have failed ... Anger at society and its attitudes.

Anger at God for not taking better care of us. Anger at parents and friends for not being more helpful. Anger at our self for not being able to manage. Our anger is a necessary and important part of the process. Anger is a stimulus to recovery. It is normal and natural.

(Spaniol and Koehler, 1994)

Like anyone who experiences loss, people who receive a diagnosis of mental health problems need space to grieve. People around who really listen, appreciate the devastating impact of what has happened, are prepared to be with us in our distress, but at the same time believe in our possibilities and worth, help us to get through set-backs and disappointments, learn from them, grow stronger because of them. Failure to address the meaning that a diagnosis has for a person and their life has 'left many people with mental illness feeling devalued and ignored and has resulted in mistrust and alienation' (Spaniol *et al.*, 1997).

Fanning the fragile flames of hope requires that people have fertile ground in which to grow (Deegan, 1996). An environment that conveys messages of value and possibility, people who can hold onto hope when you find it hard to believe in yourself. A space where you can start to make sense of what has happened ('why me?', 'who am I?', 'what's the point in life?'), recognise and develop your own resources and resourcefulness and begin to believe that a decent life and future is possible.

'The recovery process is a deeply personal process that includes two key developmental tasks: the struggle for meaning and the reconstruction of a positive identity' (Pettie and Triolo, 1999)

The answers to this quest for meaning lie not in psychiatry but in spirituality or philosophy. Having a chance to think about what matters to you, who and what is important to you, to reflect on the experiences that have shaped your life and the ideas you value.

When one looks at the language used in the literature around recovery one can see how closely it is aligned with spirituality. At the heart of the approach is a recognition and understanding of the recovery of our underlying spirit, the spark, the breath of life that gives us not just 'life' but what Jews call ru'ach or 'invigorated life'. If individual recovery is to endure then services must engage the heart and become organisations of recovery, where we all journey together.

(Gilbert, 2008)

Storytelling is also important in discovering a new sense of identity and possibility. Human beings are storytelling creatures. We know ourselves through the stories we tell of our lives. When traumatic events befall us we have to retell the stories of our lives. We connect with other people by sharing our stories. We understand our possibilities by seeing what others who have been in a similar position have achieved. 'Real life stories … are nutritious and sustaining. They feed the mind with information and the heart with hope and strength' (Pullman, 2006).

The stories of people who have faced similar challenges do much to help us feel less alone and offer images of possibility. Many people have found that some of the most important relationships that have helped them to accommodate what has happened and rebuild their lives are with people who have walked a similar path. The gift of hope that people who are a few steps ahead of you in their journey can bring should never be underestimated. Peer support also offers the opportunity to share your experiences with someone who really understands what you are going through and provides a reciprocal relationship in which both parties can grow and develop. It gives people a way of using their experience to assist others, which can be important in finding meaning in what has happened.

Taking back control

'To me, recovery means I try to stay in the driver's seat of my life. I don't let my illness run me. Over the years I have worked hard to become an expert in my own self-care' (Deegan, 1993).

Taking back control is a multifaceted journey. Often the road back into the driving seat of life involves a quest for understanding.

> He began to look around himself with new eyes, and became deeply interested in understanding all he could of the human mind, psyche and behaviour... He really has, as the saying goes, mined his own experiences for meaning and understanding, for growth and release. He has found information and inspiration from a myriad of people and sources. Of course, when one is open and intent upon learning, one finds lessons and teachers in many guises. This exploration over the past years has formed the backbone and impetus of Tim's recovery. The saying 'knowledge is power' is true, and in Tim we have watched the filtering of knowledge into wisdom, insight and a deep understanding of himself – not least in the context of the experience of schizophrenia. He worked in light of his belief that he could never change his past, but he could change his perception and reactions to it.
>
> (Gould, undated)

But such understanding must be accompanied by discovering ways of managing the vicissitudes of your mental health problems and maximising your well-being. Technical treatment and support from services may be part of this self-management plan, but only a part. People find many and varied ways of managing their mental health challenges. Each person has to experiment and do their own research, in order to work out what works best for them.

> Over the years I have learned different ways of helping myself. Sometimes I use medications, therapy, self-help and mutual support groups, friends, my relationship with God, work, exercise, spending time in nature – all of these measures help me remain whole and healthy, even though I have a disability.
>
> (Deegan, 1993)

While everyone must find their own recipe for success, many have found others who have faced similar challenges to be a rich source of ideas and inspiration. Many self-help groups and networks have grown up to enable people to learn from each other and assist each other in obtaining the help they find useful from professionals and services.

However, the journey of recovery involves more than managing your problems; it involves taking control over your destiny. Times of crisis in life offer an opportunity to take stock – decide what is important to you, rethink where you are going in life, discover and pursue your dreams and ambitions. Sometimes this may involve recognising the true value of things that you have already got, sometimes it may involve finding new sources of meaning and value.

'The greater danger for most of us lies not in setting our aim too high and falling short, but in setting our aim too low and achieving our mark' (Michelangelo, undated). Everyone needs dreams. It is our ambitions that give us a reason to get up in the morning, give us a reason to keep on going when the going gets tough. Our dreams do not have to be 'realistic': their value lies not in their realism but in their ability to motivate us. But in the face of traumatic events it is very easy to lose your dreams, lower your expectations, give up.

> I lost vital years of my life locked up, some dreams went out of the window ... but I feel stronger than ever now ... and wiser. ... I am content. I'm very into my music and

performing, making tracks, writing poetry. I am graduating this year from an Open University degree. I've passed my driving test. I have a car.

(Allen, 2010)

Identifying dreams is only the start. The next step is embarking on the journey of pursuing your ambitions. It can be tempting to wait for some magical event occur: 'When I get better I will ...', 'When I get out of here I will ...', 'When I win the lottery I will ...' Waiting for something to happen before you can do the things you want to do makes you a victim of fate. Taking back control over your destiny involves working out how you can start your journey right now. The steps you take may be small and the distance to travel may be large, but every journey starts with a single step. We may change course along the way, we may discover other sources of value and meaning, but unless we make a start we will never know what we can achieve.

Determination is important in pursuing your ambitions, but if you are to succeed you also need the opportunity to do the things you value.

The opportunity to participate

Access to those opportunities that all citizens have a right to expect is important if you are to move forward in your journey of recovery. For most people it is not enough merely to have access to the resources that are available in our communities, we also need the opportunity to contribute to those communities. Always being on the receiving end of help and support from others is a dispiriting place to be. Being able to give – to do things for others – is critical in fostering self-worth and well-being.

It can be tempting to see cure as the only route to recovery: too often we assume that unless we get better nothing is possible. But it is not possible to guess what the future holds. Some people's problems may disappear completely, some may be ever present, and some will recur from time to time. And whatever the course of your problems, a decent life is possible. The challenge is to work out ways of doing the things we want to do in the presence or absence of problems – to grow within and beyond the challenges we face. This will involve us using our own personal resources, but no man (or woman) is an island. Everyone needs support at some time or another if they are to pursue their dreams and ambitions. Sometimes this support may come from mental health services, but equally, if not more often, it comes from family, friends, neighbours and the ordinary resources available in our communities.

For example, Esso Leete (1989) describes how important work is in her life:

It gives me something to look forward to every day ... It is my motivation for getting up each morning ... As I work I become increasingly self-confident and my self-image is bolstered. I feel important and grown up which replaces my usual sense of vulnerability, weakness and incompetence.

But Leete fights what she describes as 'a daily battle with schizophrenia'. In order to work she must use her own resources. For example, she copes with the difficulty of making eye contact by looking up intermittently in conversations but looking just past the other person, copes with concentration and memory difficulties by making lists, anticipates paranoid feelings and takes preventative action. For instance, instead of worrying about the police surprising her she makes sure she sits with her back to the wall. She is also aware that her behaviour sometimes seems bizarre to other people so she takes steps to 'fit in' like not talking to her voices when other people are around.

She also needs help from others. She has worked out what sort of support she needs and seeks it from those around her. For example, she tests out reality with someone she trusts. If their perceptions differ from hers she may want to change her response and go along with more conventional ways of thinking. She finds ambiguity and vagueness difficult so asks others to communicate in a clear and specific way and copes with high levels of ambivalence by asking for extra time to make decisions. She also finds self-help groups useful as a means of accepting and dealing with her problems.

The prejudice and discrimination that a diagnosis of mental health problems attract also presents enormous problems. Many people are put off from doing the things they want to do because they fear they will be excluded or treated badly by others. Claire Allen (2008) draws on her own experience to illustrate the sort of dilemma faced by many:

> The absence of a physical mark ... presents a dilemma to those with mental health problems: whether to conceal the information or let it be known and manage the consequences ... Imagine going on a first date ... Let's say you have a diagnosis of schizophrenia. You have learned to manage your condition with the help of medication (no drink) though you've put on two stone and your favourite clothes no longer fit. Let's say that somehow, despite all this, you walk into the pub feeling fabulous. Your date agrees; the evening goes well; you see each other again. Perhaps he comes round. You've hidden your meds in the washing machine. Sooner or later you'll have to tell him – but not yet ... your secret begins to consume you. You are not the person he thinks you are. Weeks pass, months pass. You have to tell him ... Then finally, one night, you say it. He thinks you're joking. Eventually he realises you're not ... It is stigma that makes this so difficult, for while concealment denies us the possibility of being accepted as we are, being open about our mental health so often ensures that the rest of us disappears.

It can be really hard working out what to say to other people and how to deal with their reactions and there really is no 'right' answer. Some people choose to keep quiet about their problems, others prefer to say something – but not too much. For example, 'I get a bit stressed up sometimes' or 'I had a bit of a breakdown but I am fine now'. Some people choose to get it out in the open from the start, others choose to wait a while, get to know people first, 'test the water' before jumping in.

In tackling such dilemmas it is important to remember three things. First, the 2010 Equality Act outlaws discrimination and requires that employers and all providers of education, goods and services make 'reasonable adjustments' to ensure access for disabled people – and disabled people includes those with mental health conditions. These are rights we must assert. Second, since one in four people will experience mental health problems every year, it is likely that, in any situation, many people will have had difficulties themselves or have friends or relatives who have faced mental health challenges. Third, by doing things with other people you are actively breaking down prejudice and discrimination. As Esso Leete says, 'Being a member of the workforce decreases stigma and contributes to acceptance by my community, which in turn makes my life easier' (Leete, 1989).

Promoting recovery: a journey of discovery for mental health services

Recovery is a journey of individuals as they grow within and beyond what has happened to them; it is not something that mental health services do. Mental health services and the professionals who inhabit them cannot make people recover – there are no 'recovery interventions' – nor do they hold the key to recovery. The question for services is whether they assist or hinder people in their journey: whether they fan the fragile flame of hope or snuff it out; whether they help people regain their self-control and self-respect or whether they disempower and devalue those whom they serve; whether they help people to do the things they want to do or put barriers in their way.

Recovery cannot be an 'add on' to existing ways of doing things: the creation of a 'Recovery Team' or a few 'Recovery Workers'. The promotion of recovery must underpin all treatment and support provided and guides the work of every mental health worker. If this is to be achieved then a fundamental change in culture (values, beliefs and practices) is required as well as a fundamental revision of the way in which we evaluate the success of our endeavours (see Perkins, Chapter 2). There are four key elements to the transformation required:

1   A different role for mental health professionals and professional expertise.
    Instead of prescribing treatment and support and planning care for people, professionals and services must essentially form part of the self-management plans of those whom they serve. Resources need to be available for people to use in order to alleviate their distress, manage the challenges they face and achieve their ambitions. As Mary O'Hagan (2007) has said, people with mental health challenges should view mental health services as 'carriers of technologies that we may want to use at times, just like architects, plumbers and hairdressers' (O'Hagan, 2007).
2   Redefining 'user involvement' – co-production in service design, delivery and development.
    The language and practice of services is firmly rooted in a 'them' and 'us' culture. Professionals speak of 'my patients/clients/caseload' and define 'their' needs in terms of what 'we' have to offer. 'User involvement' typically means involving 'them' in 'our' services. Recovery-focused practice requires moving from 'them' and 'us' to 'we'. If services are to be of assistance to people in managing the challenges they face then they must be designed around the preferences and convenience of those whom they serve. This requires a partnership between the 'carriers of technologies' and those who may wish to use them.
3   A different kind of workforce.
    If services are to help people to rebuild their lives we must ask, 'what sort of expertise is required?' Technical treatment may be one component of this, but just how many mental health professionals do you need to run a mental health service? Are there not other sorts of expertise that may be useful? Maybe we need more welfare benefit experts, personal trainers, employment specialists, life coaches … and most especially, if peer support is central to recovery, we need the expertise of lived experience in the workforce. But peer support requires more than simply the presence of lived experience; it requires a different sort of relationship. Traditional relationships between professionals (even those who also have lived experience) and those whom they serve is hierarchical. There is the 'helper' and the 'helped' – the expert with special knowledge and the patient. Peer support is:

    - A reciprocal relationship, based on mutuality and a shared journey.
    - A way of sharing our personal story.
    - A way of being in a relationship that empowers people to recover.
    - A way of offering help and support as an equal.
    - A way of teaching, learning and growing together.
    - An attitude that values each person's experience.

    At 'Recovery Innovations' in Phoenix, Arizona, 55 per cent of the staff are Peer Support Workers, working alongside people with professional expertise on equal terms. A poster on the wall of the Recovery Education Centre that forms the hub of the service aptly describes the role of the peer workers: 'Peer support is about being an expert at not being an expert and that takes expertise.'

4   A different relationship between services and the communities they serve.

Traditionally it is assumed that the resolution of mental health problems is a task for the professional experts. People are taken out of their communities and relieved of their roles and responsibilities while experts try to resolve their difficulties. The idea is that, once their problems are resolved, they can return to whence they came and resume their ordinary social roles. For many people the reality is very different. Even though they may live in their community, they are not a part of it, and the identity of 'mental patient' eclipses all others. But life is not lived in isolation, and journeys of recovery from trauma are not travelled alone. In addition to our own personal resources and resourcefulness, the resources and resourcefulness of families and communities are central to recovery. The job of services is to support the resources of both individuals and their communities rather than to replace them.

A series of workshops conducted across England in 2008/9 reviewed the available literature and practice and identified ten key organisational challenges for mental health service networks seeking to achieve the transformations outlined above (Sainsbury Centre for Mental Health, 2010, p. 106):

1   Changing the nature of day-to-day interactions and the quality of experience of people using services and those close to them.
2   Delivering comprehensive service user led, co-produced, education and training programmes.
3   Establishing a recovery education centre to drive the programmes forward.
4   Ensuring organisational commitment – creating a recovery-focused culture at all levels.
5   Increasing personalisation and choice.
6   Changing the way we approach risk assessment and management.
7   Redefining service user involvement.
8   Transforming the workforce.
9   Supporting staff in their journey of recovery and transformation.
10 Increasing opportunities for building a 'life beyond illness'.

Training alone will not be sufficient to achieve these challenges. If whole cultures are to be transformed then training must be accompanied by a culture of innovation and effective leadership. Clearly it is not possible for organisations to change everything at once – priorities must be established. In doing this the focus should be on those areas that will have the biggest impact on culture. The organisational transformation achieved by Recovery Innovations in Phoenix, Arizona, offers an example of this (Ashcraft and Anthony, 2005). Strongly recovery-focused leadership revised the overall mission and purpose of the organisation 'to create opportunities and environments to empower people to recover, to succeed in accomplishing their goals and to reconnect to themselves, others, and meaning and purpose in life' (Johnson, 2002).

Ashcraft and Anthony (2005) described the implementation of this vision as requiring 'a huge leap of faith' – a leap based on three key changes. First, moving away from a traditional treatment basis to an educational model for promoting recovery as a way of '... reinforcing and developing people's strengths, rather than adding to the attention placed on what was "wrong" with them' (Ashcraft, 2000).

In order to make a reality of this transformation a Recovery Education Centre was established and became the core around which all other services (outreach support, crisis etc.) were organised. This Recovery Education Centre incorporated the training programme necessary to achieve the second key change. This was the recognition of the importance of lived experience by training and recruiting Peer Support Specialists – not one or two 'add ons' to existing teams, but a fundamental transformation so that over 50% per cent of the workforce were peers who had graduated from the training programme provided at the education centre. 'As the Peer Support Specialists began to work on our teams, miracles began to happen. Their recovery continued. Those with whom they worked began to recover. Our culture began to change, and we moved closer to our recovery mission' (Ashcraft and Anthony, 2005).

Third, eliminating seclusion and restraint.

> This was a huge culture shift since their use had always been seen as a necessary part of this business. Staff threatened to quit. Some threatened to call the Occupational Safety and Health Administration because they believed the company was putting them at risk. Some claimed that the company didn't care about them any more.
>
> (Ashcraft and Anthony, 2005)

> If we could stop the violence of takedowns and restraints in our Crisis Centers, that would be a demonstration that what we had thought was impossible is possible. That could begin to shift our beliefs and attitudes and jump-start the transformation of our culture ... It was a big job since we see over 1,200 people a month at our two Centers; 30% brought by police and 40% brought involuntarily ... After 18 months we got there ... Now, whenever there is something to do that is really hard, we remember that we have already done the impossible. 'Zero Restraint' has become our metaphor for transformation.
>
> (Johnson, 2002, p. 104)

The challenge in achieving recovery-focused organisational transformation is identifying those changes that will achieve this sort of fundamental cultural shift. In different organisations and circumstances different changes may be key, but it is critical to identify and tackle those talismanic challenges that can have a cascade effect on the whole culture.

There is no blueprint for recovery-focused services, any more than there is a blueprint for personal recovery. There is no single intervention or service that will prompt the first step of recovery for every individual or service. We are all on a journey of discovery – and it is one that we must travel together.

References

Allen, C. (2008) Stigma goes far more than skin deep, *The Guardian*, 6th August

Allen, S. (ed.) (2010) *Our Stories: Moving on, Recovery and Well-being*, London: South West London and St George's Mental Health NHS Trust

Ashcraft, L. (2000) META Services recovery education center business plan, Phoenix, AZ: META Services Inc.

Ashcraft, L. and Anthony, W. (2005) A story of transformation, *Behavioral Healthcare Tomorrow*, April, 12–22

Deegan, P. (1988) Recovery: The lived experience of rehabilitation, *Psychosocial Rehabilitation Journal*, 11, 11–19

Deegan, P. (1993) Recovering our sense of value after being labelled mentally ill, *Journal of Psychosocial Nursing and Mental Health Services*, 31, 7–11

Deegan, P. (1996) Recovery as a journey of the heart, *Psychosocial Rehabilitation Journal*, 19, 91–97

Gilbert, P. (2008) *Strangers in a strange land*, at http://mhspirituality.org.uk/resources.html, accessed 3 July 2011

Gould, V. (undated) *A carer's perspective on the recovery journey*, at www.scottishrecovery.net, accessed 3 July 2011

Johnson, G. (2002) META Services recovery training: Train the trainer Section 2, Phoenix, AZ: META Services Inc.

Leete, E. (1989) How I perceive and manage my illness, *Schizophrenia Bulletin*, 8, 605–609

Michelangelo (undated) cited at http://www.dictionary-quotes.com/, accessed 3 July 2011

O'Hagan, M. (2007) Parting thoughts, *Mental Notes* (Mental Health Commission, Wellington, New Zealand), 18, 4–5

Pettie, D. and Triolo, A. M. (1999) Illness as evolution: the search for identity and meaning in the recovery process, *Psychiatric Rehabilitation Journal*, 22, 255–262

Pullman, P. (2006) cited at http://www.oxfordtimes.co.uk/news/yourtown/oxford/725689, accessed 2 July 2011

Repper, J. and Perkins, R. (2003) *Social Inclusion and Recovery*, London: Balliere Tindall

Sainsbury Centre for Mental Health (2010) *Implementing Recovery. A Framework for Organisational Change*, London: Sainsbury Centre for Mental Health

Social Exclusion Unit (2004) *Mental Health and Social Exclusion,* London: Office of the Deputy Prime Minister

Spaniol, L. and Koehler, M. (eds) (1994) *The Experience of Recovery*, Boston, MA: Center for Psychiatric Rehabilitation

Spaniol, L., Gagne, C. and Koehler, M. (1997) Recovery from serious mental illness: What it is and how to assist people, *Continuum*, 4(4), 3–15

8 Drugs, drink and mental health

The impact and consequences of dual diagnosis for mental health service delivery

Liz Hughes and Peter Phillips

Introduction and background: history, context and problems

Mental health service users with co-morbid alcohol and/or drug use problems (which will be referred to as 'dual diagnosis') have presented one of the most significant challenges to British and international mental health and wider health and social care services, as well as the criminal justice system in the last two decades. The National Service Framework for Mental Health (Department of Health, 1999) and the review of implementation (Department of Health, 2005) highlighted dual diagnosis as 'the most challenging clinical problem we face', which required urgent action from mental health and substance use services, and a broad coordinated response including better collaboration between agencies, training in assessment and clinical management, preventative work and prevention of drug misuse on inpatient units.

Service users with dual diagnosis have been associated with particularly adverse clinical outcomes, high costs and problematic service utilisation issues, and this may reflect the social stigma drug users face in the wider community, mirrored by staff and other service users in the mental health service setting (Phillips, 1998).

Presentations and definitions

The heterogeneity of presentations of service users with dual diagnosis means that, in general, no one set of interventions has so far demonstrated efficacy with the population. This is compounded by a lack of consensus about which service users fall into the category and which do not, as the types of definitions reported in the research literature and those used clinically are often quite divergent (Phillips and Johnson, 2001). On the one hand the research literature would certainly define a young man with schizophrenia who regularly smokes cannabis and drinks alcohol as having a dual diagnosis, but would be unlikely to define a bereaved sixty year old drinking very heavily as a consequence/way of coping with the death of a spouse in the dual diagnosis category. The debates about definition continue and to some extent are critical in terms of service and intervention development, and access to care – surely one of the underlying critical values of a medical diagnosis?

Development of the field

The plethora of national and international work around dual diagnosis in the last twenty years has included research into prevalence and interventions; targeted staff training; the development of policies and broader education, in both mental health and drug and alcohol services; and the integration of greater security in mental health service settings. Despite these initiatives it is not uncommon to encounter professional health or social care staff who report feeling untrained, unable or even unwilling to work with service users with this very common co-morbidity (Phillips, 1998). Working with service users with drug and alcohol problems still regularly attracts statements such as 'I didn't come into mental health to work with addicts', and reference to the little educational preparation offered in most undergraduate health curricula (medicine, nursing, psychology, social work). Although there has been long overdue recognition of the role of personal experience of mental distress and ill health in those providing mental health care to others, this has yet to translate to people who have current substance use issues. When a professional knows 'too much' about drugs they can be seen as 'suspect', and their knowledge possibly indicative of personal use. Whilst modern mental health practice is rightly informed by collaborative work and extended service user involvement, it remains the norm for mental health staff never to disclose anything relating to personal experience of drugs (particularly) – and therefore claiming poor drug use knowledge can act as an extension of this defence.

Prevalence: community and residential mental health services

At first large-scale American epidemiological surveys and later European and UK studies suggested that between 30 per cent and 50 per cent of the mentally ill also have lifetime morbidity for substance use problems, and that prevalence is higher amongst inpatients and emergency service settings (Regier *et al.*, 1990). The Epidemiological Catchment Area Survey (the ECAS study) is generally still cited as the 'gold standard' work on prevalence of dual diagnosis (Regier *et al.*, 1990). It found that the 50 per cent prevalence rate was increased to 64 per cent in drug users who were engaged in drug treatment (detoxification and rehabilitation). UK community-based research tends to report lower but still significant prevalence, whilst studies of inpatient residential mental health facilities tend to report considerably higher prevalence. Three UK studies of inpatient mental health services found particularly high prevalence of dual diagnosis using research-based definitions (service users with psychotic illness, inner London) of 49 per cent (Phillips and Johnson, 2003), all acute admissions (inner London) 58 per cent (Barnaby *et al.*, 2003) and 56 per cent of all acute admissions and 90 per cent of psychiatric intensive care unit admissions (central Manchester; Schulte and Holland, 2008). Phillips and Johnson (2003) found a wide range of substances used frequently by inpatients including alcohol, cannabis, crack cocaine and opiates, including injection drug use by some of the study participants. Use *within* mental health settings was also common, with more than 80 per cent of study participants using whilst in the ward environment. Drug trading was also common in this inner London study, with 47 per cent buying drugs from other inpatients.

The impact of dual diagnosis in mental health service settings

Numerous reviews and UK national policy documents have illustrated some of the complex clinical and social problems presented by people with these problems. A common factor appears to be a higher level of 'multiple-problems', which are not solely medical, psychological or psychiatric, and this can be a serious challenge to traditional mental health care roles and services. These service users often present in crisis with problems relating to social, legal/criminal justice issues, housing, welfare and 'lifestyle' matters with which medically orientated services are not always ready or able to help directly. These problems and difficulties often reflect the social stigma that people with dual diagnosis face, in that they are not only problem drinkers or drug users, but are also mentally ill – perhaps two of the most socially stigmatised groups in society.

A number of significant clinical issues are associated with dual diagnosis, and there is equivocal evidence reported largely from North American studies that associates dual diagnosis with a wide range of poor outcomes including: relapse of psychotic illness, exacerbation of psychotic symptoms, poor medication compliance and efficacy, contact with the criminal justice system, problems with engagement and retention in (mental health or substance misuse) treatment, poor social functioning, increased prevalence of serious physical health problems such as viral hepatitis, HIV, venous thrombosis and cardiac disease in intravenous injectors, respiratory disease including pneumonia in those who smoke drugs, incidence of suicide, increased service utilisation and problems in the management of residential mental health facilities (Smith and Hucker, 1996; Dixon, 1999; Gearon *et al.*, 2001; Murray *et al.*, 2002; Cantwell, 2003). These outcomes are increasingly supported by research evidence in North America, Australasia and Europe.

Meanwhile the link between mental health inpatient facilities and drug use has meant that many mental health service providers have put stringent prevention policies in place (Wilson *et al.*, 2009). Inpatient staff have been required to adopt a more systematic approach to prevention of drug use amongst inpatient service settings – some would argue to the detriment of the therapeutic relationship with service users.

Service users admitted to acute wards are now routinely screened for evidence of substance use, by urine screening, hair or saliva testing (Gordon and Haider, 2004), and service users 'leave status' has become conditional on drug free tests. It is now also commonplace for inpatient staff to perform invasive searches of service users on admission to wards and randomly; in scenes that in the past resembled more custodial settings, staff now use puncture resistant gloves, requesting that service users empty their pockets, possessions and submit to bodily searches (Wilson *et al.*, 2009), whilst others are subjected to inspection by police style sniffer dogs in an attempt to detect the presence of illicit substances. 'Drug dog' policy generally requires that service users are asked to consent to such searches, but Gordon and Haider (2004) note that searches using dogs are not contingent on consent.

Aggression, violence, offending and dual diagnosis

Although the evidence underpinning some of the associations made between dual diagnosis and outcomes is largely North American, and is yet to be convincingly demonstrated outside these areas, one area where the research evidence is particularly strong concerns violence and aggression. As well as experiencing poor clinical and treatment outcomes, people with mental illness and co-existing alcohol problems pose an increased risk of suicide and violence. The National Confidential Enquiry into Suicides and Homicides committed by people with mental health problems (NCISHMH) reported that 27 per cent of suicides and 36 per cent homicides are committed by those with mental illness and co-morbid substance use. In a recent annual report published (University of Manchester, 2010) the NCISHMH noted that homicides committed by those with mental illness had risen and concluded: '...the likeliest explanation for the rise in homicide by people with psychosis is the use of drugs and/or alcohol' (p14).

Fazel *et al.* (2009) undertook a systematic review and meta-analysis of violence committed by people with psychosis and concluded that the link between psychosis and violence was significant, but mediated by drug and alcohol misuse. This means that those people with mental health problems who didn't have a drug/alcohol problem had a lower rate of violence. The rates of violence by those with co-morbid drug and alcohol and psychosis were on a par with substance misusers without co-morbidity. However, the direct causal relationship of how substance misuse affects violent behaviour has yet to be established. This does seem to highlight the importance of developing treatment responses and interventions that are appropriate for people with co-morbid mental health and alcohol problems.

People with mental health and alcohol problems have other social and economic challenges as well. They face social exclusion (Office of the Deputy Prime Minister, 2004); and social deprivation (East Midlands Public Health Observatory, undated) with the most deprived one fifth of the population having a 2–3 times greater loss of life attributable to alcohol and a 3–5 times greater mortality due to alcohol-specific causes. There is also a link with offending behaviour. A third of people on probation have current problems with alcohol and a third currently binge drink (National Offender Management Service, 2006). Almost half have had problems with alcohol in the past. Brooker and colleagues (2008) also found high levels of alcohol problems and mental health issues in offenders on probation in the East Midlands as part of a health needs assessment.

UK policy response

The main national policy guidance regarding dual diagnosis has been the *Mental Health Policy Implementation Guide: Dual Diagnosis Good Practice Guide* (Department of Health, 2002). It advocated an integrated treatment approach for people with mental health but rather than create specialist teams, this would be delivered within existing service structures. This was known as 'mainstreaming'. In order to deliver this, local strategies would need to be developed that required joint working and liaison between mental health and substance misuse services, as well as other sectors such as social care, housing and the criminal justice system. If the mainstream workforce was required to deliver comprehensive care for both mental health and co-existing substance misuse, then they would require the competences to do this. Training, supervision and practice development would be required particularly for services that had high rates of dual diagnosis (such as inpatient units, assertive outreach and forensic mental health). A National Dual Diagnosis Programme was established in 2005 as part of the National Institute for Mental Health (England) (NIMHE), later Care Services Improvement Partnership (CSIP), Mental Health Programme (which is now part of the National Mental Health Development Unit (NMHDU) in Department of Health). The national dual diagnosis programme commissioned a number of products to help facilitate workforce development around dual diagnosis (including *Closing the Gap. A Capability Framework* for dual diagnosis; Hughes, 2006a) as well as reviewing the progress of implementation of the *Dual Diagnosis Good Practice Guide* through a themed review (CSIP, 2007) as part of the autumn assessment in 2006–7.

The themed review aimed to identify progress in four areas: the development of local strategic plans (and locally agreed definitions of dual diagnosis), service delivery, health promotion and workforce training needs. The main findings were that 40 per cent of local implementation teams (LITs) did not have a local strategy, yet two thirds of LITs reported that people with dual diagnosis were having a severe resource impact on mental health services. Only 40 per cent of LITs collected data on user satisfaction with services. There was also a mixed picture regarding training across England, with some areas providing comprehensive training and practice development programmes and others having little or no specific training.

The themed review recommends that modern, effective provision for people experiencing dual diagnosis benefit from the following features:

- clear, designated local responsibility for the strategic development of dual diagnosis services.
- conducting a joint strategic needs assessment
- development of a clear local definition of the target population for services
- sensitive and appropriate collection of the views of users

- workforce capabilities that can be strengthened by employing resources such as the dual diagnosis capability framework and the Ten Essential Shared Capabilities: Dual Diagnosis module (Hughes, 2006b)
- assessment and care coordination including attending to substance misuse problems and physical health care needs.

The themed review focused on people with dual diagnosis, but the issues highlighted above are just as applicable in reducing alcohol related harm.

A NICE guidance on treatment for alcohol use disorders has been published (National Institute for Health and Clinical Excellence, 2011a). It acknowledges the link between alcohol and mental health, and recommends that alcohol treatment services should be able to assess for psychological difficulties as part of routine comprehensive assessments. The guidance recommends that for depression and anxiety these may remit after 3–4 weeks of abstinence from alcohol; however, if they persist then alcohol services should either be able to provide treatment for these issues or refer to appropriate services. For those with significant and complex co-morbidities with high risks (such as suicide), they should be referred for psychiatric assessment that should include effective treatment and risk assessment. The guidance also suggests that people who are dependent on alcohol may not benefit from psychological therapies, and recommends that they be abstinent or have 'significantly reduced' their alcohol consumption before embarking on therapy.

The new cross departmental government mental health strategy, *No Health without Mental Health*, was released and aims to address the importance of mental well-being and prevention of longer term mental health problems, as well as reducing poor outcomes for people with established mental health problems including improving physical health and reducing avoidable harms. Alcohol is mentioned in terms of both its impact on mental health and on physical health, and acknowledges the link between mental health and drug and alcohol use. It recommends improving coordination between mental health and drug and alcohol services, and that appropriate services should be available locally (including fully integrated care). The government will continue to promote and support commissioning and service provision for dual diagnosis.

NICE guidance for psychosis and co-existing substance misuse (NICE, 2011b) has also recently been released recently. In terms of service recommendations, all agencies should routinely screen for problems with drugs and alcohol for anyone presenting with a psychosis or suspected psychosis and, if indicated, be able to perform an assessment of drug and/or alcohol dependency. In order to do this, all professionals in secondary care should ensure that they are competent in working with co-existing psychosis and drug and alcohol. Secondary mental health services should not exclude service users from mental health services solely because of their substance misuse and there needs to be coordinated care and joint working with specialist substance misuse services for those who are severely dependent as well as having a significant mental health problem. People working in substance misuse services should be able to recognise the signs and symptoms of psychosis and undertake a mental health needs and risk assessment and to know when and where to refer to mental health services.

Evidence for effective treatments

The evidence base for effective treatment for people with co-morbid mental health and alcohol/drug problems is limited (Cleary *et al.*, 2008); however, the approaches showing most promise are cognitive behavioural therapy and motivational enhancement (including brief intervention), which are also advocated for moderate drinkers by the recently released NICE guidance for alcohol problems (NICE, 2011a). The National Treatment Agency reviewed the effectiveness of alcohol treatment (Raistrick *et al.*, 2006) and concluded that psychosocial interventions are delivered at a reasonable cost and not only result in reduced drinking, but also result in wider social benefits.

The findings of a large UK multi-site trial of motivational interviewing (MI) and cognitive behavioural therapy (CBT) plus standard care versus standard care was published recently (the MIDAS trial; Barrowclough *et al.*, 2010). Over 300 patients in London and Manchester with psychosis and substance misuse problems were recruited to the trial and randomized into two arms. In the treatment arm they received up to 26 one-hour MI and CBT sessions delivered by highly skilled and trained therapists over and above their usual care. However, despite this intensive psychological therapy, there were no significant differences in the main outcomes including admissions to hospital or death (by any means) between the two groups. There were only two significant findings – less primary substance was consumed on a substance-using day (although no overall change in substance misuse) and an increased readiness to change at 12 months, but this was not maintained after 24 months. However, there was a significant difference in percentage of days abstinent in the alcohol sub-group compared to controls, but no other significant difference in other outcomes. This does suggest that MI and CBT may have more of an impact on people with alcohol and psychosis as opposed to those who use other drugs. This was also found in other trials of psychosocial interventions reviewed in Cleary *et al.* (2008).

Training and the workforce

The traditional inpatient and community mental health workforce is not equipped to work with dual diagnosis and therefore struggles to deliver on the mainstream agenda. The last decade has seen enormous national and regional attempts to address this.

Siegfried *et al.* (1999) conducted a survey of mental health workers in Australia and found that a third had never received substance misuse training and 41 per cent had never worked clinically in substance misuse services. Maslin *et al.* (2001) undertook a training needs analysis in Birmingham mental health services and found that over 80 per cent were routinely working with dual diagnosis issues, and their training needs were more information (particularly on how substances affected mental health and vice versa), some skills training, and how to work with other agencies. This lack of training and experience may be because substance misuse is not a core part of pre-registration training for mental health professionals. O'Gara *et al.* (2005) undertook a survey of previous substance misuse training in nurse and medical training and found that mental health staff reported minimal pre-qualification training in substance misuse. Hughes *et al.* (2008) found that in a sample of community mental health case managers working substance misuse in at least a third of their caseloads, only 36 per cent had ever had any substance misuse training, and half had never worked clinically in substance misuse services. Of the training received, this was most frequently brief in-house training (typically 1–3 days).

So there is a clear gap between the level of complexity of service users receiving care in mental health services and the competence of mental health staff to address these complexities. This is especially pertinent given the national policy direction for dual diagnosis is one of 'mainstreaming', in that mainstream mental health services should be equipped to deliver comprehensive and integrated care that includes substance misuse screening; education and health promotion/harm reduction; assessments; and interventions.

Two published UK studies have examined the impact of specialist training and supervision for generic mental health staff in dual diagnosis interventions.

The COMPASS study involved training assertive outreach teams to deliver a modified integrated approach known as Cognitive Behavioural Integrated Treatment (C-BIT), which contained the philosophy of the Integrated Treatment Approach, but with a greater emphasis on applying cognitive behavioural interventions related to the interplay between mental health and substance misuse. In a quasi-experimental design, half the assertive outreach teams received training and supervision, whilst the others acted as a comparison (treatment as usual). Baseline data before training was collected on staff (attitudes, confidence and knowledge) and patients (mental state, service use and substance misuse). At follow-up there were improvements in staff outcomes, but little effect on clinical outcomes for service users. Psychopathology and severity of substance misuse remained unaffected. However, service users in the trained teams showed better engagement, and a reduction in level of conviction (how strongly they were held) of alcohol related beliefs.

The COMO trial was a cluster randomised trial in community mental health teams in South-east London. Case managers were randomly allocated to receive either a five-day skills-based training in psychosocial interventions for dual diagnosis or be in the waiting control arm (then receive training after 18 months). Case managers' caseloads were screened to identify service users with dual diagnosis of psychotic illness plus substance use at abuse or dependent levels (using DSM IV criteria). Then the service users underwent an assessment interview, completing measures on substance misuse, psychopathology, functioning and quality of life. At 18 months post training, case managers and service users repeated the measures. The training had a significant effect on case manager self-rated confidence in their skills in this area, and also knowledge about dual diagnosis. Overall attitudes failed to reach a significant improvement, although there were significant improvements on sub-scales of knowledge and adequacy of skills in the trained group. However, like the COMPASS project, there were few tangible improvements on service user outcomes, apart from scores on the Brief Psychiatric Rating Scale – symptoms showed improvement in those service users receiving care from the trained case managers. However, the level of substance use remained unchanged overall.

Conclusions

Substance misuse and mental illness have a well-established co-occurrence, but the causal link between the two has yet to be definitively established. However, a combination of social and psychological vulnerabilities is likely to interplay with environmental factors. The co-existence of substance misuse in someone presenting to mental health services is likely to be a strong indicator of a whole range of complex health and social care needs, who will incur high treatment costs, yet ultimately experience poor outcomes.

It is more than a decade since the publication of national guidance for dual diagnosis treatment, but reviews of implementation (CSIP, 2007) indicate that there is still a long way to go in terms of effective integrated care in local areas. Research evidence for effective treatments is equivocal, although there are some suggestions that brief interventions, MI and CBT may be helpful for those with mental health and moderate alcohol problems. NICE guidance has now been published (2011a, 2011b), which (like other guidance) stresses the importance of joint working between substance misuse and mental health services, particularly for those with significant and severe presentations.

In addition, new the mental health strategy recognises alcohol as a significant factor in both mental and physical outcomes. Both for psychosis and substance misuse and for alcohol problems, NICE guidance recommends that mental health and substance use services should be capable of screening and performing comprehensive assessment for people with co-morbidities. The challenge will be for commissioners and service providers to implement these guidelines in the new configurations of health and social care, as well as public health.

References

Barnaby, B., Drummond, C., McCloud, A., Burns, T. and Omu, N. (2003) Substance misuse in psychiatric inpatients: comparison of a screening questionnaire survey with case notes. *British Medical Journal*, 327(4): 783–784

Barrowclough, C., Haddock, G., Wykes, T., Beardmore, R., Conrod, P., Craig, T., Davies, L., Dunn, G., Eisner, E., Lewis, S., Moring, J., Steel, C. and Tarrier, N. (2010) Integrated motivational interviewing and cognitive behavioural therapy for people with psychosis and comorbid substance misuse: randomised controlled trial. *British Medical Journal*, 341: c6325

Brooker, C., Fox, C., Barrett, P. and Syson-Nibbs, L. (2008) A health needs assessment of offenders on probation caseloads in Nottingham and Derbyshire. University of Lincoln, http://www.lincoln. ac.uk/cjmh/publications.htm (accessed 1 April 2011)

Cantwell, R. (2003) Substance use and schizophrenia: effects on symptoms, social functioning and service use. *British Journal of Psychiatry*, 182: 324–329

Cleary, M., Hunt, G.E., Matheson, S.L., Siegfried, N. and Walter, G. (2008) Psychosocial interventions for people with serious mental health and substance misuse. *Cochrane Database of Systematic Reviews 2008*, Issue 1. Art. No.: CD001088.

CSIP (2007) Themed review report 2007: dual diagnosis. Department of Health, London, http://www. nmhdu.org.uk/silo/files/dual-diagosis-themed-review-report-2007.pdf (accessed 1 April 2011)

Department of Health (1999) *The National Service Framework for Mental Health*. Department of Health, London

Department of Health (2002) *Mental Health Policy Implementation Guide: Dual Diagnosis Good Practice Guide*. Department of Health, London

Department of Health (2005) *The National Service Framework – five years on*. Department of Health, London

Department of Health (2011) *No Health without Mental Health, a cross government mental health outcomes strategy for people of all ages*. Department of Health, London.

Dixon, L. (1999) Dual diagnosis of substance misuse in schizophrenia: prevalence and impact on outcomes. *Schizophrenia Research*, 25(S): 93–100

East Midlands Public Health Observatory (undated) Briefing: Alcohol and the East Midlands, http:// www.empho.org.uk/Download/Public/10485/1/alcoholbriefing.pdf (accessed 2 November 2011)

Fazel, S., Langstrom, N., Hjern, A., Grann, M. and Lictensten, P. (2009) Schizophrenia, substance abuse, and violence crime. *JAMA*, 301(19): 2016–2023

Gearon, J., Bellack, A.S., RachBeisel, J. and Dixon, L. (2001) Drug use behaviours and correlates in schizophrenia. *Addictive Behaviours*, 26(1): 51–61

Gordon, H. and Haider, D. (2004) The use of 'drug dogs' in psychiatry. *Psychiatric Bulletin*, 28: 196–198

Hughes, L. (2006a) *Closing the Gap. A Capability Framework for Working with People with Combined Mental Health and Substance Use Problems*. University of Lincoln/CSIP, Lincoln

Hughes, L. (2006b) *Advanced Module of the Ten Essential Shared Capabilities: Dual Diagnosis* CDROM. University of Lincoln/CSIP, Lincoln

Hughes, E., Wanigaratne, S., Gournay, K., Johnson, J, Thornicroft, G, Finch, E., Marshall, J., and Smith, N. (2008) Training in Dual Diagnosis Interventions (The COMO Study): A Randomised Controlled Trial. *Biomedical Central Psychiatry*, February 2008, 8:12

Maslin, J., Graham, H.L., Cawley, M., Copello, A., Birchwood, M., Georgiou, G., McGovern, D., Mueser, K., and Orford, J. (2001) Combined severe mental health and substance use problems: What are the training and support needs of staff working with this client group? *Journal of Mental Health*, (10), 2: 131–140

Murray, R.M., Grech, A., Phillips, P. and Johnson, S. (2002) What is the relationship between substance misuse and schizophrenia? In Murray, R.M., Cannon, M., Jones, P., Van Os, J. and Susser, E. (eds) *The Epidemiology of Schizophrenia*. Cambridge University Press, Cambridge

National Institute for Health and Clinical Excellence (2011a) CG115 Alcohol Use Disorders. Diagnosis, assessment and management of harmful drinking and alcohol dependence. http://guidance.nice.org. uk/CG115/NICEGuidance/pdf/English (accessed 1 April 2011)

National Institute for Health and Clinical Excellence (2011b) Psychosis with coexisting substance misuse. Assessment and management in adults and young people. NICE Clinical Guideline 120. National Collaborating Centre for Mental Health, London

National Offender Management Service (2006) *Working with Alcohol Misusing Offenders. A Strategy for Delivery*. National Offender Management Service, London

Office of the Deputy Prime Minister (2004) *Mental Health and Social Exclusion Report*. National Offender Management Service, London

O'Gara, C., Keaney, F., Best, D., Harris, J., Boys, A., Leonard, F., Kelleher, M. and Strang, J. (2005) Substance misuse training among psychiatric doctors, psychiatric nurses, medical students and nursing students in a South London psychiatric teaching hospital. *Drugs: education, prevention and policy*, 12 (4) 327–336

Phillips, P. (1998) The mad, the bad and the dangerous – harm reduction in dual diagnosis. *International Journal of Drug Policy*, 9, 345–349

Phillips, P. and Johnson, S. (2001) How does drug and alcohol misuse develop among people with psychotic illness? A literature review. *Social Psychiatry and Psychiatric Epidemiology*, 36: 269–276.

Phillips, P. and Johnson, S. (2003) Drug and alcohol misuse amongst in-patients with psychotic illnesses in three inner-London psychiatric units. *Psychiatric Bulletin*, 27(6): 217–220

Raistrick, D., Heather, N. and Godfrey, C (2006) *Review of the Effectiveness of Treatment for Alcohol Problems*. National Treatment Agency for Substance Misuse, London

Regier, D.A., Farmer, M.E., Rae, D.S., Locke, B.Z., Keith, S.J., Judd, L.L., and Goodwin, F.K. (1990) Co-morbidity of mental disorders with alcohol and other drugs of misuse: results from the epidemiological catchment area (ECA) study. *Journal of the American Medical Association* (264) 2511–2518

Shulte, S. and Holland, M. (2008) Dual diagnosis in Manchester, UK: practitioners estimates of prevalence rates in mental health and substance miuse services. *Mental Health and Substance Misuse: Dual Diagnosis*, 1(2): 118–124

Siegfried, N., Ferguson, J., Cleary, M., Walter, G. and Rey, J.M (1999) Experience, knowledge and attitudes of mental health staff regarding patients' problematic drug and alcohol use. *Australia and New Zealand Journal of Psychiatry*. 33 (2) 267–273

Smith, J. and Hucker, S. (1994) Schizophrenia and substance misuse. *British Journal of Psychiatry*, 165: 13–21

University of Manchester (2010) *National Confidential Enquiry into Suicide and Homicide by People with Mental Illness*. Annual report. University of Manchester, Manchester

Wilson, I., Holland, M., Mason, V., Reeve, J. and Ash, H. (2009) The management of substance misuse on psychiatric inpatient wards – a policy to promote effective good practice. *Advances in Dual Diagnosis* 2(4): 12–17

9   Gender-specific mental health care

The case for women-centred care

Louise Phillips and Ann Jackson

Introduction

It is perhaps a paradox of contemporary mental health provision that the issues of gender-specific services and practice are still largely unresolved. Given the emphasis that is placed on 'ensuring a positive experience of care and support' and 'protecting from avoidable harm and caring in a safe environment' taken from *No health without mental health* (HM Government, 2011a), then, as the authors of this chapter, we will argue again that more needs to be done to achieve inpatient services that are both safe and therapeutic for women. Ten years on, we have an opportunity to assess the extent to which services have achieved the aspiration of the Labour health minister, John Hutton, in 2001 in announcing the strategy '*into the mainstream*' to 'ensure that women are listened to and their views translated into real change…'

Our starting point is that acute inpatient services, despite the well-documented criticisms, remain a significant and expensive feature of our mental health provision. Our concern would be that little regard continues to be given to the specific needs of women: that national policy has been poorly implemented and that the barriers of implementation have been left unaddressed. The purpose of this chapter is to outline the government policy that has driven the development of UK, women-only, acute inpatient provision, provide reflections on the continued difficulties in achieving this, and suggest some ideas about future development. Let's turn briefly to what this chapter is not about. It is not an analysis of psychiatry and mental illness, nor is it a look back at historical and social origins of 'women's madness', although there is much to warrant an understanding of this in order to arrive at a gendered analysis and critique relating to the provision of contemporary mental health care. (For fuller accounts see Chesler, 1997; Ussher 1997). We are also conscious that we have only touched on the specific social issues affecting women's experiences of mental health issues, and that we are white, middle-aged and have clinical backgrounds – our lens offers a limited view.

In the UK and beyond, policy is increasingly concerned with developing strong individuals, groups and communities where fairness and social justice equality and human rights are seen to be the underpinning principles of the social world. We see the rhetoric reflected in an abundance of social and health policy, legislation in the form of the Equality Act 2010 and associated public sector duties; and a social and political imperative to 'tackle' inequalities in health. This is a useful backdrop to current mental health strategy, as it is well established that social inequality leads to health inequality (The Marmot Review, 2010) and for people who use mental health services these inequalities can be further compounded by stigma and discrimination.

This is particularly relevant for women experiencing mental health services in two important ways, which are the focus of this chapter. Firstly, women still experience inequalities in relation to earnings and income (Government Equalities Office, 2010) and, secondly, women continue to be disproportionate survivors of violence and abuse. Gender inequality is regarded as both a cause and a consequence of violence on women and girls (Women's National Commission, 2009). The evidence is compelling that these aspects of women's lives and past experiences have a direct impact on their mental health and well-being (see amongst others Itzin, 2006). In addition, women as part of the workforce, nursing as a largely female workforce, and the experience of female employees also as potential survivors of gendered violence and abuse, needs to be considered as part of the needs of all women providing and receiving care (Department of Health, 2010a). We suggest that women-centred care takes these experiences into account when designing services and providing professional care. We believe, like others (see Williams *et al.*, 2001; Tully & Gallop, 2009) that mental health nurses have a significant role in reaching a gendered understanding of nursing and promoting safe environments and compassionate responses to women receiving inpatient care. Initiatives to raise awareness amongst health professionals generally can only add to the urgency for mental health nurses to assert a professional understanding of the causes and consequences of violence against women; and prioritise responses that are informed and empowering.

This chapter will concentrate on mental health policy and practice initiatives, and asks the question: to what extent have things improved, if at all, for women since the Department of Health's strategy for women – *into the mainstream*? When the consultation was launched in 2002, there was much hope that eventually a vision for women's services had been created, based on the views and preferences of many women and based on the evidence of women's experiences. For women working in the service, it was a time of renewed optimism, that the differences between men and women would be acknowledged, agreed and accommodated into the creation of a 'gender-sensitive' or 'gender-specific' framework for women.

The following implementation guidance, *Mainstreaming Gender and Women's Mental Health* in 2003 made clear recommendations for reconfiguring services to provide safe and therapeutic spaces for women. This safety aspect was particularly important as there had been many reports of women being sexually harassed and assaulted in mixed sex environments. In 2006, the National Patient Safety Agency revealed that between November 2003 and September 2005 there were 122 incidents of sexual assault within mental health inpatient acute wards in the UK, 19 of which were rape cases. Of the 19 reports of alleged rape, in 8 cases the alleged perpetrator was another patient and in 11 cases a member of staff. In recent years this evidence has been augmented by *With safety in mind* (National Patient Safety Agency, 2006) and the policy steer of eliminating mixed sex provision in wards – this goal is still a long way from being achieved (NMHDU, 2010).

There has been a shift from the inpatient acute mental health ward as a place of treatment to a focus upon community care, with the development of crisis resolution and home treatment teams (Glover *et al.*, 2006). Consequently, acute care is largely focused on crisis and higher risk patients, and staff are arguably increasingly risk adverse. There have been a number of surveys to establish what inpatient, acute mental health services are like for service users. A survey by Mind in 2004, found that 53 per cent of patients, both men and women, said the ward surroundings did not aid their recovery, and 31 per cent stated their condition worsened (Mind, 2004). The Care Quality Commission conducted a survey in 2009 on service users' experiences of mixed sex, acute wards, and revealed that less than half (45 per cent) stated they 'always' felt safe on the ward, while 39 per cent 'sometimes' felt safe and 16 per cent did not feel safe at all. For women users of services, the traditional mixed inpatient, acute ward is particularly unsafe. Women's safety is a cause of concern for nursing staff, managers, psychiatrists, commissioners and campaigners alike. Many of the women admitted to these wards have experienced traumatic experiences including childhood sexual, physical and emotional abuse, all forms of domestic violence and sexual assault and rape. There have been many suggestions made to improve and maintain women's sexual safety in mixed-sex acute, inpatient mental health services. These include the introduction of policies to ensure consistency in the management and recording of sexual assault cases reported (Lawn and McDonald, 2009). Ward layouts have been considered to ensure that women are safer and are given specific areas that are women-only (Subotsky, 1991). Increased staffing levels are considered to bring about improvements in women's safety ensuring the presence of staff in all ward areas (Tonks, 1992). Concern about the safety of women patients led to a commitment in the NHS Plan (Department of Health, 2000) to provide gender-specific or women-only services in every health authority by 2004. The then Secretary of State, Patricia Hewitt, recently claimed on Women's Hour on Radio 4 (January 2010) that 99 per cent of all mental health wards are single sex. However, women-only mental health provision has not been achieved by all commissioners. The criteria used to define single-sex wards or women-only wards need clarification; this often means a corridor, to separate sleeping provision, toilets and bathrooms, perhaps a women's day area, and dining areas shared with male patients. It remains one of the key areas for development as highlighted by NMHDU (2010).

According to a study by Mezey *et al.* (2005), the introduction of women-only acute wards has made women less vulnerable to sexual assault by men, although women were found to be subject to threats and abuse by other women (Mezey *et al.*, 2005). A number of women-only projects have been introduced as alternatives to hospital admission, but there are surprisingly few such wards, hostels, crisis houses and contained units. In the current economic climate, we are concerned about the impact of the cuts and economic downturn for women as both public sector employees and as users of services. This concern within the context of this chapter is that women tend to use alternatives to hospital more, for a variety of reasons, and therefore any cuts to services will disproportionately impact on them and, secondly, that women become more vulnerable to violence and abuse when they are less financially independent (TUC, 2011).

Acute inpatient care for women

We argue that inpatient women-only wards are more able to provide a space that is both safe and therapeutic. However, staff need relevant education, training and supervision, particularly for the care and support of women with traumatic experiences, whether they work within mixed sex or gender specific inpatient services. In this respect, *Informed gender practice* (CSIP, 2008) is an important resource to support acute inpatient wards develop their approach to providing women-centred care. It states that:

> A high quality service will be one where everyone who contributes to the services is knowledgeable about the ways that gender, race and other inequalities can be detrimental to mental health; willing and able to help service users talk about their gendered lives and experiences and alert to and challenges the ways that gender and other inequalities undermine the safety and quality of services.

This aspiration is entirely compatible with the definition of 'quality': effectiveness, patient experience and safety embedded in future plans for an outcome-focused health care delivery (Department of Health, 2010b). Very importantly, this best practice guidance posed a fundamental reframe of a traditional (medical model) question of 'what is *wrong* with this woman?' to 'what has *happened* to this woman?'

This resource is also helpful in introducing practical ideas to support services in identifying inequalities and address the diverse needs of women.

Childhood sexual abuse and mental health

The prevalence of women in mental health services who have experienced childhood sexual abuse is well-documented: 7 to 30 per cent of girls are estimated to have been abused, which is three times higher than rates among boys (Department of Health, 2002). There are strong associations between childhood sexual abuse and mental health problems in adult life (Mullen *et al.*, 1993; Itzin *et al.*, 2008). A study by Coid *et al.* (2003) states child sexual abuse as being 'the primary abusive experience associated with the psychopathological symptoms measured in adulthood' (p336).

Many problems such as eating disorders and a diagnosis borderline personality disorder (BPD) are more frequently found among women with histories of sexual abuse (Spatoro *et al.*, 2004). Women who have been sexually abused in childhood are more likely to experience physical or sexual abuse as adults. Women with mental health problems, who have been sexually abused in childhood, have particular needs for care, treatment and support that must be addressed by mental health and other services (Department of Health, 2003). However, it is important to note that in a recent Delphi study, experts are in agreement that 'there is no single therapeutic approach that works best for every victim/survivor in this group' (Itzin *et al.*, 2010).

Women's mental health: into the mainstream (Department of Health, 2002) considered the impact of child sexual, physical and emotional abuse, all forms of domestic violence, and sexual assault and rape as significant factors in the development of mental ill health for women, clearly linking a history of child sexual abuse with higher rates in adult life of depressive symptoms, anxiety symptoms, substance abuse disorders, eating disorders and post-traumatic stress disorders (Silverman *et al.*, 1996; Itzin, 2006). It also acknowledges how survivors of child sexual abuse can experience retraumatisation during treatment including close observation, restraint, seclusion and the administration of medication for example (Judd *et al.*, 2009).

This government exercise found that mental health professionals' awareness of violence/abuse issues was very limited and that staff were not confident in acknowledging and addressing child sexual abuse experiences. It argued that specific training should be made available to all health professionals to increase confidence and competence to ask the question: 'have you experienced abuse' openly and directly, and then to respond appropriately. There are some excellent resources available to support staff learning and development on this issue; see for example: *Not mad or bad, but traumatized* DVD by Cisters (2007) and a course reader, from the Department of Health Collaborative Pilot Project, *Meeting the needs of survivors of child sexual abuse – underpinned by routine enquiry in mental health assessments* (NMHDU, 2010).

A study of survivors of childhood sexual abuse found that survivors do not object to being asked about possible experiences of sexual abuse, and those who have not had these experiences do not mind being asked the question (Nelson 2001; Stafford, 2006). The specific recommendations are unlikely to make an impact without significant changes in staff attitudes towards sexual abuse, and specific training will be essential.

Mental health staff must be adequately trained to appropriately respond to the disclosure of violence and abuse and possess the required skills to ask specific questions about these issues during the standard assessment process. Training should enable staff to identify presentations in women on wards related to a history of abuse, and to explore their responses to these. Ideally training should be incorporated with safeguarding programmes and so be mandatory, supported by regular ongoing supervision. The very best practice would ensure that women service users are co-workers in designing, delivering and evaluating this training.

Gendered violence and mental health

Despite the policy and evidence over the last decade of rising awareness around women as survivors of abuse and violence, the issues of domestic violence and other forms of violence against women and girls (VAWG) are not addressed consistently in inpatient settings (NMHDU, 2010). This is not unique to mental health services: it is a problem in all clinical settings. *Together we can end violence against women and girls: a strategy* (HM Government Strategy, 2009) highlighted many of the issues facing women survivors of domestic violence accessing services and the lack of appropriate response they receive. During the development of this cross–government strategy, it became increasingly clear in the focus groups that many women continue to experience poor attitudes from staff, who display ignorance of the issues, pay little regard to the safety needs of women and lack empathy and understanding (Women's National Commission, 2009). In the same study, the Women's National Commission made a firm recommendation in *Still we rise* that all front line workers should be trained about the causes and consequences of violence and abuse. The evidence of poor health service responses prompted the establishment of a Department of Health Taskforce. The resulting report, *Responding to violence against women and children – the role of the NHS* (Department of Health, 2010a), made 25 recommendations for comprehensive and integrated response by clinicians, service providers, commissioners, regulators and professional bodies/Royal Colleges. The first of these recommendations was to raise awareness. The report stopped short of advocating 'routine enquiry' in all health settings, but recommended its continued use within maternity and mental health services. We referred earlier to the Care Programme Approach (CPA) assessment making it compulsory to ask the following question: 'Have you experienced physical, sexual or emotional abuse at any time in your life?' And to record whether it has been asked, with an explanation to be documented if not. Obviously, this question can only be asked by 'suitably trained' staff as recommended by NMHDU (2010), to avoid the risk that it becomes another 'tick-box' exercise lacking meaning for women who use services in relation to other areas of assessment.

Most of the experience and expertise about working with women survivors of domestic violence is in the voluntary sector – but there are some useful resources to support mental health professionals develop the knowledge and skills for 'safe enquiry' and referral onto specialist services; see for example: *Sane responses: a toolkit for mental health professionals* (GLDVP, 2008). Understandably, the most useful response that can be made to a disclosure of domestic violence is one of respect and belief in a conversation that has been provided safely and with compassion and understanding (Humphreys *et al.*, 2009). The aspect of understanding is complex; women are not a homogeneous group and the diversity within different groups of women and between groups needs to be acknowledged. So, for example, services and practices must be sensitive to the specific needs of lesbian and gay women, women with disabilities, women across the age groups and women of faith, amongst other issues. In relation to black and minority ethnic (BME) women, we would recommend that services access the wealth of resources published by specialist voluntary sector providers. In particular, Siddiqui and Patel (2010) have provided a useful critique of national policy and developed a 'hybrid' model of intervention specifically designed to promote a whole-systems approach. Importantly, they draw attention to the very different risks and dangers that services often unwittingly place BME women in. Specialist services for all groups of BME women to address gendered violence in its widest forms have to be supported and developed to comply with current legislation.

The coalition government have made their commitment to continue this work programme clear by producing a *Call to end violence against women and girls* (HM Government, 2011b). In the accompanying *Action plan* a further commitment is made to the implementation of recommendations in the taskforce report (Department of Health, 2010b). Further, we note that mental health commissioning guidance highlights the need to address the mental health impact of violence and abuse (NMHDU 2011).

Reflections on education and training projects

Example: model of care, Ward A

In our first example, a large mental health trust in the Midlands developed a collaborative model of care for its first women-only ward. The model of care was developed by multidisciplinary staff, who agreed a vision and set of principles that described the purpose of the ward and set some criteria for referral to the ward. It was always anticipated that demand would be greater than the supply of beds, but that this would be an opportunity to establish a framework for future development and need, while at the same time determining best practice for caring for women on mixed sex wards.

The development of Ward A was in response to the national policy set out in *Mainstreaming gender and women's mental health* (Department of Health, 2003) with service objectives addressing privacy and dignity, and ensuring the safety of women vulnerable to the sexual assault and violence experienced on mixed acute mental health inpatient wards. In addition, the NHS Confederation briefing (2008) had provided guidance to support the development of a national policy on abuse and violence. It is well documented that a high proportion of women within mental health services are victims/survivors of all forms of emotional, physical, financial and sexual abuse and this has to be incorporated through 'routine enquiry' and included in CPA documentation. The CPA was revised in 2008 by the Department of Health to acknowledge the abuse of women (Department of Health, 2008).

This model of care was based on prerequisite standards for staffing and clarity around the patient group in terms of need and vulnerability. Immediate referral criteria, based on priority factors previously recommended within the literature for women-only provision (Department of Health, 2003) were agreed: women who are pregnant; women from BME communities with cultural preference for a single-sex ward; women with histories of abuse and violence (who state a preference to be on a women-only ward); and women assessed as vulnerable with regard to sexual health behaviours.

The model of care on Ward A was based on a set of core 'purposes' that also provided the criteria for future service evaluation:

- To provide a therapeutic and safe environment.
- To provide a focused, holistic, positive and 'distinctly different' experience of inpatient care.
- To provide a meaningful choice for women.
- To address issues of violence and abuse.
- To address specific mental health and well-being needs.
- To work collaboratively within a women-centred recovery-based approach.

The ward team set out to provide skilled care against these core purposes that was therapeutic, set the parameters for the delivery of consistent and high standards of service, and provided effective systems of inter-professional working. The emphasis was on developing an ethos and skill base for relational security, although it was anticipated at the time that this would need organisational investment and strong multidisciplinary leadership. The model went onto articulate the women-centred aspects of holistic health including physical health, with an emphasis on the specific reproductive, life cycle health needs.

Example: focus groups, Ward B

Many of the staff who took part in the education and training projects were keen to adopt a woman-centred recovery-based approach in their work with women. They wished to make a difference to their lives and help them make steps to improve their ways of relating to others, and to find and maintain safe and secure relationships. All the staff participating in the focus groups and training signed a consent form to enable the first author to write up discussions taking place and to publish the results; and the participants all gave informed consent. Time was taken during the training and workshops to ensure the views and reflections of the staff were recorded accurately. The author gained ethical approval to publish the paper (Phillips, 2009) from the Sub-Ethics Committee and final approval from the clinical director of the mental health trust.

The focus groups were held monthly with a staff team from a women-only ward in the south of England. They were a mixture of qualified and unqualified nursing staff. Within these groups, discussions took place about clinical practice in relation to work with women, such as culture and ethnicity, sexuality, women-specific mental health needs, and body image. It became apparent that this staff team did not receive training that addressed effective ways of meeting women-specific needs. For example, it was stated by some staff that some of the women service users disclosed painful experiences such as rape, and staff often did not know how to respond.

Women's spaces

Women's sexual expression was frequently discussed in the focus groups. It was very interesting – and often moving – how within the women-only space of the ward, the experiences of the women patients' sexual relationships were freely discussed. It seemed that this was comfortable for the women patients and staff and there was much laughter and joy expressed. It seemed that in this space women were able to speak. Some women patients stated to the staff that they could not discuss their sexual feelings on mixed sex wards as they did not feel safe enough to do so.

In the focus groups, issues of the women's sexualized behavior when they were unwell were also of great concern to many of the staff. Women from nearby mixed acute wards were frequently transferred to the women-only ward because their behaviour was considered by staff to be 'inappropriate'. There were reports of how women would wander into male dormitories scantily dressed. They were often perceived as being 'flirtatious' and considered highly vulnerable. Mentally ill women's sexuality seemed to be 'pathologised', as the staff taking part in the focus groups put it. The staff often felt helpless in these situations. They questioned what the most appropriate response would be to these women and it was generally considered that these women patients were being flirtatious and staff were often at a loss as to what to do. Women were often considered as 'uncontrollable' in their perceived eagerness for sex by some staff on the mixed sex wards. The issue of women's sexuality did not appear to be explored within any of the clinical areas, and the staff taking part in the focus groups claimed that these issues were not addressed at all when the women were on mixed sex wards. Consequently, women with these 'issues' were referred to the women-only ward, as the staff in the focus groups stated: 'to decrease their desires'. However, in the women-only environment, the staff were motivated to address these issues, and to make the space to do so. They expressed a need for more time in team meetings to explore these issues and further training to help them address sexuality as it impacted on the everyday running of the ward.

Experiences of gendered violence and abuse

A large majority of the women who were admitted to the women-only ward, as well as those transferred from mixed wards, had experienced sexual and physical abuse. It seemed that 'flirtatious' behaviour on the part of women who had experienced sexual abuse was often part of the process of attempting to work through the experience of abuse.

The staff on the women-only ward experienced women who were in acute distress or who were perceived as manic being frequently admitted. Consequently, 'at risk' women needing one-to-one observation, transferred from mixed sex acute wards, appeared to receive the most attention from staff. The other vulnerable women often got sidelined, which was of great concern to the staff. They were not able to effectively deal with the issue of women's abuse. They were not given an adequate opportunity to explore this issue, and they frequently spent the majority of their time responding to women in crisis. The staff believed that there was a need for another unit that would serve to meet the needs of women in crisis who were seen as high risk and requiring intensive care and observation. Many of these women did disclose experiences of sexual abuse on the women-only ward and said they would not have done this if they were on mixed sex wards.

Body image

The issue of women's sense of their bodies and in relation to the experience of mental distress (Ussher, 1997; Phillips, 2006) is well documented. The staff team on the women-only ward was aware of this and stated they would appreciate training in this subject area. They were aware that many of their women patients had experienced sexual abuse and domestic violence and they were interested in how these would affect a woman's sense of self and body. Discussions about female patients appearing to have complex and difficult relationships with their bodies were frequently raised in the focus groups.

The staff strongly stated that they would find training on eating difficulties very useful for their work with women. Interestingly, they reported that women on the ward appeared to eat openly on the ward with other patients and often in large quantities. Many of the women would become physically heavier during their stay on the ward. Obviously there are health concerns here, but it seemed that the women felt safe to take up space while on the ward. Often women feel uneasy about taking up space in the world. One of the discussions in the focus groups considered how men often presume they can take up space and for women this is much more difficult! There was an acknowledgement that women were able to take up space on the women-only ward, and they were able to be 'themselves'. One staff member said the women could walk around, wash, sit on the sofa and not worry about men being around during this time, when they were particularly in need of care and support.

Example: mixed sex acute wards – workshops

Workshops for staff working within a variety of mental health mixed inpatient services were delivered over a period of four months, and consisted of a one-day programme that was repeated every week for ten weeks. The aim of the workshops were to encourage and enable staff to work in a gender-sensitive way and develop strategies for the sexual safety of women patients in their clinical areas.

The therapeutic relationship

The staff taking part in the workshops stressed the importance of maintaining boundaries with women patients who had experienced sexual abuse, and clearly emphasised their wish to work therapeutically with them, but a number of factors prevented this. Primarily, in their view, the lack of therapeutic work and a 'space' for women was due to the demands on staff working in mixed sex wards. There were daily issues about the safety of all patients and dealing with high risk patients. There were also the responses of staff to women who had experienced sexual abuse, who frequently expressed feelings of confusion and anger. As one participant stated: 'I get so angry with the women who put themselves at risk. I do not know why they do this.' Women patients with sexual abuse histories were perceived as rather baffling and infuriating and appeared to consistently jeopardise the positive changes they made while on the wards. Staff stated that they felt hopeless, angry and intruded upon by the women, and they had limited opportunity to explore these responses. There was an overall scarcity of training and supervision given to the staff, although one particular clinical area was an exception. As staff were frequently dealing with issues of risk, particularly physical threat in relation to the male patients, they stated that in their working lives they did not have an opportunity to discuss their responses to women patients. From their point of view, there was a need to focus on the women patients and their experiences, but they felt they did not have time to do this.

The feelings encountered by staff could actually bring them closer to the experiences of their women patients, but time is essential in order to reflect on these issues. Many women patients transfer their experiences of sexual abuse onto the staff that look after them. Transference is the repetition in the present of a relationship that was significant in the person's early life. Early relationships are 'lived out' in the transference (Laplanche and Pontalis, 1988). This may be apparent in people who have experienced painful early lives such as sexual abuse, who may frequently transfer or project their feelings onto others as a way of getting rid of the anxiety it causes them. Women patients, who have experienced sexual abuse in childhood, may get rid of the painful memories, or unacceptable and disturbing thoughts associated with the abuse, and put these onto the staff caring for them. The staff may then encounter uncomfortable feelings about their women patients. They may feel sexual attraction and feel confused about the 'sexualised' behaviour of their women patients. It is important for mental health staff to distinguish between the feelings that belong to them and those that belong to their patients.

It is vital that time is spent thinking about women patients and the ways in which their early experiences may affect their relationships with others. We believe this is possible in women-only spaces, and women have reported that they are more likely to disclose abuse experiences in safe, women-only services. This may lead to the member of staff being able to think more clearly and reinforce boundaries within the therapeutic relationship. The staff stated that their often troubling responses to their women patients prevented them from establishing good therapeutic boundaries. Unclear and inconsistent boundaries have been considered to decrease a sense of safety in many patients with a diagnosis of borderline personality disorder (Geller and Srikameswaran, 2006). When good therapeutic boundaries are established, staff are less likely to feel overwhelmed and 'burnt out', and plans for the effective care of patients become clearer (NIMHE, 2003; Langley and Klopper, 2005).

There are many authors who have discussed the importance of supervision using a psychodynamic framework for understanding the experiences of patients (Evans and Franks, 1997). This theoretical perspective has the potential to enable mental health practitioners to think about and provide meaning for the anxieties they often feel about patients, thus reducing the risk of thoughtless action. Staff are very unlikely to act upon difficult responses if these are articulated in a safe and meaningful way in a supervisory relationship. It is about being given permission to say the unsayable and take hold of the reality of mental health practice. Staff should be encouraged to think about the feelings they experience that are provoked by working and caring for vulnerable women, and to put thoughts about this safely into words. What arose in the workshops was the expressed feelings of hopelessness by staff, from the experience of observing women who do not appear to help themselves and repeat destructive relationships and patterns of behaviour. Articulating the reality of our feelings and responses to the vulnerable women we care for is extremely important to their well-being.

Staff training

Staff taking part in the workshops frequently expressed how they could not make sense of why the women put themselves at risk, willingly repeating destructive behaviour and getting involved with men who might hurt them. One of the reasons why people often repeat early traumatic experiences is because these experiences are understandably reproduced or relived in adulthood in an attempt to overcome them. This is termed within a psychodynamic framework as the 'compulsion to repeat' (Laplanche and Pontalis, 1988). Theoretical understandings incorporated into training enable enhanced insight and understanding of how women who have experienced sexual abuse in early life often repeat ways of relating inherent in those early experiences.

Applying careful thought to finding out more about patients is daunting without good support. There are confusing messages in the world about women's bodies and it is worth thinking about them. Staff, and particularly male staff, may be concerned about acknowledging their responses to women patients because of the potential for being misunderstood or through fear of disciplinary action. The document, *Sexual boundary issues in psychiatric settings* (Royal College of Psychiatrists, 2007), emphasises that staff must be encouraged to recognise and acknowledge personal feelings that would actually help them to act appropriately and professionally with patients. It also states that health care workers can learn through training how to speak to patients in a gendered but unsexualised way. This is particularly important when working with women who appear to communicate in this way.

There needs to an emphasis by ward managers on actively encouraging staff 'being with' the women, which only women-only services can deliberately foster, but staff in mixed environments could focus on spending time with women during a shift, where there is not a sexualised discourse but instead positive engagement and reflection. Staff taking part in the workshops expressed how they needed capacity to think through and build up therapeutic relationships. Staff deserve training that enables them to explore ways of keeping women safe, and then to reflect on and think about their work, preferably in the context of meaningful supervision. Nurses seem to be caught up defensively in 'doing' things (the vast amount of paperwork introduced in the last decade is one example). Training is particularly useful within clinical areas on ward settings. Hardcastle (2000) argues that training could be incorporated structurally into practice, taking place within clinical areas so that it is more accessible to nurses and more cost-effective.

However, we acknowledge there are constraints within mental health clinical practice, despite the fact that the need for more staff training is often articulated by service commissioners and practitioners. Shortages of staff mean that team members cannot always undertake the training they need and reductions in central allocations as part of efficiency savings have led to trusts having less money for training.

Conclusion

The staff taking part in the model of care development, focus groups and workshops discussed in this chapter were highly motivated and dedicated nurses. They demonstrated a willingness to engage with their women patients in a meaningful way; however, they expressed that they often did not know how to respond to the women's specific experiences and subsequent health needs. This particular group of mental health nurses was deprived of the training needed to prepare them adequately to work effectively with women. They also wanted more practice supervision because while informal support often took place between staff members during breaks or outside work time, they recognized the limitations of this. The nurses found the focus groups and the workshops were very useful, affording them the opportunity to stop and reflect upon their work. Additionally they stated that they provided an opportunity to praise themselves for their hard work in working with women.

There is an obvious need for effective policies, appropriate staff levels, improvements in ward layout and a consistent approach to recording and monitoring data relating to sexual assault, and, arguably, incidences of sexual assault may decrease with these strategies in place. Women patients require acceptance, understanding, therapeutic care and guidance on how to keep safe. They need to be taken seriously by staff caring for them regardless of the 'truth' of their perceptions of others. Psychodynamic insights can help mental health professionals to understand why certain patients, particularly those with histories of sexual abuse, often relate to others in damaging ways. Staff may experience daunting and hopeless feelings about their patients and should be encouraged to speak truthfully about their reactions and responses and begin to make sense of them. Staff can then put in place therapeutic boundaries that benefit both the staff and the women in their care. For this to occur, staff need support and acceptance for this way of working from their managers and supervisors. Nursing staff are well placed to fulfil some of the lost aspects of many women patients' lives, particularly in the crucial area of the therapeutic relationship that deserves an important place in the daily running of mental health acute inpatient services.

Women patients do have particular needs. They need their mental health difficulties to be understood in light of their experiences and this includes their roles within relationships and families and in relation to their ethnic and cultural backgrounds. It is also vital that staff respect and recognise women's expression of sexuality and their experiences of their bodies. Effective training with frequent and supportive supervision will create a safe and caring environment for staff and women to work together. This requires women to have access to a therapeutic space where physical and personal boundaries are not intruded upon or misinterpreted. Gender-specific or women-only mental health services can provide this space, particularly for women who are vulnerable. Therapeutic space can be provided for women on mixed sex inpatient, acute wards, but this is more difficult when there are pressing concerns about risk and safety for all.

Finally, but most importantly, the views of women themselves should be sought. We know that some women service users prefer to be on mixed sex wards and respond very positively to the presence of male staff and patients (Travers *et al.*, 2006). Providing real 'choice' for women requires improved service-user involvement that directly impacts on service planning, delivery and evaluation, and commissioners should expect to see such approaches in place, along with outputs.

It does not cost a vast amount of money to create a safe and therapeutic space for women. While there are only very limited numbers of gender-specific services that respond adequately to women's experiences of gendered violence and abuse, this is likely to result in significant health care costs. Women with childhood sexual abuse histories are likely to repeatedly use accident and emergency (A&E) services and/or end up in the criminal justice system as they attempt to cope with their experiences. We would advocate the use of crisis homes (see Howard *et al.*, 2010 for an account of these services as viable alternatives to admission wards). They are cost-effective and have less impact on the family. We are aware that whilst this was a recommendation of *Mainstreaming gender and women's mental health*, it has not been widely adopted – although this model potentially provides an alternative pathway that may be beneficial all round. It is also interesting to reflect that there is still only one crisis house in England for women that allows them to bring their children to stay with them.

For organisations considering a whole-systems approach to developing specific mental health care for women, the Good Practice Checklist for Mental Health Trusts (NMHDU, 2009) continues to be a useful framework. This is a self-assessment tool and considers the organisational context of all service provision, the values and principles of gender equality, specific women-centred delivery, workforce development and service monitoring. There is little formal evaluation of women-only services, despite the many recommendations about the need to evaluate different models and pathways of care generally across mental health delivery. Given the rising costs of inpatient care and the desirability of increased community provision, it would seem timely to revisit the recommendations made in *Supporting into the mainstream: commissioning women-only community day services* (Department of Health, 2006).

The voluntary sector has for many years been the main provider of women-only services. They have the experience, the relationships and the expertise. For many women, mental health services are hard to access, stigmatizing and retraumatising. However, we also know that the women's sector is under increasing pressure of actual threats of cuts and withdrawal of funding. We fear for the future of women-centred services as childhood sexual abuse and VAWG affect women more – locally, nationally and globally – and continue to be prevalent in our society. Investment opportunities are being reduced, yet the rhetoric is one of prevention. A healthy mental health landscape needs multiple providers within the economy, in order to give the opportunity to all women of all backgrounds and experiences access to help when needed.

We advocate the development of infant and child mental health services – where services work to prevent and minimize the long-term effects of abuse and neglect on individuals and families. Gendered violence and abuse is widespread and the consequences to women's physical and mental health and well-being are supported by overwhelming evidence. The need for equality, fairness and justice must underpin improved responsiveness to protecting and supporting the human rights of all women who come into contact with services.

Our mental health services must reflect the continued pressure that campaigners seek, to deliver services that are women-centred, safe and effective, and that issues of violence and abuse are tackled in line with national and international legislation and best practices. It is imperative that clinical and strategic leaders commit to the human rights of women in receiving excellence in the statutory and voluntary sector services.

References

Care Quality Commission (2009) *Mental health acute service user's survey*, National NHS Patient Survey Programme, London: CQC.

Chesler, P. (1997) *Women and Madness,* New York: Four Walls, Eight Windows.

Cisters (2007) *Not mad or bad, but traumatized,* DVD, Serious Media.

Coid, J., Petruckevitch, A., Chung, W.-S., Richardson, J., Moorey, S. and Feder, G. (2003) 'Abusive experiences and psychiatric morbidity in women primary care attenders', *British Journal of Psychiatry,* 183: 332–339.

CSIP (2008) *Informed gender practice – mental health acute care that works for women,* London: CSIP.

Department of Health (2000) *No Secrets: Guidance on Developing and Implementing Multi-Agency Policies and Procedures to Protect Vulnerable Adults From Abuse,* London: Department of Health.

Department of Health (2002) *Women's mental health: into the mainstream,* London: Department of Health.

Department of Health (2003) *Mainstreaming gender and women's mental health: implementation guidance,* London: Department of Health.

Department of Health (2006) *Supporting into the mainstream: commissioning women-only community day services*, London: Department of Health.

Department of Health (2008) *Refocusing the Care Programme Approach – policy and positive practice guidance*, London: Department of Health.

Department of Health (2010a) *Responding to violence against women and children – the role of the NHS. The report of the taskforce on the health aspects of violence against women and children*, London: Department of Health.

Department of Health (2010b) *The NHS Outcomes Framework 2011/2012*, London: Department of Health.

Evans, M. and Franks, V. (1997) 'Psychodynamic thinking as an aid to clear thinking', *Nursing Times*, 93(10), 50–53.

Geller, J. and Srikameswaran, S. (2006) 'Treatment non-negotiables: why we need them and how to make them work', *European Eating Disorders Review*, 14(4): 212–217.

Glover, G., Arts, G. and Babu, K.S. (2006) 'Crisis resolution/home treatment teams and psychiatric admission rates in England', *British Journal of Psychiatry*, 189: 441–444.

Government Equalities Office (2010) *An anatomy of economic inequality in the UK: report of the National Equality Panel*, London: GEO, http:/www.equalities.gov.uk/.

Greater London Domestic Violence Project (GLDVP) (2008) *Sane responses: good practice guidelines for domestic violence and mental health services*, London: GLDVP.

Hardcastle, M. (2000) 'Real time training for mental health staff working on an in-patient setting', *International Journal of Psychiatric Research*, 6 (1): 650–656.

HM Government Strategy (2009) *Together we can end violence against women and girls: a strategy*, London: HM Government

HM Government (2011a) *No health without mental health: a cross-government mental health outcomes strategy for people of all ages*, Crown copyright.

HM Government (2011b) *Call to end violence against women and girls, Action Plan*, Crown copyright.

Howard, L.M, Flach, C., Leese, M., Byford, S., Killaspy, H., Cole, L., Lawlor, C., Betts, J., Cutting, P., McNicholas, S., Sharac, J. and Johnson, S. (2010) 'The effectiveness and cost effectiveness of admissions to women's crisis houses compared with traditional psychiatric wards – a pilot patient preference randomized controlled trial', *British Journal of Psychiatry*, 197: 32–40.

Humphreys, C., Lowe, P. and Williams, S. (2009) 'Sleep disruption and domestic violence: exploring the interconnections between mothers and children', *Child and Family Social Work*, 14: 6–14.

Itzin, C. (2006) *Tackling the health and mental health effects of domestic and sexual violence and abuse*, Department of Health, London: Department of Health.

Itzin, C., Bailey, S. and Bentovim, A. (2008) 'The effects of domestic violence and sexual abuse on mental health', *The Psychiatrist*, 32: 448–450.

Itzin, C., Taket, A. and Barter-Godfrey, S. (2010) 'Domestic and sexual violence and abuse: findings from a Delphi expert consultation on therapeutic and treatment interventions with victims, survivors and abusers, children, adolescents, and adults', Melbourne, Australia: Deakin University.

Judd, F., Armstrong, S. and Kulkarni, J. (2009) 'Gender-sensitive mental health care', *Australasian Psychiatry*, 17: 105–111.

Kmietowicz, Z. (2009) 'Patients who use mental health services in England', *British Medical Journal*, 339: b3942.

Langley, G.C. and Klopper, H. (2005) 'Trust as a foundation for the therapeutic intervention for patients with borderline personality disorder', *Journal of Psychiatric and Mental Health Nursing*, 12 (1): 23–32.

Laplanche, J. and Pontalis, J.B. (1988) *The Language of Psychoanalysis*, London: Karnac.

Lawn, T. and McDonald, E. (2009) 'Developing a policy to deal with sexual assault on psychiatric in-patient wards', *Psychiatric Bulletin*, 33: 108–111.

The Marmot Review (2010) *Fair society, healthy lives: a strategic review of health inequalities in England post-2010*, London: UCL Institute of Health Equity.

Mezey, G., Hassell, Y. and Bartlett, A. (2005) 'Safety of women in mixed-sex and single-sex medium secure units: staff and patient perceptions', *British Journal of Psychiatry*, 187: 579–582.

Mind (2004) 'Mind's report on hospital conditions for mental health patients', London: Mind.

Mullen, P.E., Martin, J.L., Anderson, J.C., Romans, S.E. and Herbison, G.P. (1993) 'Childhood sexual abuse and mental health in adult life', *British Journal of Psychiatry*, 163: 721–732.

National Institute for Mental Health in England (NIMHE) (2003) *Inside outside: improving mental health services for Black and Minority Ethnic communities in England,* London: NIMHE.

National Mental Health Development Unit (NMHDU) (2009) *Working toward women's well-being: unfinished business,* London: NMHDU.

National Mental Health Development Unit (NMHDU) (2010) *Meeting the needs of survivors of child sexual abuse-underpinned by routine enquiry in mental health assessment: Implementation of Violence and Abuse Policy,* London: NMHDU.

National Mental Health Development Unit (NMHDU) (2011) *Practical guide to mental health commissioning, Volume One,* London: NMHDU.

National Patient Safety Agency (2006) *With safety in mind: mental health services and patient safety,* Patient Safety Observatory Report, Reference number 0294, London

Nelson, S. (2001) *Beyond trauma: healthcare needs of women who survived child sexual abuse,* Edinburgh: Health in Mind.

NHS Confederation (2008) *Implementing national policy on abuse and violence, Briefing, June,* London: NHS Confederation.

Phillips, L. (2006) *Mental illness and the body: beyond diagnosis,* London: Routledge.

Phillips, L. (2009) 'The needs of staff who work with women in single-sex wards', *Mental Health Practice,* 12: 21–25.

Royal College of Psychiatrists (2007) *Sexual boundary issues in psychiatric settings,* London: Royal College of Psychiatrists.

Siddiqui, H. and Patel, M. (2010) *Safe and sane: a model of intervention on domestic violence and mental health, suicide and self harm among black and minority ethnic women,* London: Southall Black Sisters.

Silverman, A.B., Reinherz, H.Z. and Giaconia, R.M. (1996) 'The long-term sequelae of child and adolescent abuse: a longitudinal community study', *Child Abuse and Neglect,* 20: 709–723.

Spataro, J. *et al.* (2004) 'Impact of child sexual abuse on mental health', *British Journal of Psychiatry,* 184: 416–421.

Stafford, P. (2006) *Mental Health Trusts Collaboration Project,* Service User Consultation Report, London: National Mental Health Development Unit.

Subotsky, F. (1991) 'Issues for women in the development of mental health services', *British Journal of Psychiatry,* suppl. 10: 17–21.

Tonks, A. (1992) 'Women patients in mixed psychiatric wards', *British Medical Journal,* 304: 1331.

Travers, R.F., Holdsworth, P. and Edge, D. (2006) 'Not all women fancy single sex wards', *British Journal of Psychiatry,* 188(4): 396.

TUC (2011) *Bearing the brunt, leading the response, women and the global and economic crisis,* London: Trade Union Congress, www.tuc.org.uk.

Tully, T. and Gallop, R. (2009) 'The person who self-harms', in P. Barker *Textbook of Psychiatric and Mental Health Nursing* (second edition), London: Arnold Publishing.

Ussher, J.M. (ed.) (1997) *Body talk: the material and discursive regulation of sexuality, madness and reproduction,* London: Routledge.

Williams, J., Scott, S. and Waterhouse, S. (2001) 'Mental health services for 'difficult' women: reflections on some recent developments', *Feminist Review,* 68: 89–104.

Women's National Commission (2009) 'Still we rise', report from WNC Focus Groups to inform the cross-Government consultation *'Together we can end violence against women and girls',* Women's National Commission, London: WNC.

10 Race, ethnicity and mental health care

Hári Sewell

Race and ethnicity have become synonymous. The definition of institutional racism that is most commonly cited in the United Kingdom refers to 'racist stereotyping' but relates this and other failures to 'colour, culture or ethnic origin' (MacPherson, 1999, p28). This definition first appeared in the MacPherson inquiry into the racist murder of Stephen Lawrence, a black teenager in London. (The term was coined 32 years earlier by African American activist Stokely Carmichael (republished as Ture and Hamilton, 1992.)

Despite the use of the terms race and ethnicity being interchangeable they have different meanings. Race is considered to be rooted in biology and therefore genetically fixed. This notion is a misnomer as scientific evidence suggests that there are no fixed genetic pools that create races as distinct and discrete groups. There are in fact significant genetic differences within so-called races, sometimes on a par with differences across perceived racial groups (Fernando, 2002). As such, race is best understood as a social means of stratification rather than a robust scientific concept. The social utility of race is not being understated, however. There are powerful reasons for perpetuating the concept of race as a fixed and distinct form of categorisation. For example, in the United Kingdom the right wing British National Party presents a view of races as being distinct and promotes separateness on this basis. The benefit of this propaganda is that it feeds the underlying prejudices in society and perpetuates a view that others (i.e. non-white) are not just different but also deficient.

The technical definition of ethnicity encapsulates more than just race. Ethnicity is defined as the essence of self, reflecting culture, racial identity, religion, language and geographical roots (Fernando, 2009). Ethnicity is regarded as being less fixed than race. In public services, data is usually gathered on *ethnic group*, a term reserved for categories of self-identification. Ethnic group may therefore change over time if someone were to feel that another aspect of their identity becomes more salient.

There are dangers in mental health services seeing people almost singularly through the prism of race or ethnicity. Though the inequalities in service utilisation and experience based on race and ethnicity discussed in this chapter justify attention, people are more than just one-dimensional beings. Crenshaw (1994) developed the concept of *intersectionality* when discussing the relationship between race and gender in women's politics. The concept of intersectionality is useful in understanding the intersection between various forms of identity and inequality. In mental health services a Black African man who is gay and a Christian may experience poorer treatment and even explicit discrimination because of his composite identity rather than any one aspect (see Macaulay, 2010). An understanding of how different forms of discrimination intersect with each other is important in service development, otherwise one or more aspect may be overlooked.

The Equality Act 2010 (Crown 2010) identifies nine *protected characteristics* that are aspects of identity in relation to which the perpetuation of discrimination and inequality are unlawful. These are:

- age
- disability
- gender reassignment
- marriage and civil partnership
- pregnancy and maternity
- race
- religion and belief
- sex
- sexual orientation.

When considering race and ethnicity, the possibility of inequality in relation to the eight other protected characteristics needs to be considered.

Summary of the race inequality in mental health care

The types of variations and groups that are given attention are influenced by the data available either from research or the way in which national reports analyse and present information. A search of an English language online academic library using the terms 'ethnicity' and 'mental health' will yield significantly more resources with specific references to the experience and outcomes for people from African Caribbean backgrounds in mental health than for any other group. A consequence is that the findings for this group are often erroneously applied to black and minority ethnic (BME) people generally. For example the Care Quality Commission report on use of the Mental Health Act (1983) states 'Black and minority ethnic patients are more likely than white patients to be deemed incapable of consent, or capable but refusing to consent' (Care Quality Commission, 2010, p13). Elsewhere the report does, however, refer to 'some' BME groups and provides specific detail. This is a typical example of how language is used in research and reports and indicates the challenge in communicating the diversity of experience between different minority ethnic groups. Presentation of meaningful data is further hampered by the nature of ethnic coding. The term 'Asian' brings together communities with very different experiences in mental health services. In strict usage, *Asian* includes Chinese and Bangladeshi. Even the more specific term 'South Asian', which includes people from Bangladeshi, Indian and Pakistani backgrounds, groups together communities that have significant differences between them.

It is, however, not feasible to list every single minority ethnic group and the variations they experience in mental health services in this brief chapter. Further, there are differences in communities in local areas.

There are five domains in which findings from research data and service utilisation data in relation to people from BME backgrounds in mental health fall:

- disproportionate experience of factors that are linked to poor mental health (e.g. Cooper et al., 2008; Veling et al., 2007);
- higher than average rates of utilisation of services or for particular diagnoses (Care Quality Commission, 2011);

- lower than average rates of utilisation of services or for particular diagnoses (Raleigh *et al.*, 2007);
- poorer outcomes derived from the treatments and interventions in mental health services (Rathod *et al.*, 2010)
- poorer experience of relationships with mental health services and professionals (Mental Health Act Commission, 2006).

Key findings in service utilisation data and research

Domain one: disproportionate experience of factors that are linked to poor mental health

Discrimination, poverty, poorer housing, education and childhood experience of lone parenting and living in an urban area are all recognised to be contributory factors in relation to poor mental health (Marmot, 2010; Morgan *et al.*, 2008). These negative causal factors are more frequently present for most BME communities but is more accentuated for African Caribbean, Bangladeshi, Black African, Irish, Pakistani, Roma, Gypsies and Travellers (Cooper *et al.*, 2008; Fung *et al.*, 2009; Veling *et al.*, 2007).

Domain two: higher than average rates for utilisation of services or for particular diagnoses

- African Caribbean, Bangladeshi, Black African, Black other, Irish, Pakistani, Roma, Gypsies and Travellers are over-represented in inpatient services (Care Quality Commission, 2011).
- African Caribbean, Black African and mixed White/Black groups are over-represented in forensic services (Care Quality Commission, 2011).
- African Caribbean, Bangladeshi, Black African, Black other, Indian, Irish and Pakistani have raised levels of diagnosis for psychosis (Cooper *et al.*, 2008; Kirkbride *et al.*, 2008).
- All BME groups apart from Chinese, Irish and White/Black Caribbean mixed are subject to proportionately higher numbers of Community Treatment Orders (which are intended for people who have a history of non-compliance with medication) (Care Quality Commission, 2010).

Domain three: lower than average rates for utilisation of services

- Bangladeshi, Chinese, Indian and Pakistani women were less like to enter treatment under the new national model of therapy service (Improving Access to Psychological Therapies, known as IAPT) (Glover and Evison, 2009).
- Chinese, Indian, mixed White/Black Caribbean men were less likely to enter IAPT services (Glover and Evison, 2009).

Domain four: poorer outcomes derived from the treatments and interventions in mental health services

- Asian and Black groups have more repeat admissions (Singh *et al.*, 2007).
- Black Caribbean and White/Black Caribbean mixed have the longest length of stay (Care Quality Commission, 2011).
- African Caribbean and Black African people have higher drop-out rates for cognitive behaviour therapy for schizophrenia (Rathod *et al.*, 2010).

Domain five: poorer experience of relationships with mental health services and professionals

- African and African Caribbean people have poor relations with services (Sainsbury Centre for Mental Health, 2002).
- Black and Mixed groups reported higher rates of dissatisfaction for inpatient stays (Mental Health Act Commission, 2006).
- Asian groups reported lower satisfaction rates for community mental health services (Raleigh *et al.*, 2007).

These are mere summaries. For example there are sometimes significant gender differences in data. Actual numbers (too detailed for reporting here) indicate the scale of variations. Local analysis is essential.

Changes in the environment that affect race and ethnicity in mental health care

The global economic downturn has led to a contraction of resources for health and social care and related services. In such a context mental health services struggle to meet the demands for more sophisticated interventions, more expensive drugs and higher quality thresholds for the estate from which services are run. Efficiency is demanded from all areas of provision and front line services are not immune from this. Despite the politically driven mantra that front line services will be protected, trust directors of finance on a panel for the health think tank the King's Fund reported that they expect front line services to be cut as back office functions only represent five per cent of NHS trust budgets (King's Fund, 2011).

Against this background, specialist services for people from BME backgrounds have seen a significant reduction. The creation of 500 community development workers (CDW) roles was a key aspect of the strategy, *Delivering Race Equality in Mental Health Care* (DRE) (Department of Health, 2005). The national evaluation of CDWs undertaken by De Montfort University for the National Mental Health Development Unit highlighted that at December 2010 more than 32 percent of post holders were no longer in role (National Mental Health Development Unit, 2011). There have been further significant reductions in CDW numbers. The need to improve outcomes for people from BME groups remains critical, as evidenced in the report of the *Count Me In* national census of inpatients (Care Quality Commission, 2011). Managing these improvements through mainstream staff and initiatives is fast becoming the much preferred approach, driven largely by the contraction in public sector budgets. The specific funding for CDW was incorporated into NHS commissioning budgets and the cuts to posts coincide with the major programme of cost reductions rather than the end of the DRE programme.

Lighter touch regulation has also had an impact on the focus given to race equality in mental health. In 2009 the health and social care regulator, the Care Quality Commission, abandoned the performance assessment regime known as the annual health check. Along with this departure came the loss of several indicators that were explicit about the need to achieve equality, including race equality in mental health. The public sector duty in the Equality Act 2010 came into force as scheduled on 5 April 2011 but the secondary legislation to support delivery was delayed to allow for a consultation to reduce the bureaucratic burden of the legislation (Government Equalities Office, 2011). The Coalition Government's mental health strategy *No Health without Mental Health* (Crown, 2011) locates delivering race equality within an equalities framework as opposed to a discrete strategy.

Lighter touch regulation reflects a generalised changing relationship between the state and services. A consequence will be that when organisational priorities are balanced against each other, the ones to slip will be those for which there is less scrutiny and accountability. Weighed against the priorities of balancing budgets, reducing hospital acquired infections and implementing organisational reform, race equality in mental health may generate a response that remains inconsequential in relation to the level of improvement that is still required.

There have been evident changes in the language used to describe the pursuit of equality. The Equality and Human Rights Commission more frequently presents equality as *fairness* (e.g. Equality and Human Rights Commission, 2010). This change in language is also seen in publications from the Coalition Government that came to power in May 2010. As the public services editor for the *Guardian* newspaper stated 'Fairness is the Government's middle name...' (*Guardian*, 2011). The softening of tone was seen in the statement made by the chair of the Equalities and Human Rights Commission in relation to the term *institutional racism*. Mailonline, the internet-based version of the *Daily Mail* reported on 19 January 2009 that 'equality chief Trevor Phillips says the whole corrosive concept should be abandoned' (*Daily Mail*, 2009).

Alongside the softening language in relation to discrimination and equalities are changing attitudes to multiculturalism, led by the Prime Minister. 'David Cameron launched a devastating attack today on 30 years of multiculturalism in Britain, warning it is fostering extremist ideology and directly contributing to home-grown Islamic terrorism' (*The Independent*, 2011).

Commentary has begun to change. A greater respect for individual choice is cited as the reason for tolerating inequality (*Guardian*, 2010a). Individuals may be provided with opportunities to succeed but may choose alternatives. Analysis is less bold in highlighting the social, economic and psychological reasons why people struggle to avail themselves of the range of opportunities presented to them. This sets a context for mental health services where a generalised approach to fairness (with the merits of intersectionality) can now encapsulate what was previously a discretely managed national race equality agenda.

The new mantra of localism is the organisational equivalent of individual choice. The new Government's Coalition Agreement (i.e. the programme for government) used the word *local* on one or more occasions on over two thirds of the main pages in the document (Cabinet Office, 2010). Localism is the outcome of the diminution of state control in local commissioning, planning and service development and delivery. Laudable though this may be, localism has the potential to introduce significant variation across geographical areas. Priorities will largely be determined locally and areas with more diverse BME communities and a less cohesively articulated challenge are likely to find that mental health commissioners prioritise other areas of service.

Increased contestability in local government and health has been the trend for the past decade and the pace of change is now accelerating as set out in the White Paper *Equity and Excellence: Liberating the NHS* (Department of Health, 2010a). The BME mental health voluntary sector has long been cited by academics, service users and carers as providing a potentially successful alternative to statutory services (Fernando, 2003; Fountain and Hicks, 2010). These organisations tend to be smaller and have shorter contracts (Fernando and Keating, 2009). The challenges that they face put them at significant risk in the new environment of competition and contestability. There is the possibility that those that survive will be subsumed within larger generic organisations that have the resources and expertise to compete effectively, thus eroding some of the identity and unique attributes of the BME voluntary sector.

Mental health services for BME people are also affected by the loss of impact over time of the inquiries into the death of Stephen Lawrence (MacPherson, 1999) and David Bennett (a

Jamaican born patient who died whilst being restrained in a psychiatric hospital) (NSCSTHA, 2003). The national strategy *Delivering Race Equality in Mental Health Care* (Department of Health, 2005) was published inclusive of the incumbent Government's action plan to respond to the Bennett inquiry, indicating a relationship between the two.

The changes in the environment in relation to race equality in mental health are not all negative. There is now a growing awareness of the variations between different ethnic groups leading to a greater sophistication in analysis of problems (Department of Health, 2010b; Glover and Evison, 2009). Whereas in the last decade the concept of 'a BME service response' seemed credible it is now clearer that there needs to be a set of responses in relation to the different manifestations of inequality of variations.

BME lobby groups are more conscious now of the need to present evidence-based arguments and to organise not just on the basis of opposition to perceived failures but to amass the significant intellect and expertise amongst allies. In 2010 a new organization, RAWOrg (Rights and Wellbeing of Racialised Groups), was formed. They describe themselves as a 'collection of service users, campaigners, professionals and academics dedicated to ending racial inequality throughout the mental health system' (RAWOrg, 2011).

The alliances go beyond networks of those with a primary goal of pursuing race equality. The post-psychiatry movement and others challenging the orthodoxy of traditional psychiatry also work in alliance with people and organisations seeking to improve services for BME groups. For example, the first author of the book *Postpsychiatry* (Bracken and Thomas, 2005) was a signatory to a letter published by the *Guardian* newspaper challenging an article that referred to an epidemic of mental illness amongst the African Caribbean community (*Guardian*, 2010b)

Approaches to race equality in the new environment

The changed relationships between the state and local services and individuals set a tone for working towards race equality in mental health. Attention needs to be given to finding solutions rather than repeating the data and challenges of the past and acquiescing in defeat. Leaders in services need to prioritise the relationships between front line staff and those using services. Research points to the importance of relationships in improving effectiveness of interventions as diverse as therapy and medication management (Kikkert *et al.*, 2006; Shapiro and Shapiro, 1982). Solutions need to be rooted in the values and approaches of all the caring professions in mental health, including scientific management (that is, applying management theory to problem solving in relation to race inequality and mental health). Essential to progress is an understanding of the strengths and resilience of people from different minority ethnic groups (Arnold, 2011).

Those seeking solutions for the seemingly intractable racial inequalities in mental health often ask the question: what is the answer? There is, however, no straightforward, single solution.

In the pursuit of productivity and efficiency managers and staff may feel as though acknowledging and tackling issues such as power, historical legacies and unconscious prejudice is a luxury that cannot be afforded. These intangibles cannot be easily named and resolved through a management directive. Attention to them is more easily dismissed as navel gazing, dredging up the past or a sign of failure of the person who raises such matters to get on board with the new agenda. It is the ability to combine emotional intelligence with management and practice that will deliver progress in race equality in the new environment.

Figure 10.1 presents four areas in which strategies for improvement need to be located in the new environment. The three concentric circles represent the underlying features for which acknowledgement relies upon emotional intelligence.

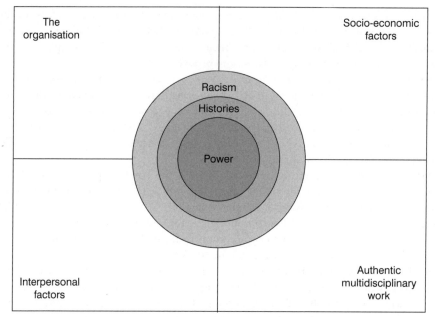

Figure 10.1 Underlying factors in the agenda for race equality.

The organisation

The culture of the organisation needs to be actively changed by those in leadership positions. Not only does there need to be a relocation of power away from professionals but also there needs to be open dialogue about the impact of power relations on people from BME groups. The values and practice of *personalisation* are consistent with the themes in the aspirations expressed by people from many BME (e.g. Mental Health Act Commission, 2006; Sainsbury Centre for Mental Health, 2002). Personalisation means that services no longer design support packages for people and retain the power to direct and provide. On the contrary, services relinquish their directing role and respect a person's right to self-determination, choice and self-actualisation (Carr, 2010). The structures of organisations need to be changed to enable people from BME backgrounds to design their own supports. Where markets are weak or absent (e.g. the BME voluntary sector) joint work will be required with commissioners to actively build capacity.

Socio-economic factors

Tackling socio-economic factors demands a public health, system-wide approach. This is consistent with the Coalition Government's mental health strategy *No Health without Mental Health* (Crown, 2011). The Equality and Human Rights Commission highlighted various forms of socio-economic disadvantage experienced by people from BME groups. These factors (such as poverty, poorer housing, education, greater unemployment), which affect various BME groups differently, are indicated as contributory factors in mental health problems (Cooper *et al.*, 2008; Morgan *et al.*, 2008; Veling *et al.*, 2007). These inequalities are passed on inter-generationally. Arnold (2011) provides a good illustration of how the negative impacts of the violence and dislocation of slavery affects generations, typified in the social inequalities faced by African Caribbean people. Darker skin has been identified as a compounding factor in relation to socio-economic disadvantage and its impact on disproportionate use of mental health services (Cantor-Graae and Shelten, 2005;Veling *et al.*, 2007).

Within system-wide approaches, the BME voluntary sector must be engaged as crucial partners in working with communities on public health, tackling socio-economic disadvantage and in building social capital (Ahmed *et al.*, 2009).

Interpersonal factors

Mental health care is delivered extensively through relationships. Kikkert *et al.* (2006) acknowledge that even the effectiveness of medication is affected by relationships between worker and service user. Modern approaches such as recovery and personalisation require an investment in relationships.The impact of race on therapeutic relationships has been investigated and explored for decades and it is established that race does matter (Moodley and Palmer, 2006). Singh *et al.* (2007) highlight that after an initial admission services are more effective at supporting white people to avoid hospitalisation than they are BME people. The researchers point to the relationship between services and those who use them as a possible cause.

The risk of poorer outcomes for BME people needs to be identified and explicitly included in care plans. Strategies will need to be put in place to reduce these risks. Introducing this requirement is likely to have a significant impact on the way of thinking in mental health.

A new way of thinking about the impact of race on therapeutic relationships, called Toxic InteractionTheory,was presented in Sewell (2009a) and Sewell (2009b).Toxic InteractionTheory suggests that the relationship between white people and BME people has a psychologically toxic effect on the latter.Toxic Interaction Theory highlights that prior experiences of racism, being stereotyped or being defined narrowly on account of race has an impact on the current relationship. Chester Pierce (1978) coined the phrase 'micro-aggressions', referring to the supposedly small but recurring episodes of stereotyping or discrimination that people of BME backgrounds face, which Alleyne (2009) describes as 'the grinding down experience'. Self-preservation and coping strategies adopted alienate white people who feel rejected and unjustifiably labelled as racist or potentially racist. Workers in mental health may wish to be forward looking for the right reasons, focusing on opportunities, recovery and capacities but the toxicity needs to be acknowledged.

Authentic multidisciplinary work

Mental health services articulate a model of multidisciplinary working and this is enshrined in policies of successive governments (e.g. Department of Health, 1999; Crown, 2011). However, Bracken and Thomas (2005) highlight the dominance of the medical profession in mental health. Esteemed psychologist Richard Bentall in his research-rich '*Doctoring the Mind*', having highlighted their humaneness, states that psychiatrists '...pursue a medical approach, in which social and psychological therapies, if they are used at all, are seen as secondary to drug treatment...' (2009). The current approach in mental health is to have standardised 'clustering' of patients using three main categories: non-psychotic, psychotic and organic (Department of Health, 2010c).This clustering of patients is regarded as a precursor to a national payment by results model. Consequently, services nationally are structuring their services accordingly. Clark (2010, p32) states that 'the intention is to have a model not purely driven by diagnosis though not completely divorced from diagnostic categories'. A challenge for mental health services in meeting the needs of people from BME groups is the establishment of a multidisciplinary approach where equal value is given to disciplines.

Professions need to give serious consideration to the evidence that the science that drives them is not always as robust as is believed. *Cultural Diversity, Mental Health and Psychiatry* (Fernando, 2003); *Madness Explained: Psychosis and Human Nature* (Bentall, 2004); *Living with Voices* (Romme *et al.*, 2009) and *Postpsychiatry* (Bracken and Thomas, 2005) all critique the evidence base for the reliability, validity and usefulness of certain diagnoses and the diagnostic process itself. The critiques in these books suggest that effective work needs to rely as much on the perspectives of the person using the service as on science, and this resonates overwhelmingly with the concerns of people from BME groups. Real progress can be achieved by giving power and authority to these marginalised schools of thinking to shape policy and service configuration.

Power, histories and racism

The power of services to define what is important needs to be acknowledged, for example tackling racial inequality or even acknowledging that race is important (Woodger and Cowan, 2010). This power is present in relationships between people from BME groups and front line staff. Workers have power to define the reality that is given credence. Insanity, risk, urgency of need are all ultimately defined or moderated by workers. It is partly this power that leads to the toxic interactions.

Psychiatry has historical roots in systemically contributing to genocide, slavery and the subjective categorisation of certain groups as mentally ill, for example homosexuals and unwed mothers (Bentall, 2004; Fernando, 2003; Read, Mosher and Bentall, 2004). This history of converting human judgements into a 'science' has been a defining feature in mental health services and all disciplines to a lesser or greater extent are agents of this legacy. The legacy of the past can be seen in the medicalisation of human distress and the inevitable response of finding solutions largely in psychopharmacology (Bentall, 2009). Stigma serves as a barrier to people from BME backgrounds making early contact with services. It is subsequent to first contact that the fear of services becomes a dominant feature (Fountain and Hicks, 2010). Organisations need to build their relationships with communities and those who use services, mindful that they are not doing so in a neutral context.

Undercurrents of blaming people for failing to do better need to be teased out in organisations, as does the often unspoken belief that investments to reduce inequality are unfairly favouring BME groups over others (The Guardian 2010b).

Talking about race, racism and racial discrimination is emotive and charged with anxiety (Singer, 2006). Despite it seeming counterintuitive, discussing race and its impact is likely to be enabling of a positive relationship. In a relationship between workers and BME people, where important and critical information is being discussed, silence about the pernicious and psychologically damaging effect of racism conveys that it is not real, relevant or important.

Solutions may be found in utilising narrative approaches (Morgan, 2000) and explanatory models (Bhui and Bhugra, 2002). Narrative approaches enable the service user story to have value alongside that of the professional (Bracken and Thomas, 2005). Explanatory models give space for the person's own definition of what they believe is happening for them with regard to a mental health problem: the actual experience itself and also the causes. Senghera (2011) illustrates for example the ways in which spiritual or religious explanations may be used by people from BME backgrounds.

Effective approaches in this cash-strapped, less-political environment are those that re-establish a connection between life experiences, and the mental health problems that bring people to the attention of services. More sustained improvements will be derived from acknowledging abuse, trauma and discrimination and tackling these explicitly in mental health treatment and care.

Conclusion

This chapter sets out the nature of inequalities for people from BME backgrounds, whilst recognising the significant degree of diversity in experience and outcome.The current operating context is of reduced resources for race-specific approaches, a softening language of race and racism and lighter touch regulation. Progress is to be made by incorporating management change alongside greater emotional intelligence in changing organisations, responding to socio-economic needs and developing effective interpersonal (therapeutic) relationships. All disciplines need to acknowledge their individual and joint obstacles to working effectively with people from BME backgrounds.

References

Ahmed, T., Jennings, Y. and Dhillon, J. (2009) 'Innovation in the Voluntary Sector'. In S. Fernando and F. Keating (eds) *Mental Health in a Multi-Ethnic Society*. Oxfordshire: Routledge.

Alleyne, A. (2009) 'Working Therapeutically with the Hidden Dimensions of Racism'. In S. Fernando and F. Keating (eds) *Mental Health in a Multi-Ethnic Society*. Oxfordshire: Routledge.

Arnold, E. (2011) *Working with Families of African Caribbean Origin: Understanding Issues Around Immigration and Attachment*. London: Jessica Kingsley Publishers.

Bentall, R. (2004) *Madness Explained: Psychosis and Human Nature*. London: Penguin Books.

Bentall R. (2009) *Doctoring the Mind: Why Psychiatric Treatments Fail*. London: Allen Lane Publishing

Bhui, K. and Bhugra, D. (2002) 'Explanatory Models for Mental Distress: Implications for Clinical Practice and Research'. *British Journal of Psychiatry*, 181, 6–7.

Bracken, P. and Thomas, P. (2005) *Postpsychiatry: Mental Health in a Postmodern World: International Perspectives in Philosophy and Psychiatry*. Oxford: Oxford University Press.

Cabinet Office (2010) *The Coalition: Our Programme For Government*. London: Cabinet Office.

Cantor-Graae, E. and Shelton, J. (2005) 'Schizophrenia and Migration: A Meta-analysis and Review'. *American Journal of Psychiatry*, 162, 12–24

Care Quality Commission (2010) *Monitoring the Use of the Mental Health Act 1983 in 2009/10*. London: CQC.

Care Quality Commission (2011) *Count Me In 2010: Results of the 2010 National Census of Inpatients and Patients on Supervised Community Treatment in Mental Health and Learning Disability Services in England and Wales*. London: CQC.

Carr, S. (2010) 'Personalisation – Choice and Control: The Issues'. In P. Gilbert (ed) *Social Work and Mental Health: The Value of Everything*. Dorset: Russell House Publishing.

Clark, M. (2010) Clusters and Pathways in Mental Health: What are the Implications for Equalities'. *Ethnicity and Inequalities in Health and Social Care*, 3, 4, 30–35.

Cooper, L., Beach, M., Johnson, R. and Inui, T. (2006) 'Understanding How Race and Ethnicity Influence Relationships in Health Care'. *Journal of General Internal Medicine*, 21, S21–S27.

Cooper, C., Morgan, C., Byrne, M., Dazzan, P. et al. (2008) 'Perceptions of Disadvantage, Ethnicity and Psychosis'. *British Journal of Psychiatry*, 192, 185–190.

Crenshaw, K. (1994) 'Mapping the Margins: Intersectionality, Identity Politics, and Violence Against Women of Color'. In M.A. Fineman and R. Mykitiuk (eds) *The Public Nature of Private Violence*. New York: Routledge.

Crown (2010) Equality Act 2010. London: Crown.

Crown (2011) *No Health without Mental Health: A Cross-government Mental Health Outcomes Strategy for People of all Ages*. London: Crown.

Daily Mail (2009) 'Why Britain is now the LEAST racist country in Europe', http://www.dailymail.co.uk/debate/article-1121442/TREVOR-PHILLIPS-Why-Britain-LEAST-racist-country-Europe.html.

Department of Health (1999) *National Framework for Mental Health*. London: Department of Health.

Department of Health (2005) *Delivering Race Equality in Mental Health Care: An Action Plan for Reform Inside and Outside Services and the Government's Response to the Death of David Bennett*. London: Department of Health.

Department of Health (2010a) *Equity and Excellence: Liberating the NHS: White Paper.* London: Department of Health.

Department of Health (2010b) *Delivering Race Equality Action Plan: A Five Year Review.* London: Department of Health.

Department of Health (2010c) *Mental Health Care Clustering Booklet 210/11.* London: Department of Health.

Equality and Human Rights Commission (2010) *How Fair is Britain? Equality, Human Rights and Good Relations in 2010. The First Triennial Review.* London: Equality and Human Rights Commission.

Fernando, S. (2002) *Mental Health, Race and Culture* (2nd edition). Hampshire: Macmillan Press.

Fernando, S. (2003) *Cultural Diversity, Mental Health and Psychiatry: The Struggle Against Racism.* Oxfordshire: Routledge.

Fernando, S. (2009) 'Meaning and Realities'. In S. Fernando and F. Keating (eds) *Mental Health in a Multi-Ethnic Society.* Oxfordshire: Routledge.

Fernando, S. and Keating, F. (2009) *Mental Health in a Multi-Ethnic Society.* Oxfordshire: Routledge.

Fountain, J. and Hicks, J. (2010) *Delivering Race Equality in Mental Health Care: Report on the Findings and Outcomes of the Community Engagement Programme 2005–2008.* Lancashire: ISCRI.

Fung, L., Bhugra, D. and Jones, P. (2009) 'Ethnicity and Mental Health: The Example of Schizophrenia and Related Psychoses in Migrant Populations in the Western World'. *Psychiatry,* 8, 9, 335–341.

Glover, G. and Evison, F. (2009) *Use of New Mental Health Services by Ethnic Minorities in England.* Durham: North East Public Health Observatory.

Government Equalities Office (2011) *Equality Act 2010: The Public Sector Equality Duty: Reducing Bureaucracy.* Policy Review Paper. London: Government Equalities Office.

Guardian (2010a) 'The Left Should Recognise that Equality is Undesirable'. 11 October. London: *Guardian.*

Guardian (2010b) 'Poor Research or an Attack on Black People'. 3 February. London: *Guardian.*

Guardian (2011) 'Fair Game for Fairness Failures'. *Society Guardian* p4, 16 March. London: *Guardian.*

Independent, The (2011) 'Cameron: My War on Multiculturalism. Independent online 5 February, http://www.independent.co.uk/news/uk/politics/cameron-my-war-on-multiculturalism-2205074.html.

Kikkert, M., Schene, A., Koeter, M. and Robson, D. (2006) 'Medication Adherence in Schizophrenia: Exploring Patients', Carers' and Professionals' Views'. *Schizophrenia Bulletin,* 32, 4, 786–794.

King's Fund (2011) *How is the NHS Performing? Quarterly Monitoring Report.* London: King's Fund.

Kirkbride J.B., *et al.* (2008) 'Psychosis, Ethnicity and Socio-economic Status'. *British Journal of Psychiatry,* 193, 18–24.

Macaulay, R. (2010) 'Just as I am Without One Plea: A Journey to Reconcile Sexuality And Spirituality'. *Ethnicity and Inequalities in Health and Social Care,* 3, 3, 6–13.

MacPherson, W. (1999) *The Stephen Lawrence Inquiry.* London: HMSO.

Marmot, M. (2010) *Fair Society, Healthy Lives*: London: The Marmot Review.

Mental Health Act Commission (2006) *Count Me In: The National Mental Health and Ethnicity Census: 2005 Service User Survey.* London: MHAC.

Moodley, R. and Palmer, S. (eds) (2006) *Race, Culture and Psychotherapy: Critical Perspective in Multicultural Practice.* Sussex: Routledge.

Morgan, A. (2000) *What is Narrative Therapy? An easy-to-read Introduction.* Adelaide: Dulwich Centre Publications.

Morgan, C., McKenzie, K. and Fearon, P. (eds) (2008) *Society and Psychosis.* Cambridge: Cambridge University Press.

National Mental Health Development Unit (2011) *National Evaluation of the Community Development Workers.* London: National Mental Health Development Unit.

NSCSTHA (2003) *Independent Inquiry into the Death David Bennett.* Norfolk, Suffolk and Cambridgeshire Strategic Health Authority. Cambridge, England.

Pierce, C., Carew, J., Pierce-Gonzalez, D. and Wills, D. (1978) 'An Experiment in Racism: TV Commercials'. In C. Pierce (ed) *Television and Education* (pp62–88). Beverly Hills, CA: Sage.

Raleigh,V., Irons, R., Hawe, E., Scobie, S., Cooke, A., Reeves, R., Petruckevich, A. and Harrison, J. (2007) 'Ethnic Variations in the Experience of Mental Health Service Users in England'. *British Journal of Psychiatry*, 191 304–312.

Rathod, S., Kingdon, D., Phiri, P. and Gobbi, M. (2010) 'Developing Culturally Sensitive Cognitive Behaviour Therapy for Psychosis for Ethnic Minority Patients by Exploration and Incorporation of Service Users' and Health Professionals' Views and Opinions'. *Behavioural and Cognitive Psychotherapy*, 38, 5, 511–533.

RAWOrg (2011) *The End of Delivering Race Equality: Perspectives of Frontline Workers and Service Users from Radicalised Groups*. London: RAWOrg.

Read J., Mosher L.R. and Bentall R.P. (eds) (2004) *Models of Madness: Psychological, Social and Biological Approaches to Schizophrenia*. Sussex: Brunner-Routledge.

Romme, M. *et al.* (2009) *Living with Voices: 50 Stories of Recovery*. Birmingham: PCCS Books.

Sainsbury Centre for Mental Health (2002) *Breaking the Circles of Fear: A Review of the Relationship Between Mental Health Services and African Caribbean Communities*. London: Sainsbury Centre for Mental Health.

Senghera, R. (2011) 'Equality and Human Rights Approaches in the NHS: Making Spirituality in Mental Health Care Count?' In P. Gilbert (ed) *Spirituality in Mental Health*. East Sussex: Pavilion Publishing.

Sewell, H. (2009a) *Working with Ethnicity Race and Culture in Mental Health: A Handbook for Practitioners*. London: Jessica Kingsley Publishers.

Sewell, H. (2009b) 'Leading Race Equality in Mental Health'. *International Journal of Leadership in Public Services*, 5, 2, 19–27.

Shapiro, D.A. and Shapiro, D. (1982) Meta-analysis of Comparative Therapy Outcome Studies: A Replication and Refinement'. *Psychological Bulletin*, 92, 581–604.

Singer, I. (2006) 'Unmasking Difference, Culture and Attachment in the Psychoanalytic Space'. In White, K. (ed) *Unmasking Race, Culture and Attachment in the Psychoanalytic Space*. London: H Karnac (Books) Limited.

Singh, S., Greenwood, N., White, S. and Churchill, R. (2007) 'Ethnicity and the Mental Health Act 1983'. *British Journal of Psychiatry,* 191, 99–105.

Ture, K. and Hamilton, C. (1992) *Black Power: The Politics of Liberation*. New York: Vintage.

Veling, W., Selton, J., Susser, E., Laan, W., Mackenbach, J. and Hoek, H. (2007) 'Discrimination and the Incidence of Psychotic Disorders Among Ethnic Minorities in The Netherlands'. *International Journal of Epidemiology*, 34, 4, 761–768.

Woodger, D. and Cowan, J. (2010) Institutional Racism in Healthcare Services: Using Mainstream Methods to Development a Practical Approach. *Ethnicity and Inequalities in Health and Social Care*, 3, 4, 36–44.

11 Age-specific service lines

Chris Fox, Siobhan Reilly, Steve Iliffe and Jill Manthorpe

Dementia care

Dementia has an estimated global prevalence of 35 million individuals (Alzheimer's Disease International, 2009). In the UK 570,000 people live with dementia – a figure that will double over the next 30 years, reflecting global predictions (Alzheimer's Disease International, 2009; Department of Health, 2009). With increasing demand and timescales of at least 5–10 years for the next possible disease modifying breakthrough, services are and have had to undergo change to cope with the increasing levels of need.

Implementation of the National Dementia Strategy

The National Dementia Strategy (NDS) was published in 2009 (Department of Health, 2009). It seeks to transform dementia services in five years. Its primary objective is to raise public and professional awareness of the need to respond to dementia as a manageable problem. A second set of recommendations focused on improving the actual response of support systems, concentrating on earlier diagnosis, peer and professional support, dementia friendly housing and technology, and (where possible) active treatment. The third set of recommendations centred on enhancing the quality of care for people with dementia and their carers, whether they are living at home, visiting hospital for treatment or living in care homes.

Whilst no one can be against such objectives, there are emerging criticisms that the strategies may be no more than a sticking plaster across some fundamental problems (Hinton *et al.*, 2007). These criticisms challenge the belief that such a strategy could produce marked change in complex systems of care within a five-year time frame. Experiences from the *National Service Framework for Older People* (Department of Health, 2001), itself a ten-year strategy, illustrate the difficulty of changing systems and care practices to reflect the fact that older people are the major patient group in the NHS. Apart from the rapid uptake of new medication and some technologies (like ultrasound and day-case surgery) most change in the NHS is slow.

Second, while the strategy is accompanied by fine words and ambitions, it has brought with it very little extra resources and these were concentrated on a few areas, such as the development of memory services and on raising public awareness. This has led to concerns that there will be greater numbers of people being diagnosed but that there will be only very limited resources with which to support them after diagnosis.

Finally, while no fault of the authors of the strategy, it would only be possible to implement its ambitions at a time of real economic growth. The economic downturn looks likely to decrease the availability of low level social care (Acton Shapiro, 2010) and the ability of public services to respond with early interventions or even to commission specialist and therefore more costly services.

All these criticisms are relevant, but the case for change is powerful and the range of pressure groups supporting a shift is growing. The standard of dementia care in England is in urgent need of improvement, with frequent failure to deliver services in a timely, integrated or cost-effective manner to support people with dementia and their families to live independently for as long as possible (National Audit Office, 2007). Putting this right demands a higher level of collaborative working across disciplines and agencies than has commonly been experienced, and a focus on creating integrated dementia care services (Bullock *et al.*, 2007), either in virtual form (through local agreements to work together) or in the shape of the joint clinical directorates as advocated by the *National Service Framework for Long Term Conditions* (Department of Health, 2006). The question is not whether we can afford to reconfigure services for people with dementia, but how best to do so.

Reconfiguring services for older people

Primary care is often the first point of contact for people with suspected dementia and most people will then be managed by primary care services. However, a diagnosis of dementia is often delayed for several years after the initial onset of symptoms and only between a third and a half of people with dementia ever receive a formal diagnosis (National Audit Office, 2007). A recent cohort study found a higher relative mortality rate in the first year after diagnosis that may be explained by more diagnostic entries being made in the primary care record at a time of crisis or late in the disease trajectory, inter-current illness, hospital admission or previous admission to an institution (Rait *et al.*, 2010).

Late recording of diagnoses of dementia in primary care means that opportunities for early intervention have been missed and increase the likelihood of crises and admissions to care. A recent cross-sectional survey of old age psychiatrists (n=318) showed that structures to deliver integrated care across the interfaces between specialist old age mental health and primary, acute and social care services were generally poorly developed (Tucker *et al.*, 2009). Indeed, a recent review has shown that much of the problem in detecting and managing dementia for GPs arises not from their own abilities but from the health systems in which they work (Koch and Iliffe, 2010). This may result from a feeling of lack of support from and communication with specialist care, and if the relationship between the generalists and specialists is dysfunctional then patients are unlikely to receive high quality care (Iliffe and Wilcock, 2005; Koch and Iliffe, 2010).

Three themes that should be considered in harmonizing approaches to the diagnosis of dementia in primary care have been identified: (1) a focus on timely diagnosis, (2) the need for the development and implementation of guidelines, and (3) the identification of appropriate referral pathways and diagnostic strategies, including multi-professional collaboration (De Lepeleire *et al.*, 2008). These researchers have also suggested that referral pathways are more effective than simple guidelines and that a clear and robust multidisciplinary infrastructure will enable diagnosis and management (De Lepeleire *et al.*, 2008) and enhance caregiver satisfaction (Hinton *et al.*, 2007; Lee *et al.*, 2010).

A decade ago only 52 per cent of GPs (n=1005) felt that early diagnosis was beneficial and only 54 per cent felt it was important to look objectively for early signs of dementia. However, this survey did indicate that there was a relationship between the presence of specific service characteristics (e.g. a memory clinic) and the strength of GPs' views on whether it was beneficial to make an early diagnosis of dementia (varying from strongly agree to strongly

---

Box 11.1 Memory services

Key service components of a memory assessment service for the early identification and care of people with dementia:

- early identification and referral of people with a possible diagnosis of dementia and
- developing a high-quality service for dementia assessment, diagnosis and management.

Key clinical issues

Key clinical issues in providing an effective memory assessment service for the early identification and care of people with dementia are:

- accurately identifying and referring all people who present with signs and symptoms of possible early dementia
- ensuring that appropriate referral pathways are in place
- providing comprehensive assessment and diagnosis of dementia, including subtype diagnosis
- providing an integrated approach to care coordination and implementation across all agencies involved in the treatment and care of people with dementia and support of their carers
- providing a quality assured service.

Source: Memory assessment service for the early identification and care of people with dementia. Commissioning guide: Implementing NICE guidance (NICE, 2007).

---

disagree) (Renshaw *et al.*, 2001). This was supported by the National Audit Office report *Improving Services and Support for People with Dementia* (2007), which emphasized a need to better develop primary care's role in dementia recognition and delivery of services.

Memory assessment services (Box 11.1) (which may be provided by a memory assessment clinic or by community mental health teams) should be the single point of referral for all people with a possible diagnosis of dementia (NICE/SCIE, 2006). The National Dementia Strategy also recognised the advantages that early assessment and intervention can have on the quality of life for people with dementia and their carers. It stated that every individual should be guaranteed access to a memory service and the support it provides, leading to the suggestion of the need for a national network of memory services (Banerjee and Wittenberg, 2009), with the implication that the development of new services is likely to increase substantially over the next five to ten years. Health care system characteristics such as the presence or absence of memory clinics are linked with both referral pathways and the way GPs and specialists work together in the diagnosis of dementia (Iliffe and Wilcock, 2005; Koch and Iliffe, 2010). It is also worth noting that this fairly recent conversion to memory clinics as the way to provide services is a departure from the UK model of social psychiatry via community-orientated services. This may represent a step (back) towards a medical model, which has been the main model in North America and much of Europe (Jolley and Moniz-Cook, 2009). Clinics were originally not seen as service components but restricted to academic centres to facilitate research (Jolley and Moniz-Cook, 2009).

Developing models of care

Overall, services do not deliver value for money to taxpayers or people with dementia and their families. In particular, spending is late with too few people being diagnosed or being diagnosed early enough (National Audit Office, 2007). Cost-effective early interventions that would improve quality of life are not being made widely available, resulting in spending at a later stage on more expensive services.

The role of Community Mental Health Trusts (CMHTs) in diagnosis and early intervention has been described as inconsistent, with most focusing solely on people with severe mental illness (National Audit Office, 2007). This, however, has been a commissioning requirement via the National Service Framework for Mental Health (Department of Health, 1999) with the rationing away from services for older people. The service mapping exercise found 131 memory services of which 38 per cent were provided in a psychiatric hospital, 27 per cent in a CMHT and 16 per cent in a general hospital. Nine per cent were located in a primary care centre and 14 per cent in other settings. It is noted that variations exist because memory services have evolved in a piecemeal fashion, often directly in response to the licensing in 2001 of acetyl cholinesterase drugs for Alzheimer's disease (National Audit Office, 2007). The National Audit Office review also found that less than a third of GPs agreed that there were satisfactory specialist services locally to meet need.

Memory clinics provided within a primary care setting may offer patients a speedier response than traditional specialist clinics. Other advantages to the patients and carers are that the setting is local, non-threatening and non-stigmatised. They also may be more affordable particularly as the numbers of dementia patients increase in the future. The assumption is that many patients and families will be better provided with affordable assessment and continued support by strengthening the activities of primary care, rather than referral of everyone to secondary care centres.

Services will inevitably develop differently, particularly as the landscape for commissioning new models of care is changing and some areas will develop more imaginative models of commissioning more quickly than others. It is clear that care for people with dementia cannot be delivered by either primary or secondary health care alone and as many older people have multiple co-morbidities, restricting their care to mental health services is inappropriate. Innovative models of care are being commissioned and these are likely to develop more rapidly over the coming years. Six examples of different models of memory services are set out below.

Example 1

A memory clinic based in and providing to a single practice in South Staffordshire with around 8,000 patients has been in operation for a number of years (Greening *et al.*, 2009; Greaves and Jolley, 2010). The contact rate has been reported at 18/1000 over-65s per annum (Greening *et al.*, 2009), which is three times that reported in a hospital-based clinic (Banerjee *et al.*, 2007) and higher than that reported at the Newbury Memory Clinic, which is primary-care-based but services a number of practices (Brooke *et al.*, 2005). This model of memory clinic has attracted a greater rate of referral than specialist, hospital-based clinics, and provides a sustainable long-term support and treatment mode (Greening *et al.*, 2009).

Example 2

Building on this model a whole service transformation across South Staffordshire has been commissioned to address inconsistent memory services. The Joint Commissioning Unit, a partnership between Staffordshire County Council, South Staffordshire Primary Care Trust and NHS North Staffordshire, commissioned in 2011 a service model that is an integral component of the South Staffordshire Dementia Strategy, modelled on the expectations of the National Dementia Strategy. Memory clinics will be based in approximately 12 practices in South Staffordshire, integrated with the Primary Care Team, they may also be based in other community-based care settings. The service will accept referrals from the 90+ practices in South Staffordshire and these can be from any registered GP, health or social care professional, third-sector agencies, or a carer or person who suspects they may have dementia. The contract has been awarded to an independent sector provider resulting in commissioners reducing their spend with the local NHS Trust.

The first contact for a patient will be an initial meeting with a dementia adviser to discuss what would happen following referral to the memory service; and to listen to the person and answer their questions. Two screening tests are also completed to be sent onto the memory service. The dementia adviser may also attend the initial meeting at the memory service to support the person with dementia and their carer. If a follow-up meeting is agreed this will involve signposting to other services, national and local, as appropriate; helping individuals and their carers with further questions after the memory service meeting; support to find and access information independently for a range of services; and looking to, and planning for, the future. This model, like many other dementia advisor services in place across England aims to provide support to people with dementia and their carers, helping them to stay at home for longer and avoiding admission to residential care or hospital.

Example 3

The local Joint Commissioning Partnership Board (JCPB) has approved the investment with matched funds from Hertfordshire Partnership NHS Foundation Trust (HPFT) to develop an Early Memory Diagnosis and Support Service (EMDASS) for Hertfordshire. By introducing this new model, the service expects to double the number of people with a diagnosis of dementia it manages within five years. The memory service will be integrated within the specialist mental health team for older people and the pathway of care will consist of four elements: primary care memory team; diagnostic memory service; early intervention and support service; and memory maintenance service. The pathway has four linked stages of care and staff will work across the whole pathway, enabling continuity of care. It is proposed that the new memory services should be run from local communities, preferably from GP practice premises and other accessible locations. The majority of clinics were formerly sited in inpatient facilities, which can be distressing for service users and their carers. By the end of September 2011 the new service will be available, through GP referral, throughout Hertfordshire.

Example 4

A recent report from ADASS (Association of Directors of Adult Social Services, 2011) has highlighted a number of initiatives that focus on improving how secondary care in hospital-based services can work in better ways for people with dementia, as well as for GPs. Programmes include i) avoiding admissions, both to general acute and to mental health inpatient wards through, for example, working more closely with care homes and ambulance services, or through the use of community-based crisis services; and ii) shortening lengths of stay through better discharge processes. Better training for hospital staff about dementia and its management, along with the use of well-coordinated person-centred plans while the person is in hospital, have proved instrumental in achieving reduced stays. ADASS describe a range of new developments, including the Sussex Dementia Partnership, which involves 11 statutory health and social care agencies, as well as the Alzheimer's Society and the South East Strategic Health Authority. Sussex Partnership Trust are the lead agency and are reported to have reduced the use of inpatient beds and to have strengthened collaboration across a range of community-based services. Another collaborative project in Darlington between health and social care providers has changed the way acute care has managed and delivered services for people with dementia, leading to their needs being met more appropriately. Early successes include the completion of mini mental state assessments within 12 hours of admission and ward staff having access to GP dementia registers, resulting in a reduced wait for patient access to all professionals involved in their treatment from 7 days to 24 hours.

Example 5

NHS Wirral in partnership with the Adult Social Care Services are redesigning and enhancing the role of the memory service. The joint commissioning strategy for dementia in the Wirral has funded Wirral Memory Service, which provides an assessment and monitoring service for people who have suspected or diagnosed cognitive impairment. Referrals come from GPs, as well as health and social care professionals. The team is made up of a consultant psychiatrist, clinical nurse specialists and administrative support staff, working closely with the Alzheimer's Society, who provide carer support, advice and outreach workers. It is anticipated that the new service will provide capacity for 800 additional referrals per annum. The memory service has been redesigned following a decision to decommission the current intermediate services and the entire service design has centred on the perspective of the person with dementia.

Example 6

The Ashton, Wigan and Leigh Memory Service have established a multidisciplinary assessment team, with a core staff base of highly skilled nurses, occupational therapists and social workers, who are supported by psychiatrists, to undertake initial assessments that form the basis of a provisional hypothesis (Page *et al.*, 2010). The service is orientated towards the lower dimensions of the step-model of dementia care. Previous old age consultant outpatient clinics have now been decommissioned. Again in this model, the Dementia Advisory Service will work in partnership within the new memory clinic adopting an 'Active Case Management Approach'. Following referral the Dementia Advisory Service maintains ongoing contact and facilitates a stratified, stepped care approach for those who use the service. The Dementia Advisor Service will harmonise with the Service Instigated Telephone Support Electronically Recalled (SISTER) Service and Family Instigated Contact (FIC) Model – both proactive self-efficacy models of support. People in Wigan who are displaying early signs of possible dementia will have access to a comprehensive memory service providing assessment, treatment and therapeutic interventions.

Additional examples

Oxford's services have: memory clinics linked closely to CMHTs, while both Norfolk and Devon have followed a CMHT integrated memory clinic model. The Oxleas Foundation Trust model has a dedicated memory service, distinct from CMHTs but with links built in. The Kent model has dedicated memory teams and both a domiciliary and clinic-based structure.

The diversity of structures we have described for memory services in dementia, either now operating or in development was predicted in the NDS, with services envisaged as developing according to local expectations and needs, as well as the right fit with service lines.

Workforce redesign to deliver the new models of service for dementia

Dementia care requires a range of flexible skills and abilities. The NDS reflects this understanding by focusing on the competencies to deliver the new services; however, service providers may still think in traditional terms of jobs and roles until they are challenged by the new commissioning environment about their approach to workforce planning and professional skill development. Old age psychiatrists will be able to focus on the complex cases where their expertise matters most if they plan to transfer diagnostic and management skills to GPs in their localities. There is also a need (clearly identified in the NDS) for in-reach support to develop hospital staff's ability to work more effectively with patients with dementia, although challenging some staff's assumptions and approaches will require careful management. Commissioners should seek to use the expertise in care home staff and social work to make dementia care work more efficiently (Iliffe and Wilcock, 2009).

Anticipatory planning – for cardiovascular disease prevention

Existing efforts to reduce the risks of cardiovascular diseases may also help to delay neurodegeneration. Cardiovascular risk factors predict the likelihood of developing dementia more than many professionals realise. Hypertension and type 2 diabetes increase the risk of developing dementia sixfold, and obesity is a risk factor for dementia independent of blood pressure and diabetes. Cognitive function changes are measurable in people with cardiovascular risk factors in middle age, making targeted primary prevention of both heart and brain disease imperative. There is the real possibility that vigorous control of cardiovascular risks at community level could postpone the onset of dementia syndrome, and there is already some evidence of this happening in the USA (Langa *et al.*, 2008). No similar pattern is obvious yet in the UK (Langa *et al.*, 2009), but this may be a time-lag effect, and we may see the incidence of dementia fall.

Evidence base for service effectiveness

Although there are many areas developing new services there is unfortunately not a strong evidence base that can guide them (Koch and Iliffe, 2010). Case management is an attractive option, but is variably defined as requiring assessment, care planning and educating, to problem solving, liaising, monitoring and counselling (Clark *et al.*, 2004; Vickrey *et al.*, 2006; Callahan *et al.*, 2006; Mittelman *et al.*, 2006; Fortinsky *et al.*, 2006). Some studies showed some positive results, although few have recorded large effects. Vickrey *et al.* (2006) recorded that case management care was more adherent to guidelines, and people received more prescribed medications and referrals to community services. Clark *et al.*'s (2004) intervention group in Cleveland, US, experienced fewer hospital and casualty admissions, and reported less embarrassment, isolation and relationship strain. Mittelman *et al.* (2006) showed that counselling caregivers could delay moves of their relative with dementia to a care home. Conversely, the caregivers in Callahan *et al.*'s (2006) trial were less stressed, but rates of hospital and nursing home admissions were unaffected, while Fortinsky *et al.* (2009) demonstrated no positive effects at all. Time-to-institutionalisation was not often measured in these studies, but, in a meta-analysis of caregiver interventions, Pinquart and Sorensen (2006) concluded that case management can lead to a reduced *risk* of institutionalisation, if not a demonstrable delay. Although the clinical, psychological and social benefits of case management hint that it may be a useful approach for people with dementia and their families, the economic benefits of this labour-intensive intervention are not yet proven (Pimoguet *et al.*, 2010).

A case for evaluation

Recognising of course that there cannot be a 'one size fits all' solution, what these models have in common is increased targeting of resources and a multidisciplinary team approach, though there is clearly variation in the roles for primary health care. The assumption underlying these developments is that the new structures and services will lead to increasingly integrated forms of care. In the current economic climate this will require focused efforts as the wider service environment undergoes change. The agencies, including primary health care, secondary health and social care and the independent sector, that support people with dementia need to work together to achieve improved patient and carer outcomes that are cost-effective. Though dementia research is currently underfunded (Luengo-Fernandez *et al.*, 2010) it is important that new models such as these are properly evaluated and robust indicators (Draskovic *et al.*, 2008) including measures of integration at both the level of the patient and the organisation (Challis *et al.*, 2006) are established.

Clearly there are multiple interacting components to these new service models and this complexity then needs to be reflected in appropriately designed research. Many successful initiatives may take years to demonstrate impact, therefore require long-term commitment to adequately reflect their results. Success in delivering high quality dementia services is dependent on primary care commissioners and local authorities agreeing a strategic plan and working together as partners to deliver it (Department of Health/NHS Finance, Performance and Operations, 2010). The challenges for the future include staying close to the new architecture of NHS and adult social care, specifically the new GP consortia and local Health and Wellbeing Boards, whose Joint Strategic Needs Assessment will inform current and future health, social care and well-being needs, in turn shaping future service plans underpinned by evidence, capable of delivering the desired outcomes.

Social care in dementia

Since 1990, social care has moved from a provider to a commissioning and information imparting role. Most social care is provided by the private sector (outside family care) and only part of this is under the control (in terms of paying for it) of local government. The NDS aspirations therefore are set within a provider and labour market that is largely outside the control of commissioners and where matters, such as the cost of staffing, the attractiveness of the service (e.g. environment, food and facilities), feature highly. Hussein, Manthorpe and Stevens (in press) have established that the profile of the social care workforce supporting people with dementia in England is different when compared to the characteristics of other workers in the social care sector.

While similar number of dementia care workers compared to other workers in social care hold no qualifications, the former are less likely to be working towards any qualifications. In terms of qualifications held and being worked towards, dementia care workers are concentrated around the very low levels of NVQ level 2/2+ and are significantly *less* likely to hold higher qualifications than other workers. Specific skills are likely to be required to deliver better quality services and more capacity may also improve job satisfaction among dementia care workers (Coogle, Head and Parham, 2006) but this is not the current situation. As Zimmerman *et al.* (2005) suggested in respect of other promising initiatives, such as developing specialist home care workers, without an ambitious and shared strategic workforce plan across all sectors, it is difficult to see how it will be possible to overcome skill and role deficits, given that each provider currently only controls a finite resource and may have no incentive to invest this differently. This makes the NDS aspirations efforts to increase training and skills particularly complex and its strategic ambitions may be thwarted by the significant skills shortage. However, pressure is growing for a radical shift: the All-Party Parliamentary Group on Dementia (2009) and members of the House of Commons' Committee on Public Accounts (House of Commons, 2010) have raised serious concerns about the slow pace of change to improve the quality of dementia care. Indeed this subject had already been identified as a matter of 'urgency' (House of Commons, 2007).

The NDS hints at a possible change in the nature of long-term residential care toward a system where such facilities are used for people reaching the end of life (so avoiding hospital utilisation), with an expectation that residents' multiple and complex needs – frailty, disability and the management of challenging behaviour – can be met by skilled nursing and care staff. This is in line with overall government policy to reduce reliance on care homes, with less places being funded. In England, researchers have recently sought the views of a panel of experts on dementia about long-term care expenditure for older people with dementia in the year 2031 (Comas-Herrera *et al.*, 2011), using a Delphi-style approach. The panel predicted a small reduction in the prevalence of dementia over the next 50 years, a freeze in the numbers of people in care homes, and an increase in the qualifications and pay of care assistants. The panel's views were incorporated into projections of future expenditure in long-term care for people with dementia, leading the researchers to conclude that projected expenditure will grow more slowly than generally feared. In this scenario we may see more people with dementia supported at home by live-in care workers as well as family members (possibly using migrant labour from Eastern Europe) and perhaps a greater development of options such as Shared Lives or Adult Placements. This is where disabled adults move to live with other people in what is sometimes referred to as adult fostering (more common among people with learning disabilities but possibly transferable). Such provision may be run by a social enterprise but more commonly it will be set up on a self-employment basis. The NDS's promotion of 'community care' confirms that home-based care is envisaged as the prominent form of support and improved access to services (Boyle, Najanathan and Cumming, 2010) may heighten demand for home care, placing resources under pressure. Indeed, the implementation of the strategy depends on £1.9 billion savings from reduced reliance on care homes and increased use of community care, even though the House of Commons (2007) cautioned against over-reliance on home care workers, seeing them as lacking understanding of dementia. Yet Hussein, Manthorpe and Stevens (in press) caution policy makers to the advice of Wellin and Jaffe (2004) and Stone (2004) that home care workers must be increasingly viewed as an important part of the dementia care workforce, recognising that in developed countries this will include large numbers of migrant workers (Spencer *et al.*, 2010). This suggests the need for greater engagement with this loose and ill-defined sector rather than further concentration on care homes and other building-based services. These developments make the aspirations of the NDS on training challenging; it is far easier to hold training in group care settings than for individuals who may be working on their own account. This flexible workforce needs to be fully engaged in the remodelling of the dementia care systems, with far less reliance on care homes as a 'default sector'. It will also prove necessary for registered professionals to offer front line carers (paid or unpaid) advice, imparting their skills directly, considering the needs of people with dementia as well as those who support them. The ability of health and social care staff to work in this way requires early fostering in educational programmes.

One of the fundamental principles of the NDS is a person-centred approach and this chimes with similar approaches in reforms to adult social care, which are underpinned by personalisation. The term personalisation is being used to describe the transformation of social care to give people greater choice, control and flexibility over the support they receive that is funded by the public sector. People who are eligible on grounds of need and income/resources are told what sums are available to them following assessment, and are assisted to devise a support plan outlining how they will meet these agreed outcomes. They can organise their own support if they wish, or have a 'virtual budget' where services are arranged by an organisation, or a mix of these approaches. 'Personal budgets' is the term generally being used to describe this system. New regulations mean people with dementia are included in this 'transformation', through permitting carers to act as proxies for receiving funding. This may be particularly attractive to some families who will be able to employ the person they choose to do the things they want; whether this is accompanying the person with dementia to the park or helping them to bake a cake. Professionals will need to understand what an individual's plan consists of, to enable them to support its delivery, while being fully aware of any risks.

Promoting choice and control involves an element of risk and balancing risks and opportunities in a managed open way redefines for some professions their scope of practice (Manthorpe and Moriarty, 2010). Health and social care organisations and professionals can sometimes face tensions between balancing risks and opportunities for individuals, alongside their duty to care for individuals deemed to be 'vulnerable', as well as the safety of the wider public (Mitchell and Glendinning, 2007; Carr and Robbins, 2009). In the case of people with dementia, vulnerability tends to be seen in increased risks in terms of their personal safety, or that of others, and their risk of being exposed to abuse or exploitation. NDS Objective 6 seeks to promote effective community support services for people with dementia and while this may presume a traditional service, such as home care agencies or day centres, the profile of these is changing. For example, it is likely that there will be fewer day centres if more people choose to use their personal budgets to employ their own relatives, neighbours and friends and to make less use of such facilities. There is general agreement that optimising support of people with dementia in their own homes is desired and desirable (see Challis *et al.*, 2010) but set in the context of wider local community options such as lunch clubs and day facilities. This changing landscape shows that the NDS needs to be implemented in the context of other transformations; and commissioners, practitioners and educationalists must be aware of this kaleidoscope.

Conclusions

Globally societies are facing enormous difficulties with coping with the needs of dementia patients and their families. With longevity increasing, dementia levels are escalating. Health and social care systems have to adapt to prevent being overwhelmed. Even if a significant breakthrough is made in treatment it is likely to be targeting the very early stages of dementia and there is no definite timescale for this with ranges of 5–20 years suggested by experts in the field. The NHS faces particular challenges due to a general reorganisation and pressures for up to seven per cent efficiency savings per annum over the next five years. Services are being asked to do much more with less resource so the way services are delivered are changing rapidly. Some of the initiatives described in this chapter will assist but much more is needed in terms of innovation and research, as argued by the Ministerial Advisory Group on Dementia Research (MAGDR, 2011).

References

Acton Shapiro (2010) *The Impact of the Economic Slowdown on Adult Social Care,* London: Local Government Association.

All-Party Parliamentary Group on Dementia (2009) *Prepared to Care, Challenging the Dementia Skills Gap,* London: HMSO.

Alzheimer's Disease International (2009) *World Alzheimer Report 2009.* http://www.alz.co.uk/research/files/WorldAlzheimerReport.pdf (accessed 1 May 2011).

Association of Directors of Adult Social Services (2011) *Response by the Association of Directors of Adult Social Services (ADASS) to 2011 Inquiry of the All-Party Parliamentary Group on Dementia: How to Save Money in Dementia Care and Deliver Better Outcomes for People with Dementia?* http://www.adass.org.uk/index.php?option=com_contentandview=articleandid=725:new-approaches-to-dementia-services-can-improve-care-in-cost-effective-way-andcatid=146:press-releases-2011andItemid=447 (accessed 28 March 2011).

Banerjee, S. and Wittenberg, R. (2009) Clinical and cost-effectiveness of services for early diagnosis and intervention in dementia, *International Journal of Geriatric Psychiatry,* 24, 748–754.

Banerjee, S., Willis, R., Matthews, D., Contell, F., Chan, J. and Murray, J. (2007) Improving the quality of care for mild to moderate dementia: an evaluation of the Croydon Memory Service Model, *International Journal of Geriatric Psychiatry,* 22, 782–788.

Boyle, N., Najanathan, V. and Cumming, R. (2010) Medication and falls: risk and optimisation, *Clinics in Geriatric Medicine,* 26(4), 583–605.

Brooke, P., Naidoo, M. and Rice, D. (2005) *The Newbury Memory Clinic Project: Final Report.* Newbury: Falklands Surgery. http://www.falklandsurgery.co.uk/memory/The%20Newbury%20Memory%20Clinic%20main%20report.pdf (accessed 28 March 2010).

Bullock, R., Passmore, P. and Iliffe, S. (2007) Can we afford not to have integrated dementia services? *Age and Ageing,* 36(4), 357–358.

Callahan, C.M., Boustani, M.A., Unverzagt, F.W., Austrom, M.G., Damush, T.M., Perkins, A.J., Fultz, B.A., Hui, S.L., Counsell, S.R. and Hendrie, H.C. (2006) Effectiveness of collaborative care for older adults with Alzheimer disease in primary care: a randomized controlled trial, *JAMA,* 295, 2148–2157.

Callahan, C.M., Boustani, M.A., Weiner, M., Beck, R., Livin, L., Kellams, J., Willis, D. and Hendrie, H. (2011) Implementing dementia care models in primary care settings: The Aging Brain Care Medical Home, *Aging and Mental Health,* 15(1), 5–12.

Carr, S. and Robbins, D. (2009) *SCIE Research Briefing 20: The Implementation of Individual Budget Schemes in Adult Social Care,* London: SCIE.

Challis, D., Stewart, K., Donnelly, M., Weiner, K. and Hughes J. (2006) Care management for older people: Does integration make a difference? *Journal of Interprofessional Care,* 20(4), 335–348.

Challis, D., Hughes, J., Berzins, K., Reilly, S., Abell, J., Stewart, K. (2010) *Self Care and Case Management in Long Term Conditions: The Effective Management of Critical Interfaces.* Report for the National Institute for Health Research Service Delivery and Organisation Programme. Southampton: National Institute for Health Research. http://www.housinglin.org.uk/_library/Resources/Housing/Support_materials/Other_reports_and_guidance/Dementia_and_domiciliary_care_-_PSSRU_full_report.pdf (accessed 26 April 2011).

Clark, P., Bass, D., Looman, W., McCarthy, C. and Eckert, S. (2004) Outcomes for patients with dementia from the Cleveland Alzheimer's managed care demonstration, *Aging and Mental Health,* 8(1), 245–251.

Comas-Herrera, A. Northey, S., Wittenberg, R., Knapp, M., Bhattacharyya, S. and Burns, A. (2011) Future costs of dementia-related long-term care: exploring future scenarios, *International Psychogeriatrics,* 23(1), 20–30.

Coogle, C., Head, C. and Parham, I. (2006) The long-term care workforce crisis: dementia-care training influences on job satisfaction and career commitment, *Educational Gerontology,* 32(8), 611–631.

De Lepeleire, J., Wind, A.W., Iliffe, S., Moniz-Cook, E.D., Wilcock, J., Gonzalez, V.M., Derksen, E., Gianelli, M.V., Vernooij-Dassen, M. and the Interdem Group (2008) The primary care diagnosis of dementia in Europe: an analysis using multidisciplinary, multinational expert groups, *Aging Mental Health,* 12(5), 568–576.

Department of Health (1999) *National Service Framework for Mental Health: Modern Standards and Service Models*, Department of Health, London.

Department of Health (2001) *National Service Framework for Older People*, London: Department of Health.

Department of Health (2006) *National Service Framework for Long Term Conditions*. London: HMSO.

Department of Health (2009) *Living Well with Dementia: A National Dementia Strategy*, London: Stationary Office. http://www.dh.gov.uk/prod_consum_dh/groups/dh_digitalassets/@dh/@en/documents/digitalasset/dh_094051.pdf (accessed 6 January 2011).

Department of Health/NHS Finance, Performance and Operations (2010) *The Operating Framework for 2010/11 for the NHS in England*. http://www.connectingforhealth.nhs.uk/systemsandservices/infogov/links/operatingframework2010-2011.pdf (accessed 28th March 2011).

Draskovic, I., Vernooij-Dassen, M., Verhey, F., Scheltens, P. and Rikkert, M.O. (2008) Development of quality indicators for memory clinics, *International Journal of Geriatric Psychiatry*, 23, 119–128.

Fortinsky, R., Kulldorff, M., Kleppinger, A. and Kenyon-Pesce, L. (2009) Dementia care consultation for family caregivers: collaborative model linking an Alzheimer's association chapter with primary care physicians, *Aging and Mental Health*, 13(2), 162–170.

Greaves, I. and Jolley, D. (2010) National Dementia Strategy: well intentioned – but how well founded and how well directed? *British Journal of General Practice*, 60, 193–198.

Greening, L., Greaves, I., Greaves, N. and Jolley, D. (2009) Positive thinking on dementia in primary care: Gnosall Memory Clinic, *Community Practitioner*, 82, 20–23.

Hinton, L., Franz, C.E., Reddy, G., Flores, Y., Kravitz, R.L. and Barker, J.C. (2007) Practice constraints, behavioral problems, and dementia care: primary care physicians' perspectives, *Journal of General Internal Medicine*, 22(11), 1487–1492.

House of Commons (2007) *Improving Dementia Services in England – an Interim Report,* House of Commons Public Accounts Committee, Nineteenth Report, London: Public Accounts Committee Publications.

House of Commons (2010) *Progress in Improving Stroke Care*, House of Commons Public Accounts Committee, Twenty-sixth report, HC405, London: Public Accounts Committee Publications.

Hussein, S., Manthorpe, J., & Stevens, M (in press) The experiences of migrant social work and social care practitioners in the UK: findings from an online survey, *European Journal of Social Work*.

Iliffe, S. and Wilcock, J. (2005) The identification of barriers to the recognition of, and response to, dementia in primary care using a modified focus group approach, *Dementia*, 4(1), 73–85.

Iliffe, S. and Wilcock, J. (2009) Commissioning dementia care: implementing the National Dementia Strategy, *Journal of Integrated Care*, 17(4), 3–11.

Jolley, D. and Moniz-Cook, E. (2009) Memory clinics in context, *Indian Journal of Psychiatry*, 51, S70–S76.

Koch, T. and Iliffe, S. for the EVIDEM-ED project (2010) Rapid appraisal of barriers to the diagnosis and management of patients with dementia in primary care: a systematic review, *BMC Family Practice*, 11, 52.

Langa, K.M., Larson, E.B., Karlawish, J.H., Cutler, D.M., Kabeto, M.U., Kim, S.Y. and Rosen, A.B. (2008) Trends in the prevalence and mortality of cognitive impairment in the United States: is there evidence of the compression of cognitive morbidity? *Alzheimers & Dementia*, 4, 134–144.

Langa, K.M., Llewellyn, D.J., Lang, I.A., Weir, D.R., Wallace, R.B., Kabeto, M.U., Huppert, F.A. (2009) Cognitive health among older adults in the United States and in England, *BMC Geriatrics*, 9, 23.

Lee, L., Hillier, L.M., Stolee, P., Heckman, G., Gagnon, M., McAiney, C.A. and Harvey, D. (2010) Enhancing dementia care: a primary care-based memory clinic, *Journal of the American Geriatrics Society*, 58, 2197–2204.

Luengo-Fernandez, R., Leal, J. and Gray, A. (2010) *Dementia 2010: The Economic Burden of Dementia and Associated Research Funding in the United Kingdom*, Cambridge: Alzheimer's Research Trust.

MAGDR (2011) *Final Report from the MAGDR Subgroup 1 on Priority Topics in Dementia Research, February 2011*. http://www.nihr.ac.uk/files/.../MAGDR per cent20S-group per cent201 per cent20final per cent20report.pdf (accessed 1 May 2011).

Manthorpe, J. and Moriarty, J., (2010) *Nothing Ventured, Nothing Gained: Risk Guidance for People with Dementia*, London: Department of Health.

Mitchell, W. and Glendinning, C. (2007) *A Review of the Research Evidence Surrounding Risk Perceptions, Risk Management Strategies and their Consequences in Adult Social Care for Different Groups of Service Users*,

Social Policy Research Unit Working Paper No DHR 2180 11.06, University of York: Social Policy Research Unit.

Mittelman, M., Haley, W., Clay, O. and Roth, D. (2006) Improving caregiver well-being delays nursing home placement of patients with Alzheimer Disease, *Neurology*, 67, 1592–1599.

National Audit Office (2007) *Improving Services and Support for People with Dementia*, London: The Stationery Office. http://www.nao.org.uk/publications/0607/support_for_people_with_dement. aspx.

NICE (2007) *Memory Assessment Service for the Early Identification and Care of People with Dementia Commissioning Guide Implementing NICE Guidance*, London: The National Institute for Health and Clinical Excellence. http://www.nice.org.uk/media/4F1/D6/Memory_assessment_service_ commissioning_guide.pdf (accessed 3 November 2011).

NICE/SCIE (2006) *Dementia: Supporting People with Dementia and Their Carers in Health and Social Care*. London: The National Institute for Health and Clinical Excellence/Social Care Institute for Excellence. http://www.nice.org.uk/nicemedia/live/10998/30318/30318.pdf (accessed 3 November 2011).

Page, S., Hope, K. and Maj, C. (2010) 'New beginnings': towards distributed responsibility in memory services, *Journal of Dementia Care*, 18, 3, 33–36.

Pimouguet, C., Lavaud, T., Dartigues, J. and Helmer, C. (2010) Dementia case management effectiveness on health care costs and resource utilization: a systematic review of randomized controlled trial, *The Journal of Nutrition, Health and Aging*, 14(8), 669–676.

Pinquart, M. and Sorensen, S. (2006) Helping caregivers of persons with dementia: which interventions work and how large are their effects? *International Journal of Psychogeriatrics*, 18(4), 577–595.

Rait, G., Walters, K., Bottomley, C., Petersen, I., Iliffe, S. and Nazareth, I. (2010) Survival of people with clinical diagnosis of dementia in primary care: cohort study, *British Medical Journal*, 341, c3584.

Renshaw, J., Scurfield, P., Cloke, L. and Orrell, M. (2001) General practitioners' views on the early diagnosis of dementia, *British Journal of General Practice*, 51(462), 37–38.

Spencer, S., Martin, S., Bourgeault, I.L., and O'Shea, E., (2010) *The Role of Migrant Care Workers in Ageing Societies: Report on Research Findings in the UK, Ireland, the U.S. and Canada*. IOM Migration Research Series No. 41, Geneva: International Organization for Migration.

Stone, R.I. (2004) The direct care worker: the third rail of home care policy, *Annual Review of Public Health*, 25: 521–537.

Tucker, S., Baldwin, R., Hughes, J., Benbow, S., Barker, A., Burns, A. and Challis, D. (2009) Integrating mental health services for older people in England: from rhetoric to reality, *Journal of Interprofessional Care*, 23 (4), 341–354.

Vickrey, B.G., Mittman, B.S., Connor, K.I., *et al.* (2006) The effect of a disease management intervention on quality and outcomes of dementia care: a randomized, controlled trial, *Annals of Internal Medicine*, 145, 713–726.

Wellin, C. and Jaffe, D.J. (2004) In search of 'personal care': challenges to identity support in residential care for elders with cognitive illness, *Journal of Aging Studies*, 18(3), 275–295.

12 Improving access to psychological therapies

Practice and policy in a changing environment

John Cape and Caroline Humphries

Introduction

In October 2007 the UK Government announced £170 million funding for a programme of Improving Access to Psychological Therapies (IAPT) for anxiety and depression in England. Three years later, IAPT services had been established covering approximately 60 per cent of the population of England, 3,660 new cognitive behavioural therapy (CBT) therapists and psychological well-being practitioners had been trained, and an estimated 282,000 people had received treatment, of whom 95,000 had recovered from anxiety and depression (Improving Access to Psychological Therapies, 2011a). In view of the success of the programme, £400 million was announced in the October 2010 UK Government Spending Review for a further four-year roll-out to cover the whole country and extend the programme.

This chapter sets out:

- The background to the establishment of the IAPT programme.
- The IAPT service and training model.
- Evidence from evaluations of the impact of the IAPT programme.
- Current developments in the programme.
- Learning from IAPT for other mental health services.

Background

Prevalence and burden of common mental health problems

The IAPT programme is designed to treat anxiety and depressive disorders, which are often termed the 'common mental health problems'. They are so called because they are indeed common in the population. The proportion of the population with at least one common mental health disorder in the most recent 2007 Office for National Statistics Adult Psychiatric Morbidity Survey of England was 17.6 per cent in the 16–64 working age group, a proportion unchanged from the 17.5 per cent found in the 2000 survey, but an increase on the 15.5 per cent found in the first 1993 survey (McManus *et al.*, 2009). Women have higher rates of common mental health disorder, peaking at a quarter (25.1 per cent) of women age 45–54; people over age 65 have lower rates (10.2 per cent). By contrast the proportion of people in the population with probable psychosis in the same survey was 0.5 per cent. Put another way, these figures indicate there are about 35 people with a common mental health disorder for each person with a psychosis.

Turning to diagnosis, the most prevalent common mental health disorders are generalised anxiety disorder (4.3 per cent of the population), depressive episode (2.3 per cent) and mixed anxiety and depressive disorder (9.0 per cent; figures from the 2007 Adult Psychiatric Morbidity Survey). Mixed anxiety and depressive disorder is an ICD-10 diagnosis for people experiencing clinically significant symptoms of anxiety and depression who do not meet criteria for any other specific ICD-10 disorder. Large-scale surveys in the USA (Kessler *et al.*, 2005) and Australia (Andrews *et al.*, 2001) give differing estimates as to which are the most prevalent specific disorders, but are broadly in agreement in the proportion of the population with at least one common mental health disorder. For example, Kessler *et al.* (2005) found phobias to be much more common than generalised anxiety disorder in the USA (the reverse of the UK survey), but found that overall 18.1 per cent of the US population had suffered from at least one anxiety disorder in the previous 12 months, which is pretty similar to the UK data.

Although 'common mental health problems' are frequently contrasted with 'severe and enduring mental health problems', they also carry significant impairment and disability (Andrews *et al.*, 2001). The overall burden of depression and anxiety disorders is significant and they are projected to be the second most common cause of loss of disability-adjusted life years in the world (World Health Organization, 2001).

Pre-IAPT treatment of common mental health problems

The 2007 Adult Psychiatric Morbidity Survey included questions about treatment for common mental health disorders. Twenty-four per cent of people with a common mental health disorder reported receiving some kind of treatment for their disorder. Medication was the most common treatment: 19 per cent reported receiving medication while 10 per cent reported receiving counselling or a psychological therapy. In terms of type of counselling or psychotherapy received, 4 per cent reported receiving counselling, 3 per cent psychotherapy and only 2 per cent CBT, although CBT was the psychological therapy most recommended by contemporaneous National Institute for Clinical Excellence (NICE) guidance (see below). Thus overall only a quarter were receiving treatment, the majority of treatment provided was medication and where psychological therapy was provided it was unlikely to be with the psychological therapy most recommended for these disorders.

In terms of location of treatment, treatment of common mental health disorders has always taken place predominantly in primary care. Treatment in secondary care mental health services is rare. The standard quoted figure is that only 5 per cent of identified cases are referred to secondary mental health care (see e.g. Goldberg and Huxley, 1980, 1992), a figure that dates back over 50 years to a study of Shepherd *et al.* (1966, 1981). With GPs identifying 50 per cent of cases of common mental health problems (again the standard quoted figure, although there is now good evidence that this is an underestimate – see Kessler *et al.*, 2002) this suggests that only 2.5 per cent of cases are seen in secondary care mental health services. Consistent with this, in the 2007 Adult Psychiatric Morbidity Survey, only 4 per cent of people with a common mental health disorder reported a secondary care mental health appointment while 38 per cent reported having talked with their GP about their mental health problem in the last year.

Pre-IAPT mental health policy regarding common mental health problems

Starting in the late 1970s, there were developments in the UK and some European countries to provide mental health services in primary care in response to the then emerging studies indicating the prevalence and burden of mental health disorders presenting in primary care (Shepherd *et al.*, 1966; Goldberg and Huxley, 1980). Psychiatrists began to provide outpatient clinics in general practices (Strathdee and Williams, 1984), mental health nurses medication advice and psychosocial treatments (Marks, 1985; Gournay and Brooking, 1994), clinical psychologists CBT (Earll and Kincey, 1982; Robson *et al.*, 1984) and social workers case work interventions (Corney, 1984). Organisational models of community mental health nurses and clinical psychologists being attached to general practices were tried out, although it was usually a select few, enterprising, mental-health-aware, larger general practices that benefited.

These developments were put on hold in the UK with a central policy directive to focus mental health services on treatment and care of people with severe mental illness (Department of Health, 1990). Common mental health problems were, in terms of national policy, not the concern of mental health services. The national policy was associated with shift from institutional to community care and significant investment in services for severe and enduring mental health problems. The 1999 Mental Health National Service Framework (NSF; Department of Health, 1999) continued this policy trend. While the NSF acknowledged the needs of people with common mental health problems in standards 2 and 3 (identification, assessment and treatment pathways for common mental health problems), there was no new associated investment to match the extensive investment in crisis, assertive outreach and early intervention teams for people with psychosis.

The developments that did occur in treatment of common mental health problems over the two decades from 1987–2007 were mostly initiated and driven at the primary care level. GP antidepressant prescribing increased three-fold (Moore *et al.*, 2009). Enterprising GPs found ways to fund counselling and psychological therapies in their general practices from primary care sources of funding. In particular two funding sources – GP fundholding from 1990–1997 and GP health promotion clinic funding from 1993–1995 – were used by GPs to employ counsellors in general practices and led to some primary care commissioners providing mainstream support for primary care counselling services.

The one central national initiative for common mental health problems that did occur in these two decades was a 2000 NHS Plan commitment to employ 1,000 graduate primary care mental health workers 'trained in brief therapy techniques of proven effectiveness' to support GPs in managing and treating common mental problems (Department of Health, 2000, 2003). This was a late addition to the NHS Plan and arose from the realisation that there was no investment for common mental health problems, the availability of keen psychology graduates and at least one study of their effectiveness in providing brief CBT-based treatments (Appleby *et al.*, 1997). These graduate primary care mental health workers and the courses designed to train them are a significant part of the IAPT story as they were the prototypes of IAPT low intensity workers and psychological well-being practitioners in the backgrounds they came from and the type of work they did.

Drivers for change in national policy

In the period of three to four years leading up to October 2007, there were a number of key drivers for a change in policy towards investment in services for common mental health problems and in psychological therapies in particular.

The first of these was NICE's publication of clinical guidelines for the treatment of depression and anxiety disorders (NICE, 2004a, 2004b, 2005a, 2005b). On the basis of their summary of the evidence for medication and psychological therapies, these guidelines recommended CBT for all anxiety disorders and depression. Some other psychological therapies (interpersonal psychotherapy, behavioural couples therapy, counselling and structured brief psychodynamic psychotherapy) were recommended in some circumstances for the treatment of depression but not for any anxiety disorders. In addition, the NICE guidance recommended low intensity psychological interventions such as guided self-help and computerised CBT for depression and some anxiety disorders, and also recommended a stepped care approach to treatment (Bower and Gilbody, 2005) in which low intensity interventions such as these are recommended to be tried first for less severe cases.

The second driver for change was consumer concern and campaigns about very long waiting times for NHS psychological therapy, often of over a year (e.g. Bird, 2006). With the increasing success of NHS policy and initiatives in reducing waiting times for treatment in other areas (Department of Health, 2009), the very long waiting times for psychological therapies within the NHS were becoming increasingly anomalous. The concerns about availability and access to psychological therapies and the need to address these were recognised for the first time nationally in the Mental Health NSF five-year review (Department of Health, 2004).

The third key driver was an economic case developed and promoted by economists and mental health researchers. Common mental health problems were calculated to cost England at least £77 billion a year, a large element of this being state funded benefits because mental health problems are the most frequent reason for people to be on disability benefits. It was therefore argued that a government programme of investment in improved access to psychological therapies could pay for itself by helping people off benefits and into work (Layard *et al.*, 2006, 2007). This argument, supported by political lobbying of its chief proponent, Lord Richard Layard, was probably a key factor in persuading the UK Treasury to fund the national IAPT programme.

IAPT pilot demonstration sites

As the case for a change in policy gained momentum, the Department of Health funded two demonstration projects to pilot what an IAPT service might consist of and its likely impact. These were in Doncaster, a post-industrial city of 300,000 people in the North of England, and in the London Borough of Newham, an ethnically diverse area of similar population. Proposals for the services were developed in 2005 with the services starting in summer 2006 and the demonstration period lasting a year. The two services, while both setting out to provide psychological therapies in accordance with NICE guidance, initially did this in different ways (Clark *et al.*, 2009; Richards and Suckling, 2009). The Doncaster service, in part because of the lack of CBT therapists locally, focused primarily on providing NICE recommended low intensity psychological therapies for depression and anxiety disorders, the majority delivered over the telephone. In contrast, the Newham service initially just provided face-to-face CBT delivered by fully trained CBT therapists, although later added low intensity interventions in a stepped care model. The eventual national IAPT service and workforce models combine features of the Doncaster and Newham service designs.

The IAPT service and training model

Principles

The national IAPT programme is based on four principles:

*   Access: Services should ensure adequate access and equity of access to psychological interventions for the populations they are commissioned to cover.
*   Evidence-based interventions: Psychological interventions provided should be evidence-based and in a stepped care pathway, in accordance with NICE guidance.

- Outcomes monitoring and focus: Outcomes of interventions should be routinely monitored on a session-by-session basis and used in discussion with service users to plan and adjust treatment.
- Service user choice and satisfaction: Service users should be given a choice between interventions where the evidence indicates that alternative interventions are effective and appropriate (this last principle was not clearly present in the initial phases of the national programme, but has become a clear principle subsequently).

IAPT service model

Central to the IAPT service model is that the psychological therapies provided should be in accordance with the evidence-base and stepped care model set out in NICE guidance.

Stepped care is an approach to organising pathways of care based on two core principles (Bower and Gilbody, 2005). First, that interventions offered should be the least restrictive that will be effective for the problems with which an individual presents. Second, that there should be 'self-correction' monitoring and feedback systems to ensure individuals are stepped-up to more intensive interventions if they are not obtaining sufficient benefit from the initially offered treatments. The definition of 'least restrictive' may refer to the impact on patients in terms of cost and personal inconvenience, but in the context of publicly funded health care systems, where specialist therapist time is a key limiting factor, 'least restrictive' is often interpreted as referring to the amount of specialist therapist time required (i.e. treatment intensity).

Figure 12.1 sets out the stepped care model in the NICE depression guideline (NICE, 2009). The stepped care model in the updated NICE guideline for generalised anxiety disorder entirely parallels this (NICE, 2011a). IAPT services focus on step 2 and step 3 of the NICE stepped model: low intensity psychological interventions are at step 2 and CBT and other high intensity psychological therapies are at step 3. The distinction within IAPT between step 2 and step 3 is both in the amount of therapist time involved (step 2 interventions requiring fewer therapeutic sessions) and in the training of the therapists involved. Thus while in principle NICE step 2 interventions could be carried out by CBT and other trained psychological therapists, in the IAPT model there are a designated group of staff (initially called 'low intensity therapists' and latterly 'psychological wellbeing practitioners') who, without necessarily having any background in mental health or psychological therapies, receive specific training (see below) in delivery of low intensity psychological interventions.

While focusing on steps 2 and 3 of the NICE stepped care model, IAPT services are also often expected to support GPs and primary care in the identification and management of people with anxiety and depressive disorders at step 1 and to support public health in mental health awareness and promotion campaigns targeted at the whole population (sometimes referred to as a missing 'step 0' of the NICE model). At the upper end of the stepped care model, IAPT services vary in the extent to which they see people with intractable disorders who might meet the criteria for step 4 interventions. In areas where secondary care community mental health services deal with a high prevalence of psychosis, which limits their ability to see more than the most high risk cases of depression and anxiety disorders, and where specialist step 4 psychological therapy services are lacking, IAPT services will see many people who in other areas would be treated in these secondary care services. Thus, individual IAPT services are always embedded in a specific wider mental health system that determines the people referred and the options for stepping people up to other mental health services.

Figure 12.2 summarises the recommended interventions at each step for all the anxiety disorders and depression for which there was NICE guidance at the time of writing this chapter

Focus of the intervention   **Nature of the intervention**

Focus of the intervention	Nature of the intervention
STEP 4: Severe and complex[a] depression; risk to life; severe self-neglect	Medication, high-intensity psychological interventions, electroconvulsive therapy, crisis service, combined treatments, multiprofessional and inpatient care
STEP 3: Persistent subthreshold depressive symptoms or mild to moderate depression with inadequate response to initial interventions; moderate and severe depression	Medication, high-intensity psychological interventions, combined treatments, collaborative care[b] and referral for further assessment and interventions
STEP 2: Persistent subthreshold depressive symptoms; mild to moderate depression	Low-intensity psychosocial interventions, psychological interventions, medication and referral for further assessment and interventions
STEP 1: All known and suspected presentations of depression	Assessment, support, psychoeducation, active monitoring and referral for further assessment and interventions

a   Complex depression includes depression that shows an inadequate response to multiple treatments, is complicated by psychotic symptoms, and/or is associated with significant psychiatric comorbidity or psychosocial factors.
b   Only for depression where the person also has a chronic physical health problem and associated functional impairment (see 'Depression in adults with a chronic physical health problem: treatment and management' [NICE clinical guideline 91]).

Figure 12.1 NICE depression stepped care model

(NICE, 2011b). A similar list has been collated for the IAPT programme from NICE guidance (Department of Health, 2011a). The recommendations cover both low intensity and high intensity psychological interventions. What is recommended differs between conditions according to the evidence, and key to delivery of IAPT services is attention to these differences, which are sometimes subtle. For example, there is a distinction between guided self-help and non-facilitated self-help (sometimes called 'pure self-help'), the latter involving no or minimal contact with a health care professional, while guided self-help involves up to six to seven short meetings to facilitate the service user making best use of the materials. While both non-facilitated and guided self-help are recommended for Generalised Anxiety Disorder (GAD) and panic disorder, only guided self-help has been found effective for, and is recommended for, depression (one likely reason for the difference being that people with significant depression have difficulty motivating themselves to use materials on their own, while people with anxiety disorders can do this).

Examination of Figure 12.2 indicates that there are conditions where more than one type of psychological intervention is recommended at a particular step. In particular, for depression but not for any of the anxiety disorders, interpersonal psychotherapy, behavioural couples therapy, counselling and brief structured psychodynamic psychotherapy are recommended as well as CBT. The choice agenda within IAPT (developed in the context of lobbying from non–CBT psychological therapists who felt that the IAPT programme initially was focused excessively on CBT) has focused on ensuring availability and choice for service users between these alternative psychological therapies for depression (Department of Health, 2010a). However, the choice agenda applies equally to choice of different low intensity interventions (e.g. for depression between guided self-help, computerised cognitive behaviour therapy (CCBT) and psychoeducational groups).

Focus of the intervention	**Nature of the intervention**
Step 3: Persistent subthreshold depressive symptoms or mild to moderate depression that has not responded to a low-intensity intervention; initial presentation of moderate or severe depression; GAD with marked functional impairment or that has not responded to a low-intensity intervention; moderate to severe panic disorder; OCD with moderate or severe functional impairment; PTSD.	**Depression**: CBT, IPT, behavioural activation, behavioural couples therapy, counselling*, short-term psychodynamic psychotherapy*, antidepressants, combined interventions, collaborative care**, self-help groups. **GAD**: CBT, applied relaxation, drug treatment, combined interventions, self-help groups. **Panic disorder**: CBT, antidepressants, self-help groups. **OCD**: CBT (including ERP), antidepressants, combined interventions and case management, self-help groups. **PTSD**: Trauma-focused CBT, EMDR, drug treatment. **All disorders**: Support groups, befriending, rehabilitation programmes, educational and employment support services; referral for further assessment and interventions.
STEP 2: Persistent subthreshold depressive symptoms or mild to moderate depression; GAD; mild to moderate panic disorder; mild to moderate OCD; PTSD (including people with mild to moderate PTSD).	**Depression**: Individual facilitated self-help, computerised CBT, structured physical activity, group-based peer support (self-help) programmes**, non-directive counselling delivered at home[†], antidepressants, self-help groups. **GAD and panic disorder**: Individual non-facilitated and facilitated self-help, psychoeducational groups, self-help groups. **OCD**: Individual or group CBT (including ERP), self-help groups. **PTSD**: Trauma-focused CBT or EMDR. **All disorders**: Support groups, educational and employment support services; referral for further assessment and interventions.
STEP 1: All disorders – known and suspected presentations of common mental health disorders	**All disorders**: Identification, assessment, psychoeducation, active monitoring; referral for further assessment and interventions

*   Discuss with the person the uncertainty of the effectiveness of counselling and psychodynamic psychotherapy in treating depression.
**   For people with depression and a chronic physical health problem.
[†]   For women during pregnancy or the postnatal period.

Figure 12.2 Recommended NICE interventions for anxiety disorders and depression

The IAPT programme mandates routine sessional outcome monitoring for all service users using standard outcome measures. These are a measure of depression, the 9-item Patient Health Questionnaire Depression Scale (PHQ-9; Kroenke *et al.*, 2001; Gilbody *et al.*, 2007), a measure of anxiety, the 7-item Patient Health Questionnaire Generalised Anxiety Disorder Scale (GAD-7; Spitzer *et al.*, 2006; Kroenke *et al.*, 2007), an ad hoc 3-item phobia scale, and a measure of functional impairment, the Work and Social Adjustment Scale (WASAS; Mundt *et al.*, 2002). These are used to help guide treatment, including whether to step up from low to high intensity treatment and whether to end treatment, and to evaluate the overall effectiveness of the service. They are supplemented by disorder-specific measures that are more sensitive to assessing change for specific disorders (especially specific anxiety disorders).

As unemployment is associated with deterioration in mental well-being and return to employment can contribute to recovery (Murphy and Athanasou, 1999), and as the economic case for impact on reducing benefits was significant to investment in the national programme, IAPT services include a focus on employment. The service model includes employment advisors supporting IAPT therapists with dedicated provision to help both employed people on statutory sick pay and unemployed people on benefits because of mental health problems. Routine outcome measurement includes service users' employment and benefits status.

Improving access and equity of access

With the origins of the IAPT programme being on improving access, approaches to making services more accessible are not surprisingly an important part of the commissioning and delivery of IAPT services. There is a target for 15 per cent of the estimated number of people with anxiety disorders and depression (adjusted for age and gender in each primary care trust (PCT) area) to enter psychological therapy each year (Department of Health, 2010a). Systems to encourage referrals and self-referrals, outreach, reducing waiting times and other barriers to access, locating services in a range of accessible venues (e.g. GP surgeries, community centres), extending clinic hours (evening and Saturday appointments), treatment by telephone and computerised treatments that people can carry out at home, are approaches that different commissioners and services use to improve access. The endorsement and emphasis on self-referrals (Department of Health, 2010a) in particular is a departure from traditional mental health services.

In addition to improving access for the population as a whole, the IAPT programme has from its inception placed a strong focus on reducing inequalities. A variety of population groups have been identified as having particular needs and barriers to access, including: black and minority ethnic communities, older people, the lesbian, gay, bisexual and transgender community, people with medically unexplained symptoms, people with disabilities and long-term physical health conditions, new mothers, offenders, veterans and people with learning disabilities (Department of Health, 2008d; Improving Access to Psychological Therapies, 2008a). Commissioners are expected to work with public health colleagues to identify local population groups at particular risk of being under-represented from the Joint Strategic Needs Assessment and factor their needs into local service specifications. This may include commissioning third-sector community organisations to deliver IAPT services to specific populations.

In order to effect improvements in access, both across the population generally and for hard-to-reach groups, commissioners and service providers work closely with Public Health teams. This joint work has three objectives: first, to combat mental health stigma, building on the national 'Time to Change' campaign, to empower people at a community level to identify their own mental health problems and seek help; second, to promote public health messages on well-being such as healthy eating, exercise, relaxation and talking about problems, to improve general well-being and resilience across the population; and third, to raise awareness of local mental health services amongst the general public and hard-to-reach groups, with a view to improving access. In particular the public health skills in social marketing are vital to identify relevant market segments, build insight, identify achievable behavioural change goals, and design an intervention mix including communications tools and service redesign to achieve the desired behaviour change.

Different services target hard-to-reach groups and adapt interventions to improve access in different ways, dependent on local needs. Options include: translation of guided self-help materials into locally relevant languages; provision of self-referral phone line services in alternative languages; provision of interpreters including British Sign Language (BSL); linking with local community development workers to encourage referrals; voluntary sector partners 'hosting' low intensity workers to facilitate local outreach; and wide-ranging communications campaigns targeting specific population groups. A key component of improving access for hard-to-reach groups is local partnership working. Partner organisations link in strategically at local IAPT board level to foster community ownership and oversight, as well as providing practical support on the ground to strengthen referral pathways and deliver high and low intensity clinics in community locations. Partners include employment agencies, social housing providers, local voluntary groups, older people's day centres, local police and safer neighbourhood teams, door-knocking services, carer's centres, black and minority ethnic (BME) community groups, faith-based organisations, alcohol and substance misuse agencies, higher education providers, children's centres and libraries.

Public health input is also valuable at the evaluation stage. Routine sessional monitoring includes a robust set of demographic data items, including age, gender, ethnicity and postcode, to enable evaluation. The Annual Public Health Equity Audit analyses service performance data to evaluate access to the service by age, gender, ethnicity, postcode, GP practice and ward, in comparison with expected access levels based on local prevalence and population distribution. This is a vital tool in identifying gaps and deciding target groups for further outreach work over the forthcoming year.

The IAPT programme encourages user involvement in service development. Many services involve patient representatives in the service design process, at IAPT board and subcommittee meetings, on tender panels and at service management meetings. After treatment, service users are often invited to join one-off focus groups, or ongoing user involvement groups, to provide their valuable feedback and input into the way the service is run. Some services also provide peer support networks for discharged patients to network, share ideas, develop social links and support each other to maintain progress and continue self-management of ongoing problems. This is a relatively new development in primary care mental health service provision. Previous practice counselling and similar initiatives have been too small scale to allow for a fundamental focus on the user perspective in the design, management and holding to account of services.

IAPT training model

In order to deliver the IAPT programme, training courses were established to train the very large additional workforce required. Existing training capacity was insufficient or unsuitable to meet the demands. The new training courses were designed to train staff in exactly those evidence-based treatments recommended by NICE for anxiety disorders and depression. As CBT and low intensity interventions drawing on CBT were the primary treatments recommended and were the skills in shortest supply, the training programmes initially focused entirely on these.

National curricula were designed for IAPT High Intensity courses for CBT therapists and for IAPT Low Intensity courses for psychological wellbeing practitioners (Department of Health 2008b, 2008c) and an accreditation system established to ensure that courses were delivering training in accordance with the prescribed curricula. Both are one-year courses with a mixture of university-based teaching and workshops and supervised on the job learning in IAPT services. The Low Intensity courses are one day a week in college; the High Intensity courses two days a week.

Later, training funding was made available for courses in other NICE recommended treatments for depression – interpersonal psychotherapy (IPT), couples therapy for depression, counselling for depression and dynamic interpersonal psychotherapy (DIT), a structured brief psychodynamic psychotherapy for depression (Improving Access to Psychological Therapies, 2011b). These are all brief 5–10 day courses designed for psychological therapists already trained in related therapeutic approaches. So while the one-year CBT-based courses were designed to train a new workforce, these later courses were designed to adapt the skills of existing trained therapists to be able to provide NICE consistent therapies.

Evaluation

There are three main sources of data to evaluate the IAPT programme:

- Data from the two pilot demonstration sites.
- Audit of the first wave of IAPT services.
- Key performance indicator data submitted by all IAPT services over the first two years of the roll-out of the national programme.

Pilot demonstration sites

An evaluation of the two demonstration sites has been reported by Clark *et al.* (2008, 2009) with additional information and data on the Doncaster site published by Richards and Suckling (2008, 2009). Both these evaluations are by IAPT 'insiders': David Clark is national clinical lead for the IAPT programme and David Richards and Rupert Suckling were responsible for establishing and running the Doncaster service. An independent evaluation commissioned by the Service Development and Organisation (SDO) Research Programme is still awaited at the time of writing this chapter.

The evaluations were conducted a year after the services started and primarily used data collected by the services on dedicated clinical information systems designed for the pilot services. Data completeness was impressive in both services (for example 99.6 per cent of Doncaster and 88.3 per cent of Newham service users who were seen at least twice before discharge had both assessment and end of treatment clinical outcome measures completed). Various built-in characteristics of the clinical information systems enhanced data completeness and these two systems have subsequently been used by most IAPT services.

The Doncaster service, focusing on low intensity interventions, saw more people but for fewer sessions (an average of 4.9 sessions for people who attended more than once) compared to the Newham service in which the majority of people seen received a high intensity psychological therapy (average of 8.2 sessions). In each service 55–56 per cent of people recovered (had scores at assessment on the PHQ-9 or GAD-7 in the clinical range and below the clinical threshold on both these measures post-treatment), which was slightly above the 50 per cent recovery figures anticipated in the design of the programme from extrapolation from recovery rates in clinical trials of psychological therapies. A postal and telephone follow-up of all people discharged after two sessions of treatment indicated that, on the whole, recovery rates were maintained at follow-up.

The Newham service included the option of self-referral. An analysis of self-referrals indicated that they were equally as severe as GP referred cases, but had been depressed or anxious for longer and were representative of the Newham population in terms of ethnicity compared to GP referrals, which were more likely to be white. This finding of better access of ethnic groups through self-referral led to self-referral being encouraged nationally within IAPT services.

Audit of year one services

The North East Public Health Observatory was commissioned by the IAPT programme to analyse audit data from the first year of operation of the first wave of IAPT services established following establishment of the national programme (Glover *et al.*, 2010). Thirty-two services submitted data on patients seen between October 2008 and September 2009. The main analyses were on 79,310 patients who were seen at least once.

Services varied considerably in their staffing and the interventions delivered. While the median site had 45 per cent low intensity and 55 per cent high intensity staff (compared to the IAPT standard of 40:60), the interquartile range (IQR) was 36 per cent – 57 per cent low intensity staffing with the most extreme sites having 13.6 per cent and 100 per cent high intensity. A median proportion of 13.1 per cent of service users (IQR 6.4 per cent to 17.8 per cent) were stepped up from low to high intensity interventions. In terms of high intensity therapies, 58 per cent of service users received CBT and 50 per cent counselling (with 2 per cent receiving other therapies), a higher proportion of counselling than expected in the IAPT service model. Again there was variation between services with the proportion receiving CBT versus counselling varying from 100 per cent to 20 per cent.

The median recovery rate of people treated by the wave 1 sites, calculated in the same way as for the demonstration sites, was 42.2 per cent, which was lower than that for Doncaster and Newham. Services varied in their recovery rate from 30.3 per cent to 63.0 per cent. This, while suggestive, does not necessarily mean that there was a difference between services in the effectiveness of their treatments as there could have been differences between sites in their case-mix (people with higher initial depression and anxiety scores not surprisingly were much less likely to recover and the Glover *et al.* (2010) analysis did not report on case-mix differences between sites). Glover *et al.* (2010) did check on whether there were site factors that related to differences in recovery rate and found that services with a higher proportion of high intensity staff were more likely to have higher recovery rates; no other site factors were related to recovery rate but with only 32 sites the statistical power of any comparison was low.

Headline figures from key performance indicators

The original three-year IAPT Implementation Plan (Department of Health, 2008a) set out the expectation that the IAPT programme nationally should deliver:

*   Steady roll-out nationally, with at least 20 sites in 2008/09 and increasing coverage in 2009/10 and 2010/11.
*   3,600 trained therapists by 2010/11.
*   900,000 people accessing treatment, with half of those completing treatment moving to recovery and 25,000 moving off sick pay and benefits by 2010/11.

In relation to these commitments, key performance indicator (KPI) data submitted by IAPT services from inception of the national programme in October 2008 up to December 2010 indicated (Improving Access to Psychological Therapies, 2011a) that:

*   147 of the 151 primary care trusts in England had a service in at least part of their area, covering approximately 60 per cent of the adult population of England.
*   3,660 therapists have been trained.
*   491,000 people started treatment, 282,000 completed it, 95,000 moved to recovery and 18,200 came off sick pay or benefits.

A snapshot of London IAPT performance between October 2008 and August 2010 is available from the NHS London website (NHS London, 2011). In the first year, the five London wave 1 sites (Camden, City and Hackney, Ealing, Haringey, Southwark) delivered the following outcomes between October 2008 and August 2009:

*   8,787 people entered IAPT psychological therapies.
*   220 people moved off sick pay and benefits having completed IAPT treatment.

In the second year, a further ten London wave 2 sites joined the IAPT Programme (Greenwich, Hammersmith and Fulham, Islington, Lambeth, Lewisham, Newham, Sutton and Merton, Tower Hamlets, Wandsworth, Westminster). The London wave 1 and 2 sites delivered the following outcomes between September 2009 and August 2010:

- 33,972 people entered IAPT psychological therapies.
- 1,280 people moved off sick pay and benefits having completed IAPT treatment.
- 42 per cent average recovery rate amongst patients entering the service at the clinical threshold for 'caseness' and completing two or more treatment sessions (January to August 2010).

Current developments

Roll-out nationally and new areas

The original IAPT programme three-year investment was to cover half the country. The UK Government's October 2010 Spending Review settlement committed £400 million to completing the roll-out of IAPT across the rest of England. *Talking therapies: a four year plan of action* (Department of Health, 2011a) issued on 2 February 2011 as a supporting document to the new public mental health strategy *No health without mental health* (Department of Health, 2011b), gave details of the roll-out. The additional investment in PCT baselines and Strategic Health Authority (SHA) Multi professional Education and Training (MPET) budgets would provide the investment for services to cover the rest of the country and to train therapists for this. However, coming at a time of unprecedented cuts in other NHS expenditure and the new funding not being earmarked for IAPT services (unlike in the first two years of the programme), there have been doubts expressed as to whether this funding will be used by NHS commissioners to invest in IAPT services and training. Public questioning of this led to the dismissal by the government of one IAPT national advisor (*Guardian*, 2011).

Talking therapies: a four year plan of action (Department of Health, 2011a) also set out new areas for IAPT. The programme is to be expanded to include children and young people, people with long-term health conditions and medically unexplained symptoms, and people with severe mental illnesses. In each case this involves an extension of IAPT beyond its original focus on anxiety disorders and depression. For example, for children and young people, conduct disorders, self-harm and eating disorders are mentioned as well as anxiety disorders and depression. The most radical departure in the expansion is the inclusion of psychological therapies for severe mental illness, given the origin of IAPT to invest in treatment of common mental health problems neglected for two decades when mental health strategy focused on severe mental illness. However, in all these areas of expansion, any new funding from the £400 million investment is likely to be limited to training programmes in these areas. Service development is likely to be more limited and will build on existing IAPT, CAMHS, and secondary care mental health services rather than developing new services.

Data reporting

From the beginning of the IAPT programme, all services were required to collect a minimum data set (Improving Access to Psychological Therapies, 2008b). This was collected locally, with commissioners providing high level data returns only on a few national KPIs.

In April 2011 the Information Standards Board approved a revised version of the IAPT data set as a National Operational Standard (Department of Health, 2011c; Improving Access to

Psychological Therapies, 2011c). 2011/12 is a transitional year, giving time for all IAPT service providers to prepare for mandatory electronic returns of 50 data items on each service user seen to a central reporting system from April 2012. This new process will provide detailed IAPT data for central analysis, benchmarking and feedback to services, commissioners and to the public through publication of IAPT data reports on the NHS Information Centre website. The information provided to the public on issues like comparative recovery rates between services will be a first for mental health services.

Competition

The July 2010 White Paper *Equity and excellence: liberating the NHS* affirmed the government's support for competition in the NHS and set out the policy intention to extend patient choice to 'any willing provider' (Department of Health, 2010b). Plurality of providers is already a reality in IAPT provision, with commissioned IAPT services in 2011/12 being divided between different types of NHS trusts and third-sector organisations (voluntary and charitable bodies) with a very small number of private sector providers. The nature of IAPT services, without major fixed capital costs such as inpatient beds or requirement for any medical staff means they are more open to competition between providers than most mental health services. There is also a very large potential pool of psychological therapy providers – third-sector organisations providing counselling and psychological therapies and private psychological therapy group practices as well as NHS providers. Retendering of IAPT service contracts is already common and payment by results (PbR) cost per case tariffs (see below) may increase this trend. Potential benefits of increased competition and plurality of providers are value for money, access to hard-to-reach groups through third-sector providers with strong community networks, increased quality and accountability for delivery of outcomes through strengthened tendering processes, and increased patient choice in multi-provider partnership IAPT services.

Payment by results

The Department of Health is committed to the introduction of payment by results to IAPT. It is conducting a feasibility study in 2011 to test how this could best be achieved. It will also seek to ensure alignment with the 'care clustering', using diagnostic groupings for the purpose of payment by results in mental health (Department of Health, 2010c, 2011a). With the now well established use of outcome measures in IAPT services, the intention is that IAPT PbR will make use of data on clinical improvement and/or recovery in the payment mechanism, making it at least in part a true payment by results (outcomes) rather than payment by activity. Moving to an outcomes-focused payment mechanism will radically change the commissioning landscape and in principle open up the IAPT provider market to an increasing range of providers.

Learning from the IAPT programme – implications for other mental health services

In our conclusion to this chapter, we set out aspects of the IAPT programme that we consider may have learning points for other mental health services. The IAPT programme stands on the shoulders of one and half centuries of learning about the delivery of public mental health services, but as the new kid on the block may have one or two things already in its early years to pass on. We suggest four interrelated areas for attention:

- Protocolised care based on evidence.
- Stepped care.
- Assistant practitioners and their supervision.
- Outcomes focus.

The IAPT service model is highly protocol-based. The way services are structured, the treatments provided and the number of treatment sessions (and so when to end treatment) are based on evidence from NICE guidance, defined in treatment protocols. These are what are covered in IAPT training programmes and are the focus of supervision. The purpose of these protocols is to ensure that what is provided is similar to the treatments provided in successful research trials. This is not to say that the multiple co-morbidities and complex social problems that many people present are ignored, but that within such complexity it is all the more important to have a clear central target of treatment and treatment protocol to reach that target so that therapeutic efforts are not diluted in pursuing multiple goals. Clinicians are inevitably influenced by all sorts of factors in what they are drawn to deliver to an individual service user and clear protocols help keep focus and reduce variation in what is provided. By contrast, other mental health services, while they may have many clinical policies, are often lacking in clear protocols for intervention.

Stepped care is central to the IAPT service model, trying less intensive interventions first and calibrating programmes of care and the grade and skill of worker delivering the intervention to the changing needs of the service user. While there are clearly elements of calibrating care to service user needs in all mental health services, the steps are not usually so clearly defined. Also, over the past two decades, there has been a strong gate-keeping element in UK secondary mental health services leading to an all or nothing approach to care.

The majority of people seen in IAPT services will be treated, at least part of the time, only by staff with minimal mental health training (i.e. they never see, or only during some of their treatment see, a trained mental health professional). The work of these staff is guided by very clear intervention protocols and weekly intensive case supervision that focuses on adherence to the intervention protocols. This system of unqualified or minimally qualified staff working independently to highly structured protocols supervised by experienced trained staff may have pointers for how assistant practitioners might be used in other mental health services.

The focus on clinical outcomes, measured every session, is at the heart of the IAPT model. The focus on outcomes orients staff and IAPT service users to the goals of treatment and progress towards these goals. While clinical change and ultimately clinical recovery, as in IAPT services, may not be the focus of some services and service users, the approach and technology of focusing on outcomes is equally applicable to service user-defined recovery goals or other service-defined goals.

These four areas are interrelated. The outcomes focus determines the evidence-based interventions that are most likely to achieve these outcomes, and detailed protocols for delivery of these interventions make it possible for well supervised assistant practitioners to deliver many of them in a stepped care system. While these are the key message from the new IAPT kid on the block, they are also messages that will be recognised by readers from many other sources and in other chapters of this volume.

References

Andrews, G., Henderson, S. and Hall, W. (2001). Prevalence, comorbidity, disability and service utilisation: overview of the Australian mental health survey. *British Journal of Psychiatry*, 178: 145–153.

Appleby, L., Warner, R. and Faragher, B. (1997). A controlled study of fluoxetine and cognitive-behavioural counselling in the treatment of postnatal depression. *British Medical Journal*, 314: 932–936.

Bird, A. (2006). *We need to talk: the case for psychological therapy on the NHS*. London: Mental Health Foundation.

Bower, P. and Gilbody, S. (2005). Stepped care in psychological therapies: access, effectiveness and efficiency. Narrative literature review. *British Journal of Psychiatry*, 186: 11–17

Clark, D.M., Layard, R. and Smithies, R. (2008). *Improving access to psychological therapy: initial evaluation of the two demonstration sites. LSE Centre for Economic Performance Working Paper No. 1648. London: London School of Economics.*

Clark, D.M., Layard, R., Smithies, R., Richards, D.A., Suckling, R. and Wright, B. (2009). Improving access to psychological therapy: initial evaluation of two UK demonstration sites. *Behaviour Research and Therapy, 47: 910–920.*

Corney, R.H. (1984). The effectiveness of attached social workers in the management of depressed female patients in general practice. *Psychological Medicine*, 47: Monograph Supplement 6

Department of Health (1990). *The Care Programme Approach for people with a mental illness. Joint Health and Social Services Circular HC(90)23/LASSL(90)11.* London: Department of Health.

Department of Health (1999). *National service framework for mental health: modern standards and service models.* London: Department of Health.

Department of Health (2000). *The NHS Plan: a plan for investment, a plan for reform.* London: Department of Health.

Department of Health (2003). *Fast-forwarding primary care mental health: graduate primary care mental health workers.* London: Department of Health.

Department of Health (2004). *National service framework for mental health – five years on.* London: Department of Health.

Department of Health (2008a). *IAPT implementation plan: national guidelines for regional delivery.* London: Department of Health.

Department of Health (2008b). *IAPT implementation plan: curriculum for high intensity therapies workers.* London: Department of Health.

Department of Health (2008c). *IAPT implementation plan: curriculum for low intensity therapies workers.* London: Department of Health.

Department of Health (2008d). *Commissioning IAPT for the whole community.* London: Department of Health.

Department of Health (2009). *NHS referral to treatment (RTT) waiting times statistics for England: 2009 annual report.* London: Department of Health.

Department of Health (2010a). *Realising the benefits: IAPT at full roll out.* London: Department of Health.

Department of Health (2010b). *Equity and excellence: liberating the NHS.* London: Department of Health.

Department of Health (2010c). *Payment by results draft guidance for 2011–12.* London: Department of Health.

Department of Health (2011a). *Talking therapies: a four year plan of action.* London: Department of Health.

Department of Health (2011b). *No health without mental health.* London: Department of Health.

Department of Health (2011c). *Improving Access to Psychological Therapies (IAPT) data standard. London: Department of Health.*

Earll, L. and Kincey, J. (1982). Clinical psychology in general practice: a controlled trial evaluation. *Journal of the Royal College of General Practitioners*, 32: 32–37.

Gilbody, S., Richards, D. and Barkham, M. (2007). Diagnosing depression in primary care using self-completed instruments: a UK validation of the PHQ9 and CORE-OM. *British Journal of General Practice*, 57: 650–652.

Glover, G., Webb, M. and Evison, F. (2010). *Improving access to psychological therapies: a review of the progress made by sites in the first roll-out year.* Durham, UK: North East Public Health Observatory.

Goldberg, D. and Huxley, P. (1980). *Mental illness in the community: the pathway to psychiatric care.* London: Tavistock.

Goldberg, D. and Huxley, P. (1992). *Common mental health disorders: a bio-social model.* London: Tavistock.

Gournay, K. and Brooking, J. (1994). Community psychiatric nurses in primary health care. *British Journal of Psychiatry*, 165: 231–238.

Guardian (2011). Health adviser sacked for speaking out in the Guardian.7 February. Available at http://www.guardian.co.uk/society/2011/feb/07/david-richards-health-adviser-sacked (accessed 14 May 2011).

Improving Access to Psychological Therapies (2008a). Equality and Diversity Toolkit. Available at http://webarchive.nationalarchives.gov.uk/20090706163455/http://www.iapt.nhs.uk/2008/10/equality-and-diversity-toolkit/ (accessed 14 May 2011).

Improving Access to Psychological Therapies Programme (2008b). *Improving Access to Psychological Therapies (IAPT) outcomes toolkit 2008/9.* London: Improving Access to Psychological Therapies Programme

Improving Access to Psychological Therapies (2011a). About IAPT. Available at http://www.iapt.nhs.uk/about-iapt/ (accessed 14 May 2011).

Improving Access to Psychological Therapies (2011b). High Intensity Therapies. Available at http://www.iapt.nhs.uk/workforce/high-intensity/ (accessed 14 May 2011).

Improving Access to Psychological Therapies (2011c). Measuring outcomes. Available at http://www.iapt.nhs.uk/services/measuring-outcomes/ (accessed 14 May 2011).

Kessler, D., Bennewith, O., Lewis, G. and Sharp, D. (2002). Three year outcome of the detection of depression and anxiety in primary care: a longitudinal study. *British Medical Journal*, 325: 1016–1017.

Kessler, R.C., Chiu, W.T., Demler, O. *et al.* (2005). Prevalence, severity, and comorbidity of 12-month DSM-IV disorders in the National Comorbidity Survey Replication. *Archives of General Psychiatry*, 62: 617–627.

Kroenke, K., Spitzer, R.L. and Williams, J.B. (2001). The PHQ-9: validity of a brief depression severity measure. *Journal of General Internal Medicine*, 16: 606–613.

Kroenke, K., Spitzer, R.L., Williams, J.B.W., Monahan, P.O. and Lowe, B. (2007). Anxiety disorders in primary care: prevalence, impairment, comorbidity, and detection. *Annals of Internal Medicine*, 146: 317–325.

Layard, R., Bell, S., Clark, D.M., Knapp, M., Meacher, M., Priebe, S. *et al.* (2006). *The depression report: a new deal for depression and anxiety disorders.* London School of Economics, Centre for Economic Performance. Available at http://cep.lse.ac.uk (accessed 4 November 2011).

Layard, R., Clark, D.M., Knapp, M. and Mayraz, G. (2007). Cost-benefit analysis of psychological therapy. *National Institute Economic Review*, 202: 90–98.

Marks, I. (1985). Controlled trial of psychiatric nurse therapists in primary care. *British Medical Journal*, 290: 1181–1184.

McManus, S., Meltzer, H., Brugha, T., Bebbington, P. and Jenkins, R. (2009). *Adult psychiatric morbidity in England, 2007: results of a household survey.* Leeds: The NHS Information Centre for Health and Social Care.

Moore, M., Yuen, H.-M., Dunn, N., Mullee, M.A., Maskell, J. and Kendrick, T. (2009). Explaining the rise in antidepressant prescribing: a descriptive study using the general practice research database. *British Medical Journal*, 339: b3999.

Mundt, J.C., Marks, I.M., Shear, M.K. and Greist, J.M. (2002). The Work and Social Adjustment Scale: a simple measure of impairment in functioning. *British Journal of Psychiatry, 180:461–464.*

Murphy, G.C. and Athanasou, J.A. (1999). The effect of unemployment on mental health. *Journal of Occupational and Organisational Psychology*, 72: 83–99.

NHS London (2011). Mental health data. Available at http://www.london.nhs.uk/your-nhs-in-london/publishing-nhs-data/mental-health-data (accessed 14 May 2011).

NICE (2004a). *Depression: management of depression in primary and secondary care (clinical guide 23).* London: National Institute for Clinical Excellence.

NICE (2004b). *Anxiety: management of anxiety (panic disorder, with and without agoraphobia, and generalised anxiety disorder) in adults in primary, secondary and community care (clinical guidance 22).* London: National Institute for Clinical Excellence.

NICE (2005a). *Obsessive-compulsive disorder: core interventions in the treatment of obsessive-compulsive disorder and body dysmorphic disorder (clinical guideline 31).* London: National Institute for Clinical Excellence.

NICE (2005b). *Post-traumatic stress disorder (PTSD): the management of PTSD in adults and children in primary and secondary care (clinical guideline 26).* London: National Institute for Clinical Excellence.

NICE (2009). *Depression: the treatment and management of depression in adults (update) (clinical guideline 90).* London: National Institute for Clinical and Health Excellence.

NICE (2011a). *Generalised anxiety disorder and panic disorder (with or without agoraphobia) in adults: management in primary, secondary and community care (clinical guideline 113).* London: National Institute for Clinical and Health Excellence.

NICE (2011b). *Common mental health disorders: identification and pathways to care (clinical guideline 123).* London: National Institute for Clinical and Health Excellence.

Richards, D.A. and Suckling, R. (2008). Improving access to psychological therapy: the Doncaster demonstration site organisational model. *Clinical Psychology Forum, 181: 9–16.*

Richards, D.A. and Suckling, R. (2009). Improving access to psychological therapies: phase IV prospective cohorts study. *British Journal of Clinical Psychology,* 48: 377–396.

Robson, M.H., France, R. and Bland, M. (1984). Clinical psychologist in primary care: controlled clinical and economic evaluation. *British Medical Journal,* 288: 1805–1808.

Shepherd, M., Cooper, B., Brown, A.C. and Kalton, G. (1966). *Psychiatric illness in general practice.* Oxford: Oxford University Press.

Shepherd, M., Cooper, B., Brown, A.C. and Kalton, G. (1981). *Psychiatric illness in general practice.* 2nd edn. Oxford: Oxford University Press

Spitzer, R.L., Kroenke, K., Williams, J.B.W. and Lowe, B. (2006). A brief measure for assessing generalized anxiety disorder: the GAD-7. *Archives of Internal Medicine,* 166: 1092–1097.

Strathdee, G. and Williams, P. (1984). A survey of psychiatrists in primary care: the silent growth of a new service. *Journal of the Royal College of General Practitioners,* 34: 615–618.

World Health Organisation (2001). *The world health report 2001– mental health: new understanding, new hope.* Geneva: World Health Organization.

Part III
The new territory

13 Delivering new services
Changes in professional roles

Sally Hardy and Neil Brimblecombe

Introduction

This chapter considers how best to predict and influence the future public mental health and social care models of service as a means of determining what will be required of mental health professionals. We draw from existing literature in exploring the contemporary debate about achieving 'healthy' communities with mentally healthy individuals who are sustained and supported by a mental health and well-being workforce. Within the chapter the implications of an evolving approach to contemporary public mental health and social care delivery are explored. We consider the elements that influence how health care is delivered, and how they influence health professional roles. The education and training requirement for new mental health professional roles capable of delivering new services is touched upon. How these political debates promote and enable mental health and well-being of individuals, living and working within 'healthy' communities, will be used to further a critical debate on future-proofing the mental health professions.

Professional boundaries and service delivery

In recent years the concept of 'competency', as a fundamental building block to providing safe standards of practice, has been both a boon and threat to professions; offering on the one hand a way of clearly defining skill levels and associated knowledge requirements that, in turn, informs standards of professional training. However, dividing a profession's activities into myriad small competencies offers a challenge to the professions. First, in being able to articulate clearly the core components of a professional's specific contribution, then, second, the potential for this very process in allowing other groups of workers to be able to identify selected individual competencies and point out that, with suitably focused training, they too could undertake that role, perhaps more cheaply and without the legal restrictions that professionals have to apply on condition of their registration. Some welcome the demise of professional demarcations, whilst others document a strong objection to losing professional identity with the associated risk of stress and anxiety due to a lack of role clarification (Sainsbury Centre for Mental Health, 1997; Brown *et al.*, 2000).

According to Masterson (2002), each professional group undertakes a separate training (often within separate institutions) defining their own particular perspective on health and illness. This in itself has been linked to how a further separation occurs in service delivery and organisation. This separation is further witnessed in how different professions undertake specific forms of assessment and then prescribe or undertake various treatment or intervention modalities. It is perhaps this professional segregation that has led to concern that patients are frequently finding themselves having to negotiate a gap between these different service specialties, particularly when a person's care requires the engagement of services across professional or structural boundaries in services. For example, whilst waiting for a referral the patient may have treatment delayed whilst integration between letters, records and service times are negotiated. It can be compounded by the need to attend different services on different sites. Once at the appointment, the person is then expected to complete new sets of documentation (often with very similar information being recorded on each), and then being exposed to new terminology, cultures and approaches, which can all slow down a patient's progression through a complex health and social care system. In cancer care, for example, these types of processes have been recognised to increase a patient mortality, and as a result the introduction of a navigator role has been introduced to specifically help patients quickly access the care they require (Steinberg *et al.*, 2006; Freund *et al.*, 2008). This approach is now being extended and tested in other health services (Griswold *et al.*, 2010) in an attempt to improve patient experience and health outcomes.

There are in fact very few health care related tasks or activities that are specifically restricted to any one professional group, particularly as medical prescribing and other 'extended roles' have led to a widening scope of practice for nursing. Government policy continues to promote inter-professional and interagency working as its preferred option of delivering patient-focused clinical care pathways and best value for money. As a result, over the last decade professional boundaries are becoming blurred as opposed to rigidly defined. Is this the beginning of the end for professional distinction and what lessons can be learnt about professional role development?

Lessons from the past

Psychiatry emerged as a medical speciality at the end of the 18th century and found a secure power base within the county asylums from the middle of the 19th century. Medical superintendents (doctors in charge of asylums) had strict control over the activities of attendants (a group later to evolve into psychiatric/mental health nurses), the justification for which was the need to protect patients from cruelty and neglect. The medical superintendents' desire for their own enhanced professional status led to formalised training for attendants at the end of the 19th century (Nolan, 1993). In the first part of the 20th century trade unions demanded improved pay and conditions, whilst professionalising mental health nursing was a secondary priority. Reorganisation following the creation of the National Health Service in 1948 lessened the superintendents' authority and with it came a shift in the management of mental health nursing. The leadership role for psychiatrists was less clearly defined outside the hospital setting; indeed other professions often claimed greater specialist knowledge in relation to the wide range of needs that were referred to community-based services. In the community setting the professions thus joined the inter-professional jostling for 'space, attention and independence' (Coppock and Hopton, 2000).

The move towards community care allowed mental health nurses to develop greater independence, which was supported by changes in nurse education. The growth of the community mental health team in the 1980s also gave a new arena for many professions, such as clinical psychology and occupational therapy, where prior to this they had narrowly defined roles within institutional settings. In this new environment, professions needed to make claims to their expertise in particular specialist clinically focused areas. However, with more radical reviews of what mental health services should provide coming from the political arena, professional groups were again challenged about their self-defined areas of expertise.

Change and professional role developments

Following the release of the *National Service Framework for Mental Health* in 1999 (Department of Health, 1999) the government supported a range of developments to create change in the roles of mental health staff so that they could meet the requirements of the National Service Framework (NSF) specifically, such as person-centred care. Mental health professionals were challenged by the user movement, which suggested that they had established services that were often reflective of the needs of staff rather than meeting service needs. Community mental health teams worked Monday to Friday 9–5 and large numbers of individuals were seen in outpatient clinics (often by junior doctors whom they did not know).

Significantly the first major changes were proposed by psychiatrists, who were dissatisfied with their caseload size and the broad, poorly defined responsibility that they felt they had for other professionals' cases as well as their own. As a result of reviewing the situation, proposals were made (often rolled out painstakingly slowly) that led to a greater shared ownership of decision making in, for example, the community-based teams and as a result the abandonment of large outpatient clinics. Psychiatrists began to focus their attention to seeing service users with the most complex needs and offering their support to other professions to manage less complex cases (Care Services Improvement Partnership *et al.*, 2005).

The Chief Nursing Officer's (CNO) review of mental health nursing (Department of Health, 2006) advocated for a changing focus in day-to-day practice, with emphasis placed more on supporting a recovery approach rather than a traditional focus on psychiatric measures of illness. A range of new roles were also supported, in particular nurse prescribing (Dobel-Ober *et al.*, 2010).

What can be learned from this review of the history of the mental health workforce is that change is more likely to take place if professions are convinced that changes benefit workers, as well as the people they care for.

Political influence as a lever for change

The NSF (Department of Health, 1999) preceded the CNO review for mental health nursing (Department of Health, 2006) as the first document to establish mental health as a major population risk and which challenged conventional values and beliefs around how and where mental health care should or could be delivered. Mental health was for the first time positioned alongside medical conditions such as cancer, heart disease and diabetes. The NSF (Department of Health, 1999) altered the focus of care away from a 'specialist' hospital-based inpatient bias to that of a more generalist approach delivered through community-based provision. As a direct result, the value base of mental health care was challenged. First identified in the famous Water Tower speech (Enoch Powell, 1961) it was only in 2000 (some 40 years later) that a national large-scale process for closing the last few large public institutions (including mental health hospitals, orphanages and care homes) took place. These changes were sustained by a political emphasis on the contestability of public services and a need for modernisation and reform that continues as a theme in today's coalition.

Alongside this major organisational reform came a recognition that the service user, family and carer voices mattered. Service provision had previously been medically defined and organised, and how things got done revolved around professional demands and expectation. Another lesson appears to be that political interest during the decade prior to the publication of the CNO's 2006 report was around 'how to' deliver mental health care (i.e. via a rapid process of de-institutionalisation of hospital-based care to community provision). Emphasis more recently is seen to be shifting towards concern around 'how much?' in terms of cost-effective and outcome-based interventions. This continues alongside a more consistent 'who', in terms of efficiency and effectiveness of service delivery, which has moved towards consideration of inter-professional and interagency working practices.

The NSF (Department of Health, 1999) was introduced in an attempt to tackle growing population risk and subsequent economic impact on health and social care. Although this 'top down' approach was criticised, it did support major change. In attempting to develop new roles, the NSF (Department of Health, 1999) was useful in a number of ways in that it was:

- Specific: describing certain types of service to be present everywhere in England.
- Prescriptive: services being mandated with targets that had to be met.
- Supported centrally: via the establishment of the National Institute of Mental Health to actively work with services and professions to implement change.

In June, 2010 a Coalition Government was elected in England. A new mental health outcomes strategy document was launched on 2 February, 2011. The strategy emphasises what the NSF outlined through an explicit interconnectedness between the physical health and well-being of the nation's population and impact on productivity, alongside a burgeoning economic demand (estimated at between £77 billion to £110 billion per annum, when considered as a public mental health orientated intervention cost analysis).

An ethos of public mental health care outcomes

The current political emphasis remains focused on health outcomes: for the individual and subsequently for the whole nation. Mental health is therefore being relabelled as public mental health.

The quotation presented in Box 13.1 offers a clear indication of how and what the implications are for future-proofing mental health care professional roles, and how services will need to be shaped to deliver this 'socially inclusive' public mental health agenda.

No health without mental health (Department of Health, 2011), the new mental health strategy, contains many desirable goals and the change agenda will be achieved in an entirely different way from its predecessor, the NSF. *No health without mental health* has no prescriptive models or targets. Instead, change will be created through a focus on outcome measures and NICE guidance, all set within a commissioning framework. Service providers will be commissioned with the expectation that they meet measurable outcomes and comply with a range of NICE guidance. It is likely that this will need to be done within a specific financial envelope, which is likely to be a powerful force in producing change in professional roles.

In response to the 2005 government manifesto to improve access to psychological therapies the Department of Health in 2006 launched its Improving Access to Psychological Therapies (IAPT) programme. A number of related policy initiatives within the Department of Health have emphasised the importance of psychological therapies in mental health (Department of Health, 2004, 2007). Service users increasingly demand psychological therapies in a variety of forms (Sainsbury Centre for Mental Health, 2006).

Policy directives have resulted from evidence of the effectiveness of manualised psychological therapies (such as cognitive behavioural therapy (CBT) in randomised controlled trials (summarised in numerous NICE recommendations) and the evidence of the likely cost-effectiveness of investment in this area (Layard, 2006; Layard *et al.*, 2007). Early results from the IAPT pilot sites are encouraging, not only from a clinical perspective

---

Box 13.1 Public mental health and well-being

Good mental health and well-being are associated with improved outcomes for individuals including longevity, physical health, social connectedness, educational achievement, criminality, maintaining a home, employment status and productivity.

Although future costs of mental illness will double in real terms over next the next 20 years, some of this cost could be reduced by greater focus on whole-population mental health promotion and prevention, alongside early diagnosis and intervention. So what can we do?

- Use a life course approach to ensure a positive start in life and healthy adult and older years.
- Build strength, safety and resilience: address inequalities and ensure safety and security at individual, relationship, community and environmental levels.
- Develop sustainable, connected communities: create socially inclusive communities that promote social networks and environmental engagement.
- Integrate physical and mental health, reduce health-risk behaviour and promote physical activity.
- Promote purpose and participation to enhance positive well-being through a balance of physical and mental activity, relaxation, generating a positive outlook, creativity and purposeful community activity.

Source: Department of Health, 2011.

---

but also in terms of return to work and, therefore, economic effectiveness (Clark, Layard and Smithies, 2008). For further discussion see Chapter 12 (Cape and Humphries).

Within their workforce training manual, the Care Services Improvement Partnership (CSIP) and the National Workforce Program (NWP) for the National Institute for Mental Health (England) (NIMHE) (CSIP/NIMHE 2007b) consider workforce development for IAPT training, specifically the introduction of primary care graduate mental health workers and how these posts have increased in number across the country to deliver the IAPT programmes. As more services merge into the private and independent sector, the issue of retaining well trained staff of this calibre may become even more complex, particularly when social enterprise organisations are part of the commissioning and delivery of integrated services.

The IAPT programme is directly focused on NICE guidance, which describes both advised therapeutic interventions and a service model to deliver it. The service has become structured on two levels: high intensity and low intensity. Interestingly the high intensity workers come from a range of disciplines including nursing, psychology and allied health professionals taking on an entire new role, whilst the low intensity workers are not from professional health care backgrounds at all. This is a clear example where individual professionals have responded to service need and the low intensity workers suggest a future where a wider range of defined and competency-based trainings will deliver wide sections of services. The continued concern about non-regulation of 'non-professionally qualified' staff is likely to need resolution before this development reaches its maximum potential.

Future-proofing the mental health workforce

Mental health nurses make up the largest professional group in mental health services, with 48,000 registered mental health nurses working in the National Health Service in England from a total of 660,000 registered nurses (Nursing and Midwifery Council, 2011). There are also over 30,000 non-professionally qualified staff working with nurses who make a vital contribution to health care teams. Nurses work in every area of practice, and are numerically predominant in many organisations, and yet do not represent the largest salaried professional group.

Over the last few years, a number of new roles have been introduced, for example modern matrons and nurse consultants, and associated new 'advanced practice' skills (e.g. prescribing and psychosocial interventions) have been developed. These changes provide opportunities for new ways of working that can help services become more service-user-centred and effective.

Significant training and education opportunities are being identified in the literature that ten years ago were not available. Evidence around the introduction of new roles for the mental health workforce (particularly community based, prescribing and team or service leader roles) are now more readily available. Continuous professional practice development opportunities have increased in terms of choice for nurses to work and learn alongside other health practitioners that can be used to further hone and enhance knowledge and skill development post initial registration. There is uncertainty about how much funding will remain available for practitioners to access post-registration development, which will be the responsibility of NHS trusts from 2012.

Brimblecombe (2009) outlined how mental health nursing has the fastest growing number of senior practitioners attaining professorial academic posts, working both within and across higher education institutions and service providers as clinical chairs. Consultant nurse posts are increasingly being appointed, allowing highly specialised practitioners to work alongside other specialist and advanced practitioner roles. The career trajectory for mental health nurses is progressive and strong. At the same time there is a growth in training nurses to undertake psychological interventions following the success of IAPT, alongside interest in workers taking on this platform of knowledge. There is also interest in exploring the scope for non-medical prescribing. All of these developments have helped to widen the spectrum of knowledge development for a mental health profession that should be enabling a mental health nursing workforce to remain fit for purpose. Yet it remains difficult to accredit these role changes with tangible evidence of patient outcomes or improvements in service user and carer experiences with very few new roles having an integrated evaluation approach. Brimblecombe (2009) concludes that the profession has further to go in maximising the added value and patient benefit attributed from these new roles. All professions are required to identify and articulate their contribution to health care, particularly at a time when cost-efficiency and outcomes-based delivery modes align themselves well to research.

A new form of professionalism

The social inclusion and equality elements of policy directives have led to some innovative role developments being introduced in mental health. For example workers being employed specifically for their personal experience of mental health services is increasingly common, bringing particular benefits to nurse training recruitment whilst simultaneously addressing stigma and promoting core values of inclusion. Patient advocacy, responsibility for population health, the forging of new partnerships and the evidence-based health care culture, have all worked to consider what might be needed to constitute new forms of professionalism. As consumers of health care become more articulate, informed and engaged in their health care, professionals need to respond and provide care that satisfies and even retains that person's interest, trust and opinion, particularly if and when incentive payments begin to follow patient satisfaction results and their health care outcomes. Creating a new professionalism therefore includes value and attitudinal changes, as the balance of power shifts from self-serving elitism to inclusive partnership working and collaboration (as discussed by Simpson, Chapter 3) (Mechanic, 2000).

With the introduction of mental health care support workers, apprenticeships and a large reliance on non-professionally registered health care assistant roles comes a high level of cynicism that these new posts are being created as merely a cheaper workforce. What these new posts have also potentially added to is a growing concern that senior nurses are being further removed from clinical activity, taken away from the clinical context through high level demand for their time in resource management, office-based roles and associated meetings. Yet, despite this move from the clinic to the committee, few senior nurses are drawing on policy to influence strategic plans at trust board level (Callaghan *et al.*, 2010).

Increasingly there is a shared multidisciplinary focus on change, with nursing and other disciplines being asked to unite and engage together in a process of interagency working. This requires staff to be trained with a set of transferable skills that will enable them to work within different contexts of care as services move towards ensuring care can be achieved 'closer to home' (Department of Health, 2008).

Building on the capabilities framework, first introduced by NIMHE in 2004, the *Capabilities for inclusive practice* (Department of Health, 2007) has identified separate capabilities for inclusive organisation/service and for an inclusive practitioner. There is a separate capability identified for promoting recovery, but this is relatively brief, reflecting the thinking of the time. The package is comprehensive, but its guidance will only have any impact if it is taken up by the workforce, with ongoing and effective clinical supervision as a mechanism to ensure ongoing development and to help embed new skills and evidence-based practices for the new functions and roles.

Clinical supervision is identified in a lot of the literature of the last decade as a means of achieving effective practice. What effective clinical supervision means is not supervision as a process of line management, but a process for providing regular space and time in the workplace setting to allow staff to achieve a level of high support and critical reflection that is needed to counterbalance the high level of challenge experienced by staff engaged in the daily clinical activities, as well as in the organisational, structural and national change agenda (Hyrkas and Paunonen-Illmonen, 2008).

One concern with working in and across integrated multidisciplinary teams is that leadership can become diffuse (Øvretveit, 2009). Leadership is a key element that arises again and again when considering the literature on enabling sustainable innovation and improved practice change. The literature cites numerous definitions of 'leadership' and what constitutes a good and effective 'leader'. A useful working definition as a means to explore clinical leadership is: 'Leadership is seen in terms of unifying people around values and then constructing the social world for others around those values and helping people to get through change' (Stanley, 2009).

New ways of working for mental health nursing

Mental health nurses can influence health care through their sheer number: nurses being the largest single professional workforce in the health services; through being a conduit between the service users and service provision; and given their ability to provide a holistic approach to care delivery, including a bio-psychosocial approach to recovery.

Nurses throughout history have adapted to change and have influenced all aspects of health care. They are able to respond well to the changing health care needs of individuals, groups and whole communities. Below are two examples taken from the New Ways of Working (NWW) website where mental health nurse practitioners are responding flexibly to both policy reform and local population need:

> An innovative nurse consultant role provides a clinical focus for mental health workers and practice nurses working within primary care over a large geographical area (1,000 square miles). The role is to improve access to psychological interventions through training staff in the use of patient-empowering models of care, such as guided self-help and depression case management, and to provide consultation on developing computerised CBT, psycho-education and bibliotherapy services. Advice on the development of new (graduate and gateway workers) and established (practice nurse and community mental health nurse) roles has supported new ways of working within a stepped model of care.

> A nurse-led clinic, where a community psychiatric nurse (CPN), has set up a lifestyle clinic for service users. Training as a supplementary prescriber made the CPN more aware of the need to work with service users on issues such as smoking, diet and exercise, and to have discussions about medication and optimising prescribing practice in order to minimise side effects. In the clinic, Mary is able to undertake basic measurements, including blood tests, and to liaise with colleagues in primary care to manage physical health problems, such as diabetes, collaboratively.

> (NIMHE National Workforce Programme (NWP) 2009)

Critical questions

Some of the key questions for both organisations and service providers of a public mental health care agenda and the professions delivering that care will be:

* What staff competencies are needed to deliver the outcomes that we are to be measured against?
* What staff competencies are needed to provide services in a way determined by evidence such as NICE standards?
* Which professions currently have those competencies?
* Who can deliver those competencies as effectively and efficiently?
* How will those competencies be evaluated in terms of health outcome sustainability?

Meanwhile, the professions may rightly be asking themselves:

* How do/can we as a profession define, evaluate and measure our contribution to health care?
* What do we need to be able to do in the future that we do not or cannot do now?
* Is that a route that the profession wishes to take?

The future of the mental health workforce is a critical issue, as with nurse prescribing in the past. However, with a plethora of new commissioning bodies and a greater number of service providers operating, it is likely that many such debates will be at a micro level. However, if coordinated through schemes of work that collate all of these micro level debates, such a collective data set may influence and inform ongoing service developments, role evaluations and improve outcome data that can further influence the developing professions. Nursing is large enough to provide a coordinated approach, such as that achieved through the Chief Nursing Officer review (Department of Health, 2006), which can help to further shape, influence and promote new values, professionalism and evidence of the key contribution nursing can offer to contemporary health service delivery.

Summary

The factors influencing whether professional roles can and will continue to change new service delivery are complex. Looking back, history reveals that change for professions is often a slow and difficult process. The history of individual professions, the relationship between professions, the nature of the professions themselves and the availability of potential levers for change are just some of the factors that impinge on the equation. Undoubtedly, what is also highly significant in considering the possibility for future change is the specificity of what these new services will actually look like, and the attributes, competencies and attitudes that are needed from people working to deliver them.

References

Brimblecombe, N. (2009) *Is there a future for mental health nursing?* Eileen Skellern Memorial Lecture. City University. London.

Brown, B., Crawford, P., and Darongkamas, J. (2000) Blurred roles and permeable boundaries: the experience of multidisciplinary working in community mental health. *Health and Social Care in the Community* 8 (6) 425–435.

Callaghan, P,. Repper, J., Lovell, K,. Playle, J., Baker. J., Clifton, A., Shaw, T., Stacey, G., Nelson, P,. Minshull, S., Swarbick, C., Schnieder, J. and Watkins, M. (2010) *Evaluation of the Chief Nursing Officers Review of Mental Health Nursing England.* Research Report. University of Nottingham, Nottingham

Care Services Improvement Partnership, National Institute for Mental Health in England Care Workforce Programme and Royal College of Psychiatrists (2005) *New ways of working for psychiatrists: enhancing effective, person-centred services through new ways of working in multi-disciplinary and multi-agency contexts. Final report 'but not the end of the story.'* London: Department of Health.

Care Services Improvement Partnership, National Institute for Mental Health in England Care Workforce Programme and Royal College of Psychiatrists (2007a) *New ways of working for everyone: a best practice implementation guide.* London: Department of Health.

CSIP/NIMHE (2007b) *Mental health: New ways of working for everyone, developing and sustaining a capable and flexible workforce.* London: Department of Health.

Clark, D.M., Layard, R., and Smithies, R. (2008) *Improving Access to Psychological Therapy: Initial Evaluation of the Two Demonstration Sites.* LSE Centre for Economic Performance Working Paper No. 1648. http://www.iapt.nhs.uk/silo/files/improving-access-to-psychological-therapy-initial-evaluation-of-the-two-demonstration-sites.pdf Accessed xxxx

Coppock, V. and Hopton, J. (2000) *Critical perspectives on mental health.* London: Routledge.

Department of Health (1999) *National Service Framework for mental health: modern standards and service models.* London: Department of Health.

Department of Health (2004) *The NHS Improvement Plan: putting people at the heart of public services.* London: Department of Health.

Department of Health (2006) *From values to action: the Chief Nursing Officer's review of mental health nursing.* London: Department of Health.

Department of Health (2007) *Capabilities for inclusive practice.* London: Department of Health, www.socialinclusion.org.uk.

Department of Health (2008) *Delivering care closer to home: meeting the challenge.* London: Department of Health.

Department of Health (2011) *No health without mental health.* London: Department of Health.

Dobel-Ober, D., Brimblecombe, N. and Bradley, E. (2010) Nurse prescribing in mental health: national survey. *Journal of Psychiatric and Mental Health Nursing* 17, 487–493.

Freund, K.M., Battaglia, T.A., Calhoun, E., Dudley, D.J., Fiscella, K., Paskett, E,. Raich, P.C .and Roetzheim, R.G. (2008) The NCI Patient Navigation Research Program Methods, Protocol and Measures. *Cancer* 15 113 (12) 3391–3399.

Griswold, K.S., Pastore, P.A,. Homish, G.A. and Henke, A. (2010) Access to primary care: are mental health peers effective in helping patients after a psychiatric emergency? *Primary Psychiatry* 17 (6) 42–45.

Hewison, A. and Griffiths, M. (2004) Leadership development in health care: a word of caution. *Journal of Health Organization and Management 18 (6) 464–473.*

Hyrkas, K. and Paunonen-Illmonen, M. (2008) The effects of clinical supervision on the quality of care: examining the results of team supervision. *Journal of Advanced Nursing* 33 (4) 492–502.

Layard, R. (2006) The case for psychological treatment centres. *British Medical Journal* 332, 1030–1032.

Layard, R., Clark, D,. Knapp, M. and Mayraz, G. (2007) Cost–benefit analysis of psychological therapy. *National Institute Economic Review, 202, October.*

Masterson, A. (2002) Cross boundary working: a macro-political analysis of the impact on professional roles. *Journal of Clinical Nursing* 11, 331–339.

Mechanic, D. (2000) Managed care and the imperative for a new professional ethic. *Health Affairs* 19 (5) 100–111

NIMHE National Workforce Programme (NWP) (2009) *New Ways of Working for Mental Health Nursing.* http://www.healthcareworkforce.nhs.uk/nimhe/content/view/49/460/

Nolan, P. (1993) *A history of mental health nursing.* London: Chapman and Hall.

Nursing and Midwifery Council (2011) Useful information. http://www.nmc-uk.org/Registration/Useful-information/ (accessed 27 July 2011).

Øvretveit, J. (2009) *Leading improvement effectively: a review of research.* London: The Health Foundation.

Powell, E. (1961) The Rt. Hon. J. Enoch Powell. Minister of Health. Address to the National Association of Mental Health Annual Conference, 9 March 1961

Sainsbury Centre for Mental Health (1997) *Pulling together: the future roles and training of mental health staff.* London: The Sainsbury Centre for Mental Health.

Sainsbury Centre for Mental Health (2006) *Briefing 31: choice in mental health care.* In association with Kings Fund. London: Sainsbury Centre for Mental Health, http://www.centreformentalhealth.org.uk/

Stanley, D. (2009). Leadership: behind the mask. *ACORN: the Journal of Perioperative Nursing in Australia* 22 (1) 14.

Steinberg ML *et al.* (2006) Lay patient navigator programme implementation for equal accesss to cancer care and clinical trials. *American Cancer Society* 31 October, www.interscience.wiley.com.

14 Delivering physical health care in modern mental health services

What works and why we all have to bother

David P. Osborn

Introduction

The association between physical and mental health is well established and unquestionable. Yet people with mental health problems continue to suffer scandalous rates of physical health conditions, over a decade into a new millennium. People with schizophrenia or bipolar disorder die between 10 and 25 years earlier than their counterparts without mental health problems.

This chapter briefly describes the factors responsible for this premature mortality in people with mental health problems. The biggest cause of this mortality gap is cardiovascular disease as well as its modifiable risk factors, namely smoking, diabetes, hypertension and high cholesterol. This problem is further compounded by high rates of unhealthy lifestyles and the weight gaining side effects of some psychotropic medications. Although the link between cardiovascular disease and mental disorder serves as a useful paradigm for this chapter, all types of physical health care (including sexual health) should be assessed routinely in all mental health settings, from community to inpatient, across all ages and in conditions as diverse as depression, personality disorder, substance misuse and learning disability.

Mental health services must now make a difference, by consistently assessing physical health and by working closely with primary care services to manage physical conditions.

This work is at the core of the UK Government's mental health policy: *No health without mental health* (Department of Health, 2011). Modern services must prioritise this physical screening, should be familiar with which interventions can work for people with poor mental health, and the NHS must demonstrate improvement in physical health outcomes over the next five years. This chapter highlights some of the initiatives that underpin this challenging but rewarding work. We have to become more holistic, more efficient and deliver care that will consistently improve both physical and mental health, without expecting an increase in the resources – it needs to become core business.

The mortality gap

The latest Department of Health mental health strategy is reassuring in its commitment to the physical health of people with severe mental illnesses. Governments certainly have a duty to act given the high quality, alarming research evidence from around the globe. Death rates are devastating in people with schizophrenia, bipolar disorder and other long-term mental health conditions. The scale of the problem varies from study to study, but most authorities agree that the difference in life expectancy is about 10–25 years. The main cause of excess deaths is cardiovascular disease, in other words heart attacks and strokes. This is an inequality that remains frustratingly persistent.

An example of mortality findings from the United Kingdom is our own study using the General Practice Research Database (GPRD), (Osborn *et al.*, 2007a). This database includes anonymised clinical data from hundreds of real life general practices across the UK. It is a powerful resource for answering important clinical research questions, using accurate NHS records. Whilst the database is complicated to manage and to analyse, it does allow us to draw conclusions from thousands of patients without placing a huge research burden on participants. We identified around 50,000 people with severe mental illnesses such as schizophrenia in general practices. We obtained an average of five years follow-up data on these patients between 1990 and 2002. We compared their death rates from cardiovascular disease to the death rates in approximately 300,000 people without schizophrenia. The results were shocking, especially regarding young people with severe mental illness, who were three times more likely to die from a heart attack or stroke. Similarly, people aged 50–75 with schizophrenia or similar disorders were twice as likely to have died from cardiovascular disease.

The causes of poor physical health

Smoking

People with mental health problems are far more likely to smoke than the general population. All mental health professionals are aware of this link from their clinical experience. Smoking probably underpins much of the association between poor mental health and cardiovascular disease. It also explains high rates of respiratory disease, including pneumonia, and, given the price of cigarettes, smoking also renders people with mental health problems economically even poorer. Rates of smoking are between 50 and 80 per cent in people with schizophrenia, while the general population rate is now less than one in four.

Smoking is one of the most important health considerations for people with long-term mental health conditions. Nicotine dependence can be a challenge when people require admission to hospital since all mental health units in the UK must be smoke free by law. The law was introduced in 2008, and many people working in services thought it would be an impossible change to impose in mental health settings (Ratschen *et al.*, 2009). In fact, smoke free policy is now fully implemented in UK mental health care, with far fewer problems than predicted by cynics. Most units are smoke free and many do not have smoking areas available. This demonstrated that cultural change is achievable in mental health services, despite stigmatising attitudes that it is impossible with this group of patients. The smoking ban means that mental health professionals in inpatient settings need the skills to support people with mental health conditions to stop smoking, either temporarily or in the long term. Smoking also acts as an enzyme inducer in the liver. This means that smoking may increase the rate at which the body breaks down some medications including antipsychotics such as clozapine. Nursing staff need to be aware of this fact when patients stop or start smoking, for instance if they are admitted to a psychiatric inpatient unit. For example, if a patient stops smoking, their liver will no longer be stimulated into breaking down clozapine. As a result, the levels of clozapine in the bloodstream will increase, despite the oral dose remaining the same. This may have an impact on side effects for the patient. All patients have their smoking status recorded on admission as part of the screening process. This also acts as an opportunity for a brief discussion regarding smoking, which may also increase an individual's motivation to seek help quitting. The impact of smoking cessation interventions for people with severe mental illnesses is reviewed later.

Obesity

Weight gain is one of the biggest concerns raised by people with mental health problems. For some, it is a result of the psychotropic medication that they take for treatment and long-term maintenance of their disorders. Weight gain is a side effect of some mood stabilising medications such as lithium and valproate, which are used in bipolar affective disorder, as well as some antidepressants such as mirtazepine and the tricylics. An element of this weight gain is driven by increases in appetite. This is compounded by the fact that people with disorders such as schizophrenia are more likely to eat unhealthily and take less exercise.

Our general practice research in inner city London highlighted the problem: we invited people with and without long-term mental health problems to complete standard and validated diet and exercise questionnaires. People with schizophrenia stated that they were more likely to eat fatty foods and ate far less fibre-containing foods such as fruit and vegetables. Meanwhile they were also far less likely to take even mild exercise such as walking somewhere slowly for 15 minutes at a time (Osborn *et al.*, 2007b).

This research took place almost a decade ago, and since that time the bigger story has been the advent of the second generation antipsychotics (SGAs) from the mid to late nineties. The SGAs were hailed as an advance on account of their decreased likelihood to cause Parkinson-like side effects, including rigidity and tremor. By 2002, the SGAs were recommended as first line treatment for schizophrenia by the National Institute for Health and Excellence (NICE), in their schizophrenia guideline (National Institute for Clinical Excellence, 2002). However, it quickly became apparent that these medications had the potential to induce rapid weight gain. Patients taking medications such as olanzapine and clozapine may put on up to 5kg in the first five weeks of a prescription. The effects of this weight gain may be seen many years down the line and can extend to diabetes and hypercholestrolaemia, each with their own impact on rates of cardiovascular disease. Obesity also affects multiple domains of physical health as well as impacting on both mental health and well-being. It is therefore the business of all mental health professionals to be aware of weight gain, to measure it and to help overweight patients to access interventions to decrease their weight. The first step is to ensure that patients are offered a measurement of body mass index (BMI) when medication is commenced and at regular in intervals thereafter, preferable monthly for the initial three months. This should be accompanied by a glucose measurement, assessment of total cholesterol and high density lipoprotein (HDL) cholesterol. Random samples are fine, over and above fasting levels, at least in the first instance.

Diabetes and abnormal lipids and mental health

The relationship between diabetes and poor mental health is of huge clinical significance. People with diabetes are far more likely to suffer with common mental disorders such as depression and anxiety (Barnard *et al.*, 2006; Das-Munshi *et al.*, 2007). There is also compelling evidence that when the two conditions co-exist, patients have far worse outcomes in terms of both their mental health but also their physical health. This is true in terms of both long-term glycaemic control and cardiovascular events. For this reason, primary care services are expected to screen people with diabetes for mental health conditions and there has been a concerted research effort to find interventions that will improve physical and mental health in this group of patients.

There is also an important relationship between severe mental illnesses, such as schizophrenia and diabetes. This has been described anecdotally in the literature for over a century, but better epidemiological research has recently estimated that people with schizophrenia have a two to fourfold increased risk of diabetes (Osborn *et al.*, 2008). Various hypotheses have been cited, including possible common genetic pathways for the conditions, unhealthy lifestyles that predispose to diabetes as well as the roles of SGAs and indeed poverty and social deprivation. It certainly seems that SGAs may play a part in the high rates of diabetes, but the main message is that all people with severe mental illnesses should be screened for diabetes. Similarly it seems that rates of abnormal lipids and of hypertension are worryingly high in people with poor mental health (McEvoy *et al.*, 2005). When we have explored the roles of smoking and social deprivation in our own research, we find that all these factors are important, but none of them totally explains the relationship between poor mental and physical health (Osborn *et al.*, 2007a). This question is of academic and aetiological importance, but in the context of service design, there is one important message: many (if not all) of the modifiable risk factors for cardiovascular disease are present in excess in people with poor mental health. Services must therefore ensure that these risk factors are assessed and then managed appropriately.

Sexual health and infectious diseases

The importance of sexual health in people with mental health problems is finally gaining the attention it requires. This is partly on account of the high rates of sexual side effects that may occur with medications including both antidepressants and antipsychotics. Some antidepressants may impair ability to achieve orgasm, while antipsychotics may also induce menstrual abnormalities and erectile dysfunction. This is particularly true for the antipsychotics most likely to cause hyperprolactinaemia, through their central blockade of dopamine. These include most of the first generation antipsychotics, as well as the SGAs risperidone and amisulpride. It is essential that staff routinely enquire about sexual function in people prescribed these agents, since dose adjustment or a change in agent can often overcome the problem. Prolactin levels should be taken where appropriate with advice given regarding the implications of raised prolactin levels in the short and longer term (Peveler *et al.*, 2008). While some staff may not always feel comfortable exploring these side effects, if they are ignored it is unreasonable to expect service users to adhere to the prescribed medication regime.

Blood borne viruses

Infectious, blood borne conditions (including HIV and hepatitis B and C) are a further important, yet frequently ignored, focus. In the UK *physical health* care services, routine (opt out) testing is often offered for these infections in certain localities, on account of the high density of people who come from populations with a high risk of infection. In mental health services, especially those in inner city areas, it is often the case that many patients come from these higher risk communities. Yet screening for blood borne viruses is rarely routinely offered within mental health services. There is evidence that many mental health practitioners lack confidence in offering such services to their patients, while acknowledging the importance of this work (Hughes and Gray, 2008). However, all contacts with services offer an opportunity for early detection of infection, which can in turn lead to increased survival through effective treatments.

The key is effective training, incorporating routine offers of screening within general mental health practice as well as primary care. This requires suitable arrangements with pathology laboratories and close liaison with local HIV and infectious disease services for aftercare and support.

I will now turn to some of the barriers to the provision of adequate physical health care for people with severe mental illness, before addressing the most important question for mental health services: what works in terms of preventing and decreasing rates of poor physical health?

Access to physical health care and stigma

The stigma of mental health care is one of the highest priorities in helping people with poor mental health over the next decade. It is one of the six objectives of the UK Government's 2011 mental health strategy (Department of Health, 2011): namely that fewer people will experience stigma and discrimination and that public understanding of mental health will improve. The latter goal is tied into the successful Time to Change campaign, led by Rethink, the severe mental illness charity (Rethink, undated).

Stigma may play a potent part in the negative experience of some service users when accessing services for their physical health. The Disability Rights Commission used the term 'diagnostic overshadowing' to describe the way that people with mental health problems or learning difficulties experience care. When they consult for physical problems, they find that the health professional only concentrates on their psychological symptoms such as hearing voices or feeling suicidal, and that their physical health is ignored (Disability Rights Commission, 2006). Despite attending to discuss a chest problem or screening tests, they feel short-changed by their interaction and the care they receive. This story is too commonly repeated by service users when I attend meetings to discuss physical health research.

This term, diagnostic overshadowing, is usually used to describe interactions with the providers of emergency services or primary care services. We do know that people with severe mental illnesses may be less likely to be screened for physical conditions in primary care. Roberts *et al.* (2007) examined the GP notes of 195 people with schizophrenia in Birmingham and found that recording of blood pressure weight and lipids are much lower than in the general population.

This either means that GPs are not offering tests to people with severe mental illness, or that service users are declining the tests. However, although professionals may assume that people with mental health problems are not interested in their physical health, we have shown this really is not true.

We explored this hypothesis by inviting people in general practices to attend their surgery for a healthy heart check test, including a cholesterol and glucose measurement and a calculation of their overall cardiovascular risk. We aimed to assess whether people with schizophrenia were less likely to attend the check. Contrary to stereotypical attitudes, people with illnesses like schizophrenia were not less likely to attend the test than the general population. The difference in attendance rates differed by less that 6 per cent between the two groups (Osborn *et al.*, 2003).

Addressing some of these negative beliefs about people with mental health problems is an important focus for modern mental health services. We have a duty to ensure that service users are accessing primary care and also that they receive basic screening when they are admitted to our services or when we are prescribing medications that may cause adverse side effects, such as weight gain.

The roles and responsibilities of primary and secondary care mental health services in providing physical care

Since people with long-term mental health problems have high rates of physical health problems, they require routine screening for these conditions. The interface between primary and secondary care services is a crucial consideration in service delivery.

The NICE guidelines for both schizophrenia and bipolar affective disorder are clear in respect of responsibilities. Both documents recommend that people with severe mental illnesses receive an annual physical screen from their GP, and that this focuses on cardiovascular risk (NICE, 2006, 2009).

The schizophrenia guidelines of 2009 also state that the GP should send the physical health results, such as blood tests and BMI, to mental health services. However, NICE guidelines do not necessarily produce immediate changes in routine clinical practice; the lag between publication of guidelines and implementation may stretch for many years. In primary care, the other driver for improving care has been the GP contract of 2004 and the associated Quality and Outcomes Framework (QOF), which remunerates GPs for the care of specific conditions. In mental health, GPs are expected to keep a register of all people with severe mental illness under their care. They are also expected, and remunerated, for providing an annual review.

We recently completed a national study exploring whether there had been improvements in physical health care since the introduction of QOF in England, namely since 2004. We identified almost 20,000 people with severe mental illnesses, including schizophrenia and bipolar affective disorder, in a primary care database called the Health Improvement Network (Osborn et al., 2011). We compared annual rates of screening for blood pressure, glucose, blood pressure and cholesterol between 2000 and 2007, before and after QOF, in approximately 400 general practices across the country and representing diverse areas in terms of deprivation. There were reassuring improvements in the rates of screening for all these risk factors over the follow-up period, year on year. At the beginning of the decade, there were systematic inequalities where people with severe mental illness were less likely to be screened for BMI and other risk factors. But by 2007 people with severe mental illnesses were *more likely* to be screened by their GP than their counterparts in the general population without major mental health problems. However, there was a worrying finding for the subgroup of people over 60 with schizophrenia or bipolar disorder. They were still less likely to receive screening, again compared to a general population comparison group. Our conclusion was that rates of screening are at their highest in the general population over 60 since it is this group who are most at risk of heart disease. When these age groups were considered, people with mental health problems again appear to suffer inequitable care in the UK. In a sub-analysis, we explored whether inequalities were more pronounced in areas of the UK that were more socially deprived. In fact we found no differences in rates of screening for cardiovascular risk factors such as BMI in these more deprived areas, suggesting that GPs in those areas seem to be serving their patients with schizophrenia equally well.

So while primary care is expected to provide physical health care, and QOF has delivered tangible improvement in the quality of care for people with severe mental illness, there are still important roles for secondary care mental health services in the domains of physical health.

These responsibilities include making sure that people with mental health problems are accessing appropriate screening and once screened that they receive support in accessing interventions that are effective, personalised and free from stigma. This may require key workers to act as advocates for people with mental health problems, arranging and attending meetings and helping to ensure the user's perspective is taken on board. Many mental health professionals express that they are interested in physical health care, but that they lack the skills to intervene if they detect abnormal risk factors such as high blood pressure or high cholesterol. It is here that the mental health professional (MHP) has a facilitator role, ensuring that the patient accesses the GP for up-to-date treatment and advice, and supporting them in accessing this care.

Furthermore, mental health services have a role in the provision of adequate screening and physical assessment within their own services. The following section describes how mental health services can contribute to basic physical health care when people use their services. It also addresses some of the evidence regarding interventions for weight gain, for smoking and other physical health problems in people with the most severe mental health problems.

What physical care can specialist mental health services provide in a climate of efficiency?

Routine physical assessment is part of the holistic care that modern mental health services should be providing across the board, whatever the clinical, political and economic climate. Patients die on mental health wards and in the community, often without receiving adequate standards of basic screening and health interventions. As the NHS expects greater quality, and productivity, we must all ensure that standards of physical health care retain their priority within our services.

Modern acute services

Acute admissions have always offered an incredible opportunity for the identification of physical health problems that may be related, or coincidental, to the mental health presentation. All service users' carers and families expect physical health to be routinely considered.

Where medical input is available, a full medical history and examination should always be offered, as soon as possible and as an emergency if there are signs or symptoms of acute physical need. Sadly, examinations are often neglected in acute settings, and not necessarily because the patient refuses them. Although an acute, agitated presentation occasionally means that a full exam is not possible within the first few hours of admission, it is essential that physical health is revisited later on (Iwata *et al.*, 2011). We know that patients who lack insight to their condition are more likely to refuse examinations, but we need systems that ensure that physical health is revisited regularly among patients who initially refuse. I have spent the last decade stressing that physical examinations and investigations should be performed in isolation; they must be targeted and based on a physical history. This is where most medical diagnoses are made.

All patients should be offered physical observations including BMI, blood pressure, pulse and temperature. This requires up-to-date training packages for staff and systems to ensure that equipment is adequate, modern and well maintained. Other investigations should be tailored to peoples' age, physical condition and history (including metabolic and sexual dysfunction) as well as the possible side effects of any psychotropic medication they are taking. This is standard good mental health care.

Incentivising physical health monitoring in secondary care

Rates of physical examinations are now being maintained in many NHS localities by including them in Commissioning for Quality and Innovation (CQUIN) targets, on which trusts depend for a percentage of their financial remuneration. The CQUIN indicators (which reward trusts for excellence) often include a minimum rate for physical examinations on inpatient wards within certain time frames, for example the first 72 hours (perhaps setting a target of 85 per cent). In other NHS mental health trusts CQUIN indicators have included payments for recording all patients in community mental health teams who are also on primary care registers for chronic physical health problems such as cardiovascular disease or indeed chronic obstructive pulmonary disease. Only by knowing this information can the key worker support that person in obtaining high quality care.

Physical assessments in settings where medical or nursing input is less readily accessible

As our services diversify and modernise, there are elements of the service that have rightly moved away from the medical model. Some services are increasingly staffed by non-clinical support workers, and clinical and medical time may be more limited. However, it is inconceivable that people using these modern services should expect inferior standards of physical health care. Planners, commissioners and service managers must ensure that physical health care is always embedded within these new services, in terms of policy, staffing, training and availability of equipment.

A first example is crisis resolution teams, whose aim is to provide an alternative to inpatient admission for people experiencing acute mental health crises. Inpatient care is unpopular with service users and expensive, and the option to offer intensive treatment at home is highly valued for many. However, it must not be at the expense of robust holistic care. If crisis teams are truly an alternative to admission, they must provide similar quality services including physical assessment, examination and monitoring. They should ensure that this assessment is performed on admission, be it by the GP, the junior doctor in accident and emergency, or whoever else refers to the team. The team must be flexible, according to each individual's needs and care pathway, but they must be systematic in ensuring each assessment is complete. This includes completing a physical care plan for ongoing monitoring, depending on the findings of the initial assessment.

The same is true for other alternative services to admission such as crisis houses, which are increasing in frequency throughout the UK. These houses are usually smaller units outside general medical or mental health trusts, and several do not routinely offer physical assessments (Johnson *et al.*, 2009). Given the inequalities in physical health suffered by this population, lack of physical facilities may be a missed opportunity in modern alternatives such as crisis houses. Each provider needs to consider their role in facilitating both assessment and access to ongoing physical health care.

Tools are available for physical health assessment and screening that can be employed in acute and community settings. I am a huge proponent of the Physical Health Check tool, which was developed by Rethink, the severe mental illness charity, and is freely available to download from their website (Rethink, 2008). The tool assists non-clinicians to enquire regarding 1) current physical problems, and 2) access to preventative health care including screening for cardiovascular risk factors, cancer and oral health. Finally it allows the clinicians to make a plan to act on any findings of omissions. With tools as straightforward and helpful as this, there is no excuse for anyone working with people with mental health problems to avoid asking about physical health, whatever their level of clinical training or confidence.

What interventions could improve physical health in modern mental health settings?

There is a consensus that most physical health care for service users with mental health problems should be delivered by the experts in primary care. In the current NHS climate of efficiency and quality, mental health staff must equip themselves with the knowledge to steer and signpost their clients to the best services available. This means being able to offer brief interventions regarding smoking, diet and exercise, and guide patients towards healthier lifestyle options. This is true in inpatient settings as well as in the community. It is particularly important for people who require longer term residential care, where access to primary care may be more limited.

We know that interventions for smoking and weight reduction can be successful in people with severe mental illnesses (Faulkner *et al.*, 2007; Banham and Gilbody, 2010). One challenge is to overcome the negative thinking and stigma about people with severe mental illness. Many of them rate their physical health as important. There is some evidence that people with psychosis are more likely to perceive the influences on their physical health as external to their own locus of control (Buhagiar *et al.*, 2011). If this research is true, then all mental health staff might have an impact by routinely assessing simple physical health outcomes and helping their clients to regain a sense of agency regarding their own health. This work fits neatly within the philosophy of recovery: it is collaborative and holistic and free of extra cost.

Can we expect extra specialist services for improving physical health in mental health services?

It seems unlikely that extra staffing costs will be forthcoming for physical health care within modern health services, in an era of austerity and efficiency. We must now show that we are delivering simple physical care as part of our core holistic business along with our excellent psychological treatments, positive risk taking and modern person-centred care. Perhaps it is stigmatising not to expect all mental health professionals to possess essential physical health competencies. We would not allow such omissions in other areas of health care. We expect all health visitors to be able to detect post-natal depression, we expect practice nurses to detect depression in their diabetes clinics and we expect GPs to detect early psychosis. Why shouldn't we expect mental health professionals to be able to discuss smoking, to record weight changes, to ask about sexual function, to screen for common medical conditions and to request tests for side effects alongside their other, wide-ranging skills?

Much intervention research in the last decade has focused on the addition of specialist staff into mental health teams, either receiving referrals to deliver well-being work with people with psychosis (Smith *et al.*, 2007), or organising screening for all people in community teams (Osborn *et al.*, 2010). The problem is that when these staff move on from their teams, their impact is probably not maintained. They have not instilled skills in their team mates because they have done the work *on their behalf* rather than *alongside them*.

Physical health must remain on the agenda of mental health trusts and this means managers, policy makers and commissioners must focus on whether basic physical assessments and interventions are being provided throughout their services. The rest will fall into place. Professionals should not be expected to perform care outside their expertise, but everyone should be capable of forming a basic physical care action plan. We can't rely on other staff to come in from elsewhere to perform these straightforward tasks for us.

So how do we maintain quality in physical health care? There are several local options, including the incentivisation of physical health care in wards, crisis teams and community settings. Repeated audits of basic physical health care across all services remain essential. These audits must be locally determined and tailored to the setting, for example blood borne infections for some people who misuse substances or malnutrition in people with dementia.

One cheering, national intervention, which is relatively cost neutral, has been the work of the Prescribing Observatory for Mental Health (POMH-UK), based at the Royal College of Psychiatrists centre for care and quality improvement. Mental health trusts can sign up to a variety of basic audits aimed at improving aspects of psychiatric prescribing, and these trusts receive feedback on their performance as well as benchmarking against other trusts. One example is the impact of their audits on measurement of side effects of the SGAs, which were described earlier in this chapter. Measurement of glucose, cholesterol, blood pressure and BMI was assessed in assertive outreach teams across the country. The results were fed back to the teams and when POMH-UK organised their re-audit, rates of measurement of risk factors had increased across the board (Barnes *et al.*, 2008). In other words, simple interventions can make a huge difference to behaviour within mental health services. They need to be sustained, audited and they need to be rewarded. We must not allow diagnostic shadowing to return to mental health services, but we must keep our guard. The mind–body divide has been around for centuries, and most mental services are now organised and delivered separately from services for the 'body'. But we have begun to win the battle whereby physical health outcomes are seen as importantly as mental health outcomes in the people who use our services. We must not allow a return to the dark days where mental health services viewed physical health care as an 'add on' rather than its core business.

References

Banham, L. and Gilbody, S. (2010) Smoking cessation in severe mental illness: what works? *Addition*; 105: 1176–1189.

Barnard, K.D., Skinner, T.C. and Peveler, R. (2006) The prevalence of co-morbid depression in adults with type 1 diabetes: systematic literature review. *Diabet Med*; 23: 445–448.

Barnes, T.R.E., Paton, C., Hancock, E., Cavanagh, M.R., Taylor, D. and Lelliott. P., on behalf of the UK Prescribing Observatory for Mental Health (2008) Screening for the metabolic syndrome in community psychiatric patients prescribed antipsychotics: a quality improvement programme. *Acta Psychiatrica Scandinavica*; 118: 26–33.

Buhagiar, K., Parsonage, L. and Osborn, D.P. (2011) Attitudes towards physical health in people with severe mental illness: a cross-sectional comparative study. *BMC Psychiatry*; 11:104.

Das-Munshi, J., Stewart, R., Ismail, K., Bebbington, P.E., Jenkins, R. and Prince, M.J. (2007) Diabetes, common mental disorders, and disability: findings from the UK National Psychiatric Morbidity Survey. *Psychosom Med*; 69: 543–550.

Department of Health (2011) *No health without mental health*. London: Department of Health.

Disability Rights Commission (2006) *Equal treatment: closing the gap. A formal investigation into physical health inequalities experienced by people with learning difficulties and mental health problems*. London: Disability Rights Commission.

Faulkner, G., Cohn, T. and Remington, G. (2007) Interventions to reduce weight gain in schizophrenia. *Schizophr Bull*; 33: 654–656.

Hughes, E. and Gray, R. (2008) HIV prevention for people with serious mental illness: a survey of mental health workers' attitudes, knowledge and practice. *Journal of Clinical Nursing*; 18: 591–600.

Iwata, K., Strydom, A. and Osborn, D. (2011) Insight and other predictors of physical examination refusal in psychotic illness. *J Ment Health*; 20 (4): 319–327.

Johnson, S,. Gilburt, H., Lloyd-Evans, B., Boardman, J., Leese, M., Osborn, D.P,. Shepherd, G,. Thornicroft, G. and Slade, M. (2009) Inpatient and residential alternatives to standard acute wards in England. The Alternatives Study 1. *British Journal of Psychiatry*; 194: 456–463.

McEvoy, J.P., Meyer, J.M., Goff, D.C., Nasrallah, H.A., Davis, S.M., Sullivan, L., Meltzer, H.Y,. Hsiao, J., Stroup, T.S. and Lieberman, J.A. (2005) Prevalence of the metabolic syndrome in patients with schizophrenia: baseline results from the Clinic Antipsychotics Trials of Intervention Effectiveness (CATIE) schizophrenia trial and comparison with national estimates from NHANES III. *Schizophrenia Research*; 80:19–32.

National Institute for Clinical Excellence (2002) *Schizophrenia: core interventions in the treatment and management of schizophrenia in primary and secondary care. Clinical Guideline 1*. London: NICE. www.nice.org.uk.

National Institute for Clinical Excellence (2009) *Schizophrenia: core interventions in the treatment and management of schizophrenia in primary and secondary care (update). Clinical Guideline 82*. London: NICE. www.nice.org.uk/cg82.

National Institute for Health and Clinical Excellence (2006) *The management of bipolar disorder in adults, children and adolescents, in primary and secondary care. Clinical Guideline 38*. http://guidance.nice.org.uk/CG38.

Osborn, D.P.J., King, M.B. and Nazareth, I. (2003) Participation in cardiovascular risk screening by people with schizophrenia or similar mental illnesses. A cross sectional study in general practice. *BMJ*; 326: 1122–1123.

Osborn, D.P.J., Levy, G., Nazareth, I., Petersen, I., Islam, A. and King, M. (2007a) Relative risk of cardiovascular and cancer mortality in people with severe mental illness from the United Kingdom's General Practice Research Database. *Archives of General Psychiatry*; 64: 242–249.

Osborn, D.P.J., King, M.B. and Nazareth, I. (2007b) Physical activity, dietary habits and coronary heart disease risk factor knowledge amongst people with severe mental illness. A cross sectional comparative study in primary care. *Social Psychiatry and Psychiatric Epidemiology*; 42(10): 787–793.

Osborn, D.P.J., Wright, C.A., Levy, G,. King, M.B., Deo, R. and Nazareth, I. (2008) Relative risk of diabetes, dyslipidaemia, hypertension and the metabolic syndrome in people with severe mental illnesses. Systematic review and metaanalysis. *BMC Psychiatry*; 8: 843.

Osborn, D.P.J., Nazareth, I., Wright, C.A. and King, M.B. (2010) Impact of a nurse-led intervention to improve screening for cardiovascular risk factors in people with severe mental illnesses. Phase-two cluster randomised feasibility trial of Community Mental Health Teams. *BMC Health Services Research*; 10: 61.

Osborn, D.P.J., Baio, G., Walters, K., Petersen, I., Limburg, H., Raine, R. and Nazareth, I. (2011) Inequalities in the provision of cardiovascular screening to people with severe mental illnesses in primary care. Cohort study in the United Kingdom THIN Primary Care Database 2000–2007. *Schizophrenia Research*; 129(2–3): 104–110.

Peveler, R.C., Branford, D., Citrome, L., Fitzgerald, P,. Harvey, P.W., Holt, R.I.G., Howard, L., Kohen, D., Jones, I., O'Keane, V., Pariante, C., Pendlebury, J., Smith, S. and Yeomans, D. (2008) Antipsychotics and hyperprolactinaemia: clinical recommendations. *J Psychopharmacol*; 22(Suppl): 98–103.

Ratschen, E., Britton, J. and McNeill, A. (2009) Implementation of smoke-free policies in mental health in-patient settings in England. *The British Journal of Psychiatry*; 194: 547–551.

Rethink (2008) The Physical Health Check. http://www.rethink.org/how_we_can_help/research/research_themes/physical_health_chec.html.

Rethink (undated) Time to Change. http://www.time-to-change.org.uk/home.

Roberts, L., Roalfe, A., Wilson, S. and Lester, H. (2007) Physical health care of patients with schizophrenia in primary care: a comparative study. *Family Practice*; 24(1): 34–40.

Smith, S., Yeomans, D., Bushe, C.J., Erikkson, C., Holmes, R., *et al.* (2007). A well-being programme in severe mental illness. Reducing risk for physical ill-health: a post-programme service evaluation at 2 years. *European Psychiatry*; 61(12):1971–8.

15 Commissioning new mental health services

David Jobbins

Introduction

This chapter aims to set out how mental health commissioning has developed over the last 25 years in order to give an understanding of how services have developed over that time. The chapter then concludes by considering the impact of changes occurring in 2011 and how this may impact on the way that services may further develop and also the type of services these may be.

In 2011 the NHS is probably undergoing its most profound changes since its inception in 1948. As well as being fundamental in their concept the changes envisaged in the current Health and Social Care Bill (Department of Health, 2011a) have still to be enshrined in law as this chapter is being written. There is still considerable discussion about the possible amendments to be considered in the legislation as it continues its journey through parliament and also about what this will mean in terms of translating the legislation into implementation across the country.

It is within this context that this chapter considers what could happen in the commissioning of mental health services and what new types of service may emerge. It is therefore important to state that this is a piece that discusses possible options but has no unique knowledge of what is intended to come into place over the next two years. Before considering these options and what they might look like it is worth reviewing what is already in place and the changes that have occurred over the last 20 years.

The development of mental health commissioning between the 1980s and 2010

Commissioning in the NHS first commenced as part of the 1990 NHS reforms (Department of Health, 1990) that saw the creation of NHS trusts and the purchaser–provider split. Previously district health authorities directly managed hospital and community services for their area. What was known as the purchaser–provider split was the process where provider units became separately managed NHS trusts, with contracting functions together with other functions like public health remaining in district health authorities as the first part of creating a commissioning environment in the NHS. Whilst this was applied to all services provided by the NHS except primary care, it was clear that the main focus at that time was general acute services where there were more immediate cost pressures. For mental health a much more important development was the introduction of Care in the Community. Care in the Community was the policy by which patients with serious mental health problems and physical and learning disabilities moved from long-term care in institutions to more community- or home-based care. The policy was developed in the Department of Health White Paper *Caring for People: Community Care in the next Decade and Beyond* (1989) and passed into legislation in the 1990 Act. This played a fundamental role in the change and evolution of UK mental health services and ensured continued momentum in the drive to close the old long-stay mental illness institutions that then sat at the core of mental health provision. It was also the case that mental health was often not the focus of the other key plank of the 1991 Health Act. This was the introduction of GP fundholding, which gave GPs the opportunity to take on commissioning responsibilities for particular service areas for their patients. In general, fundholding practices focused on particular areas of general acute activity rather than mental health services although it is worth noting that many practices established a variety of counselling services from the savings derived from fundholding commissioning activity.

It can therefore be argued that less time and resource was committed to the development of mental health commissioning during the 1990s and meant that the contractual relationship between the commissioner and the provider developed in a very different way to that for general acute services. The principle at the heart of the mental health service level agreement, or contract, has been to meet local service requirements, if not all local need, within a total sum of money. This made it challenging for both the commissioner and the provider to define what good performance actually looked like or for consensus to be reached on where a contract was over or underperforming.

To some extent the developments in mental health from the mid-1990s to the mid-2000s may have hidden this issue. The key changes during this period were the *Mental Health National Service Framework* (NSF; Department of Health, 1999) and the growth of joint commissioning in mental health across the country. Whilst it is true that not all areas of the country have a joint commissioner who manages both health and social care contracts, this appears to be the case in most of the country and there is a general acceptance that you cannot successfully commission either health or social care in isolation of the other. Indeed, in the early part of the century a considerable amount of effort was spent by the NHS and local authorities in trying to encapsulate the joint commissioning and joint purchasing arrangements in Section 75 agreements (Department of Health, 2006). Section 75 refers to the relevant section in the NHS Act (2006) that set out a range of approaches to the written agreements between an NHS body (primary care trust (PCT), NHS trust or NHS foundation trust) and a local authority to cover joint commissioning or joint provision arrangements or the creation of a pooled budget between the NHS and the local authority.

Whilst this process was useful in encouraging the NHS and local authorities to think in some detail about how they worked together it is debatable whether this work achieved as much as was hoped in actually improving the commissioning and contracting functions either singly or jointly.

It could be argued that the implementation of much of the mental health NSF was a centrally driven commissioning initiative in that it determined what new services needed to be established and commissioned across the country. It also provided health authorities and, from 2002, PCTs with additional funding to ensure that they were put in place. Although these additions were reflected in service level agreements and, latterly, contracts, it was more commonly in the form of a changed contract value than from a detailed description of the range of services to be provided. Whilst the NSF looked at a wide range of areas in mental health, the part that had the greatest impact on secondary mental health services was the introduction of crisis resolution and home treatment, assertive outreach and early intervention teams to augment and build on the existing community mental health teams (CMHTs).

Individual commissioners needed to consider how much they wanted to invest. However, there were target sizes set for each area across the country against which they were monitored. Targets served to ensure that a focus was maintained on mental health through this period and although there was a feeling in many areas that the approach to monitoring these targets was overly prescriptive and did not recognize variations in need across the country the overall impact was positive in bringing considerable new investment and a real focus to mental health. Unfortunately, because the changes were delivered with new money there was not always a real concentration of effort on thinking about the changes that would be needed to the rest of the mental health system to ensure there was no duplication of provision, nor a process to ensure best use of resources. This meant that rather than redesigning CMHTs so that they complemented the roles of the new specialist teams, in many areas CMHTs continued to operate in much the same way they always had done. In some areas this led to duplication between CMHT and new team roles or led to some confusion for service users in trying to navigate the system.

The other impact of change being delivered through new investment was that when there was no more new money mental health started slipping down the agenda in many parts of the country. This may not have been important if, during the period of growth, there had been a strengthening of mental health commissioning and a strengthening of its position within the strategic thinking of commissioning organisations. This did not generally occur and a major contributor to this may well have been the introduction of payment by results (PbR) as a payment mechanism for a number of areas of provision in general acute services. PbR began in a limited way in the NHS in 2003/04 and is the hospital payment system in England by which commissioners pay providers a national tariff or price for the number and complexity of patients treated or seen. The currency, or unit of payment, is the Healthcare Resource Group (HRG). HRGs are clinically meaningful groups of diagnoses and interventions using similar levels of NHS resources. The resultant tariffs (of which there are currently more than 1,000) each cover a spell of care, which is the period from admission to discharge.

This was because PbR introduced a direct relationship between volume of activity delivered and levels of payment due to the provider. In order to manage financial flows it would thus need considerable commissioner focus and resource. This meant that acute services needed more focus by commissioning directors, with the result that less focus went on mental health where there was no currency or tariff that could increase costs to the commissioner in a year.

One part of the system that seems not as influenced by the NSF was primary care. It would be wrong to think that the NSF has nothing to say about primary care. Indeed two of the seven standards (standards 2 and 3) covered primary care and access to services. However, because subsequent targets were related to establishing new teams for people with severe mental illness, much of the rest of the NSF became somewhat overlooked. Whilst there was a consensus that people with a common mental illness and depression were primarily cared for in primary care, it was often felt that anything more serious needed to be referred into specialist mental health services. It may be the case that this dated back, in some instances, to the days of the old long-stay hospitals when there was a general expectation that people with long-term and profound mental health problems were sent to long-stay hospitals where it was expected that many could stay for many years. It seemed to be felt that there was little that primary care and other NHS services had to contribute to their care and recovery within this arrangement.

Perhaps the physical locations of many of these long-stay facilities, often walled and isolated in the countryside or the edge of towns or cities, compounded a perception amongst those managing and providing care that these services sat outside the mainstream of the NHS. It could be argued that this arrangement not only compounded the stigma directed towards people with serious long-term mental illness but also seemed to stigmatise mental health services in the thinking of the rest of the NHS so that the services, as well as the people using these services, became distant and separated from the mainstream.

An additional consequence of these arrangements was the lack of confidence experienced by many in the rest of the NHS in being able to respond to the needs of this part of the population. As well as a lack of confidence, which made referral on much more likely, there was also a real lack of experience, knowledge and expertise in how to provide effective care. This often extended to a lack of awareness of other services, in health, social care, the non-statutory sector and a wide range of other organisations that can play an important role in the recovery of people with serious mental illness. This may also have had the effect that when commissioning was introduced there was often only very limited understanding and knowledge of mental health services by the commissioning organizations, making it more difficult to commission mental health services effectively. It has largely remained the case that the majority of specialist understanding of mental illness and mental health services resides within the specialist mental health trusts.

Of course, it would be completely wrong to say this is universally the case and indeed many mental health commissioners have become expert in their knowledge and understanding of mental illness and services and have often had a role in educating colleagues in the rest of their organisation. It has also been the case that a number of GPs and other members of the primary care team across the country have developed particular mental health interests and expertise that has manifested itself in practitioners taking on roles such as GPs with a Special Interest (GPSIs). However, this is still more the exception than the norm and many in primary care, general acute services and other non-mental health parts of the NHS would not describe themselves as being hugely familiar with serious mental illness and mental health services.

The impact of PbR

The implementation of PbR for general acute services provided a framework for the introduction of a tariff and currency to determine the level of funding to be paid for a range of services. This had the advantage of being able to be much more specific about contracted activity levels for those services but, when attached to the government agenda of driving down waiting lists and waiting times for those services, also became a cause of enormous increases in expenditure and, increasingly, cost pressures as the availability of funding to cover the resultant increases in activity and cost became increasingly limited. This meant that as well as there being a need for PCTs to bolster their acute commissioning resources to keep abreast of these developments, together with associated finance, public health and analytical resources, there was also a tendency for board level priorities being on those areas and in finding potential solutions to these challenges in primary care. It is also worth noting that a number of general acute service areas, such as coronary heart disease and diabetes, also had their own NSFs that drove service development in those areas and thus, to some extent, provided additional competition to mental health achieving greater focus and priority in the commissioning agenda.

Thus, at a time when the NSF could have led to a much greater emphasis on mental health strategy and commissioning, other technical changes in acute commissioning and the enormous amount of emphasis on waiting lists meant that mental health did not move to centre stage. This was compounded by there being no tariff for mental health services, only the block contract as described earlier, and also the exclusion of mental health from the waiting list agenda. Indeed, the lack of a national mechanism to cost mental health activity meant that there was limited incentive to look at further service redesign in mental health as a route to reducing costs or referrals to secondary mental health services. This was because unless the commissioner was able to decommission the whole service it has proved difficult to agree what percentage of the funding should be removed when there is a partial reduction in that service.

It is arguable that this combination of factors culminated in an environment where the greatest resource challenges to the NHS lay in the general acute sector and that whilst addressing this through service redesign and commissioning has been very challenging it is felt that the mechanism of PbR presents a vehicle that can be used to work to a resolution. It is probably also the case that there are a number of procedures that require a defined, time limited intervention and have a clearly discernible outcome, which means that it is easier to define when an episode of care has come to an end. It is thus probably rather easier to measure progress and success in delivering change.

In mental health there is currently no PbR and an 'episode' of secondary care is often much longer and difficult to say when that care has fully come to an end. This can give the perception that delivering change is difficult and it is hard to demonstrate the success of that change. This can lead to a belief that making changes is too difficult or will take too long and therefore it becomes a lower priority than other areas where it is felt that success is easier to achieve.

Over the last four years the Department of Health has been considering how PbR could be extended to mental health services. The existing acute PbR methodology does not work for establishing currencies for the treatment of mental illness so a new methodology and approach was necessary for mental health commissioning. This paper will not discuss this in any detail but instead will focus on the opportunities offered by this mechanism and other changes in the NHS environment following the 2010 general election.

The model of PbR due to be implemented for mental health services from April 2012 may not provide national tariffs for each service from that date but it has established a currency for many services: the care clusters. The mental health care clusters are what is called a type of Category Valued Person Observation. A service user is assigned to a care cluster, which is based on symptoms and associated needs, rather than diagnosis, using a decision tree or algorithm based on a score derived from using a national mental health clustering tool. There are currently 20 care clusters ranging from Common Mental Health Problems (Low Severity) – cluster 1 – to Cognitive Impairment or Dementia (High Physical or Engagement) – cluster 21. Clusters have currently only been developed with adults although work is currently underway to develop clusters with children and adolescents as well as for people with substance misuse problems and people in forensic mental health services.

This enables a mechanism for agreeing contract values that are more closely related to activity levels than is currently possible with the block contract approach. The key benefit of the tariff is that it makes meaningful the commissioning and contracting process and provides a much more focused approach to the negotiation and contract setting process. Given that progress has been slow in setting up this new commissioning mechanism it is likely that this meaningfulness will develop over the course of the next few years. This would be sensible because an immediate shift from a very loosely specified block contract to a very specific contract based on care clusters could be very destabilizing, particularly if there is a difference in perception between the commissioner and provider about whether the existing service is over or undercharged in the block contract. Whilst this could lead to some rather fraught negotiation and discussion these are discussions that need to happen as part of setting in place more sophisticated and detailed contract rounds that are much more precise about the range and volume of provision to be commissioned and provided in any year.

The challenges of mental health commissioning

It was widely recognised that as well as the services that the NHS has commissioned and provided for mental health service users, there was also a considerable amount of activity and provision that was the responsibility of local authority social services departments. For many years local authorities and the NHS planned, commissioned and provided these services largely separately but it was clear that this was not the best way to either use resources or provide the best services and best outcomes for the people using those services, as described earlier with regard to Section 75 agreements.

The approach taken in many areas for resolving this was to bring together the health commissioner and social care commissioner roles in a single officer or team who were jointly funded by, and jointly accountable to, the PCT and the local authority. This was an arrangement that generally worked well when the two organisations were in agreement or there weren't pressures, financial or otherwise, on the system. However, when there was a difference in priorities between the two funding agencies the commissioner was often not of sufficient seniority to be able to resolve the disagreement themselves. This sometimes left issues not fully resolved and potentially left the commissioner in a somewhat isolated position in that they were not fully seen as belonging to either organisation. This could often make it difficult for the mental health commissioner to influence colleagues in their organisation and they struggled to keep mental health high in the commissioning priorities of the organisation.

The block contract also meant that mental health was seen as less of a financial risk because there was not necessarily a relationship between cost and change in activity levels. In general the only exceptions to this were more specialist, tertiary services such as eating disorders or forensic services where there is a combination of cost and volume contracts or named patient contracts, but these are smaller very specialist services. Cost and volume contracts are generally used for specialised mental health services such as forensic services when there is a contract with an NHS provider for a number of patients. Named patient contracts are individual contracts for the care of a particular patient, often in forensic services. These are usually rolling one year contracts based on a weekly or monthly rate. These are usually for patients' care in the independent sector.

Payment is based on the unit cost of providing care for one patient for one month multiplied by the number of patients. These contracts are agreed annually.

These arrangements do not apply to the mainstream secondary mental health services that make up the majority of the activity of mental health trusts and foundation trusts.

This range of factors, and there are probably more, have led to a situation where expertise in commissioning mental health services is generally less developed than many other parts of health service delivery and provision. It is important to consider the changes over the last 20 years and the arrangements and environment in which mental health is currently commissioned because these factors will play an important part in the shaping of new commissioning structures and the move to design and commission new types of mental health services.

A new era of mental health commissioning?

The Health and Social Care Bill, currently making its passage through parliament, provides significant opportunities to revisit the current situation and the mechanisms through which mental health services are planned and commissioned. The proposed introduction of clinical commissioning offers the opportunity for much greater clinical engagement in all aspects of the commissioning process, including mental health. The proposal to introduce health and well-being boards to provide greater local authority input into health strategy could mean that services, again like mental health, that are jointly commissioned and provided could achieve a higher profile in health priorities than perhaps is always the case currently.

It is probably fair to say that where there have been previous initiatives to develop GP involvement in commissioning, such as practice-based commissioning (PBC), that mental health has often not been high on priorities. PBC was a mechanism introduced in 2005 to devolve responsibility for commissioning a number of services from PCTs to groups of GPs. Whilst this did not mean actual devolution of budgets, there was meant to be an incentive for GPs to engage in the form of any savings being available for the groups of GPs or PBC groups to either commission additional services or activity or develop new services in primary care. The limited level of savings realised meant that this agenda never fully gained popularity with primary care. This policy was introduced by the Department of Health (2005) in the document *Commissioning a Patient-led NHS*.

This is perhaps due to the difficulties in delivering savings and incremental changes in provision due to the block contract but also due to a key difference between mental health provision and that of pretty much all other services. There has often been an expectation that secondary mental health services will take on the management of the care of their patients for sizeable periods of time, years in some instance, with comparatively little input from primary care or other health services where there are instances of severe mental illness beyond something like an annual health check. As described earlier, this could lead to a lack of understanding about how mental health services are managing the care and recovery of their patients and also can lead to a lack of confidence by others in taking on the primary management of that care. This could mean that there is a lack of familiarity about how best to take forward change and as a result to leave much of the development and change agenda with the specialist provider.

By extension it could be assumed that the intention to establish clinical commissioning groups to take on the majority of commissioning would not change this situation but it appears that this is not going to be the case in all areas. This is because although many GPs do not feel expert or confident in managing serious or enduring mental illness they do see a lot of people with mild mental illness. They also recognise that there are a number of people on their patient lists who may currently have their care managed by a mental health trust but who will often be discharged back to their care and, if there are subsequent problems, it may not be easy to set in place arrangements whereby they can rapidly get specialist advice from secondary mental health services or refer the patient back to them quickly. A failure to ensure changes in the way that this interface operates can lead to very real and practical challenges for general practice in best meeting the needs of people with serious mental illness, particularly at a point where the patient is in crisis and needs urgent help and care.

As a result a number of GP pathfinder organisations and individual GPs have identified mental health as a priority area on which they would like to see a real focus. GP pathfinders are self-selecting groups of GP practices, of a wide range of size, selected to take on commissioning responsibilities from PCTs as a mechanism for testing the policy direction of the Department of Health White Paper (2010) *Liberating the NHS: Equity and Excellence*. So far there have been four waves of pathfinders announced by the current Secretary of State for Health, Andrew Lansley. It is more likely than ever before that this interest will be sustainable because of the introduction of mental health PbR in April 2012.

This could lead to very different types of services than are currently generally in place because once there is a much greater level of leadership in delivering change from the commissioning organisations then it is likely that the options for a range of providers and how these services would work will be much wider than is currently the position. A key reason for this is that in an environment where change is driven by the existing provider, it is likely that those change proposals would position the existing provider as a likely provider for the new services. The argument to support this, with some justification, is that the existing providers employ most of the clinical expertise and experience in providing these services and have the ready-made infrastructure for taking on any new services. This is evidenced by the frequently voiced views by many existing mental health providers that they are well placed to vertically integrate to undertake primary mental health provision.

Whilst this is probably the case this may serve to limit the potential options for the ways that services could be provided and could serve to widen what would be defined as specialist mental health services further and also limit the amount of care provided by generalist, or primary care, health providers. This could also serve to keep the role of the non-statutory sector as mental health providers, as opposed to advocates, lobbyists, information and pastoral support providers, quite small and underdeveloped.

Thus, a significant change in the prioritisation and level of interest in mental health change and redesign could lead to services that may look very different to many of those already in place. It may also open up many more opportunities for bringing together the other services critical to successful recovery for patients such as housing, employment services and other areas related to the personalisation agenda. The personalisation agenda was launched by the government in 2007 and was encapsulated in the Department of Health ministerial concordat document *Putting People First: A Shared Vision and Commitment to the Transformation of Adult Social Care*. The aim is to enable everyone who receives support, whether provided by statutory services or funded by themselves, to have much greater choice and control over the support they receive through the use of direct payments and individual budgets. The agenda has been maintained by the Coalition Government and it is planned to introduce individual health budgets.

This could also be an opportunity for joint ventures between the NHS and the non-statutory sector and other independent sector providers to develop totally different and new services focused on the needs of patients and support them towards recovery.

It is also an opportunity to widen the range of primary mental health services that could either be managed wholly within primary care or potentially as a joint venture with secondary mental health services. These developments could play an important role in breaking down the stigma around mental health services and the belief held in some quarters that there should be separate provision for mental health patients. This would undoubtedly help develop the level and breadth of mental health expertise across primary care.

It is perhaps where primary and secondary care comes together that services could change the most over the coming years. Work that is currently being finalised by the mental health team at London Health Programmes (LHP) proposes an approach that brings primary care and specialist mental health services together in order for existing services to work in a different, more joined up way. LHP is an organisation funded by London PCTs and the Department of Health to provide a range of services to support the NHS in London. It leads the development of proposals to improve health and health care services for Londoners. LHP works with patients and clinicians to review NHS services to propose changes to improve outcomes. It includes a mental health team that has developed best practice models of care to support local redesign of mental health services across the capital. This could manifest itself as new teams or services that bring together those currently working in different organisations as new integrated services. The project to develop this model of care (London Health Programmes, 2011) has been predicated on taking best practice and the advice of professionals, people using mental health services and their carers to propose ways of increasing quality and productivity, but it also recognises that existing services and strategies vary enormously across London and the country as a whole. This has meant that service change and development needs to be in that context and an approach that seeks to set in place the same configuration across the country runs the risk of duplicating existing work or, perhaps worse, contradicts and confuses existing initiatives.

The process of planning and implementing this work across London is still at a very early stage and it is unclear what this might look like but it is envisaged that the design and working practices of services would increasingly become ones that had a much greater focus on ensuring that patients only use secondary care or specialist mental health services when they need to. This work also aims to support primary care or general acute services to care for those patients when they do not need to be under specialist mental health care. This change could be a challenge because in a number of areas there is an acceptance that mental health care is often not the preserve of non-mental health providers. Changing this attitude and approach across all services is likely to lead to fundamental changes in the ways that services are planned and delivered, but this probably calls for changes in thinking by all agencies with responsibilities for the mental well-being of the population.

Although this is potentially more of a change in approach and perspective than in the specifics of the treatment provided it is likely to take time to see this model of care widely in place across the country because behavioural change takes longer to embed than technical changes. This could be a challenge in commissioning terms because there could be incremental change in the way that teams and services operate rather than something that would require a totally new specification in one go.

This changed way of working is called 'shared care' in the model and, in essence, that is what the approach is about: secondary and primary care practitioners across health and social care in both the statutory and non-statutory sectors working together much more closely and in a more integrated way. Shared care is a key component of the model of care for people with long-term mental health conditions. It is important to note that this is not a new term but, instead, describes a transfer of clinical responsibility to primary care with the support and collaboration of secondary care. By improving the competence and capacity of primary care services, the model is designed to ensure that other health problems, such as physical health, are not neglected. This article does not intend to consider this model in any detail but discusses it as an example of the sort of changes likely to occur across the system that will lead to the evolution and development of services that could look very different to the ones in place in 2011.

It would be wrong to ignore that this level of change is without risk because whenever you introduce significant change there is always going to be some level of risk. Therefore it is essential that commissioners and providers, primary and secondary health services, health and social care services and statutory and non-statutory services agree a shared vision and are willing to work together to ensure that the person using the services remains at the heart of planning, commissioning and provision.

Conclusion

The ways that mental health services have been commissioned over the last 20 years have probably not changed significantly because the tools and mechanisms for undertaking this commissioning have not really changed much and this has meant that there have been few incentives or opportunities for commissioners to drive change whilst using a block contract backed up by only very basic levels of information and detail of outcome.

The combination of the imminent introduction of PbR for mental health and the levels of financial challenge currently in the system now make the need to change unavoidable.

This is due to the need to radically change the ways that all health services are planned and delivered if they are to remain affordable in the face of considerably increased life expectancy. The financial and economic challenges facing western economies also mean that it is unlikely that mental health will avoid close scrutiny by commissioners and decision makers. This level of scrutiny could be seen as a threat by the mental health community but should be viewed as an opportunity to get mental health into the mainstream of both commissioning and delivery of services because in this way quality will best be driven up by being looked at in much more detail. This has got to be better for patients by not considering their physical and mental health needs separately in planning and delivery terms. This is emphasised by the current focus on this by the Department of Health as part of the new mental health strategy (Department of Health, 2011b). The strategy has six shared objectives. Objective 3 is that more people with mental health problems will have good physical health.

The proposed changes to the way that mental health services are commissioned can thus act as a catalyst both for improvements in the ways that mental health is commissioned and also opens up opportunities to really innovate and change the ways that services are delivered. This can significantly widen the roles of primary care, general acute services and the non-statutory sector in providing high quality care and contributing to the recovery and greater well-being of the people who use those services.

References

Department of Health (1989) *Caring for People: Community Care in the next Decade and Beyond*, London: Department of Health.

Department of Health (1990) *National Health Service and Community Care Act*, London: Department of Health.

Department of Health (1999) *Mental Health National Service Framework*, London: Department of Health.

Department of Health (2005) *Commissioning a Patient-led NHS*, London: Department of Health.

Department of Health (2006) *NHS Act*, London: Department of Health.

Department of Health (2007) *Putting People First: A Shared Vision and Commitment to the Transformation of Adult Social Care*, London: Department of Health.

Department of Health (2010) *Liberating the NHS: Equity and Excellence*, London: Department of Health.

Department of Health (2011a) Health and Social Care Bill, London: Department of Health.

Department of Health (2011b) *No Health without Mental Health*, London: Department of Health.

London Health Programmes (2011) *Mental Health Models of Care for London*, London: London Strategic Health Authority.

16 Working in mental health

Practice and policy in a changing environment – conclusions

Tom Sandford, Claire Johnston and Peter Phillips

This book is based on the premise that the long-term trend in the UK towards community-based care for people with mental health problems can only be sustained if it is founded on services that are appropriate and desirable to mental health service users. This population, freed from the impositions of institutional services, will assert increasing discretion over their involvement with the mental health service. How well placed are we to manage this transition?

The book has described how a paradigm shift in the ways in which mental health services are delivered is happening – both for service users and for professional mental health care workers. These include: a better organised and more influential user movement; substantial hospital bed closures and less dependency on hospital-based service delivery models; a plethora of new programmes of community-based mental health care delivered by an increasing plurality of providers; new mental health policy and legislation; the changing of professional roles; and more robust human rights. All this is set in a current context of economic downturn and pressure to reduce public sector spending.

The authors have also set out a vision of how mental health services and the staff who work in them should respond to this scenario. New providers – especially in the third sector – have already challenged the culture and the cost base of the public sector mental health system in areas such as drug and alcohol services and secure services. Meanwhile the commissioning of mental health provision echoes this demand for greater plurality to meet the Lansley principle of 'any willing provider', driving transformation of services across whole care pathways as Dr Tang (Chapter 4) highlights. The book sets out how the reader can operate and develop a relevant contribution in this environment.

Many of the fundamental foundation stones are in place and are already making this happen. Parsonage (Foreword) notes that the increase in expenditure on NHS mental health services over the past ten years mirrors that for other areas in the NHS. His analysis confirms that the sector shared fully in the extra provision made available to the NHS, which was underpinned by strong economic growth during much of the last decade. Cape and Humphries (Chapter 12) illustrate how this resource has, for example, significantly changed the type of service on offer through improved access to psychological therapies. They examine the benefits of increased competition, arguing its potential to access hard to reach groups through third-sector providers with strong community networks and increased patient choice in multi-provider partnerships.

Looking ahead, Parsonage (Foreword) suggests that the prospects for all health services, including mental health are very different. Public expenditure will be constrained for a number of years as the need for deficit reduction impacts the volume and value of services being commissioned over a period when the recovery from the 2008 recession is likely to be slow and protracted. He notes how continued pressures from demographic change, new technology and the tendency of health costs to increase more rapidly than general inflation can only be contained by services becoming much more efficient. Dr Tang (Chapter 4) takes up this theme, highlighting the benefits of delivering more for less, through the adoption of care pathways, using the needs-based clustering tools for mental health payment by results – although others view this as payment by activity. Cape and Humphries (Chapter 12) contribute further to this debate, explaining how the established use of outcome measures in IAPT services will make use of data on clinical improvement and/or recovery, making it a true payment by results.

Parsonage's analysis of the economic context affecting mental health is that there will be upward pressures on the demand for services just as budgets become increasingly constrained. He cites the persistence of high unemployment, which is well established as a risk factor for mental ill health, as are other aspects of a weak labour market such as job insecurity, debt problems and housing repossessions. Additional demands on mental health services are also likely to arise from the knock-on effects of cuts in other public spending programmes such as social care, welfare benefits, housing and criminal justice. Meanwhile Fox and colleagues (Chapter 11) consider the success to date of putting into place the ambitions of the National Dementia Strategy, which, while only published in 2009, was the product of a different economic climate. Despite this the authors demonstrate that cost-effective early interventions for people with dementia, through the provision of memory services, have made modest progress, though not at a fast enough pace.

Quality and outcomes will increasingly be the government's drivers for this new world, and public sector commissioners will be looking for service providers who are innovative, adopt interventions that work and who also have a focus on prevention. Service user experience will be more highly valued, as will patient safety. These priorities and focus will challenge many existing providers, who may not be best qualified to survive in the new world of competition and the increasing demands of Monitor and the Care Quality Commission as regulatory dynamos. At its heart, as Perkins argues cogently (Chapter 2) meaningful mental health practice starts with 'the person in their life' and builds toward a future of their own design, providing hope, control and opportunity.

The role of the workforce in contemporary mental health is a theme throughout the book, with a plethora of case examples from new service models about the emerging evidence for more competent practitioners, along with models of supervision and leadership based on best evidence. Nolan (Chapter 5), Hughes and Phillips (Chapter 8) and Hardy and Brimblecombe (Chapter 13) all consider what needs to be done to deliver complex therapeutic interventions in multi-skilled teams, while reducing the overall resource and using assistant practitioners and peer support workers as part of the team's make-up. The role of professionals is taken to task by Repper and Perkins (Chapter 7), with Perkins (Chapter 2) quipping from Winston Churchill that professionals should be 'on tap' and not 'on top'.

Jobbins (in Chapter 15) describes how GPs will be at the heart of commissioning these services, and he also discusses some of the challenges of getting new commissioning relationships and decisions right. McCulloch and Lawton-Smith warn (Chapter 1) that this will not be easy. They note how, for example, prisons and secure units could simply continue the history of asylums and there is real concern that secure services could be seen as 'non-discretionary' and take a disproportionate slice of increasingly tight mental health budgets.

The demand for increased efficiency will enhance the need for better integrated care – care that is integrated around the service user rather than around the provider. Perkins (in Chapter 2) describes just how fundamental this change needs to be and Perkins and Repper (Chapter 7) describe how the opportunity to participate has to be totally embedded in services if they are to effectively foster self-worth and well-being. These strategies are reinforced by

Simpson (Chapter 3). Tang (Chapter 4) describes how application of the care pathway approach can help achieve the increased efficiency demanded in a financially austere environment and Nolan (Chapter 5) emphasises how community rather than hospital-based approaches will underpin this. Killaspy (Chapter 6) reminds us of the strategic importance of rehabilitation in service provision. Securing these changes will not be easy, and Hardy and Brimblecombe (Chapter 13) describes how challenging this will be for staff working in services of the future, who will need different skills and a new commentary.

We should be in no doubt that these changes are essential. For example, Osborn (Chapter 14) describes how the association between physical and mental health is well established and unquestionable, yet people with mental health problems continue to suffer scandalous rates of early death and morbidity from physical ill health – he evidences how people with schizophrenia or bipolar disorder die between 10 and 25 years earlier than their counterparts without mental health problems. Mental health services must now make a difference, by practitioners consistently assessing physical health and by working closely with primary care services to manage physical conditions when they are detected. The reluctance of mental health staff to equip themselves to steer and signpost service users to the best services available and to offer brief interventions for smoking, diet and exercise has to be overcome – after all we expect district nurses to detect depression in their diabetes clinic.

These changes can be secured and there is evidence of the sector having managed aspects of service change well in the past that augers well for the future. For example, mental health was one of the first clinical areas to make community nursing more attractive for service users and nurses alike. Likewise, case management has a strong history in mental health care and could be developed much further in terms of securing outcomes. Cape and Humphries (Chapter 12) tell the IAPT story, which has had astonishing success using four interrelated areas: protocolised care based on evidence, stepped care, the use of assistant practitioners who are appropriately supervised and a strong focus on outcomes. These services may be the new kid on the block but, as the authors suggest, they do have some learning that other mental health services could benefit from.

Whilst the combination of severely constrained budgets and continuing cost and demand pressures clearly creates a difficult environment for the development of mental health services, one could also argue that they create the opportunity of a lifetime to do things differently. Doing things differently is a recurring theme throughout the chapters of this book.

Some of the most welcome changes in mental health service provision have been the increasing commentary from women and black and ethnic minority cohorts amongst the service user population. Phillips and Jackson (Chapter 9) elaborate on what needs to underpin gender specific mental health care. The changes they describe, whether they be in culture or in respect to practice and security, simply have to happen on a widespread basis if our mental health services are to be safe and fit for purpose for women and are to justify funding in a more austere economic environment. The stigma and discrimination experienced by women in mental health services is powerfully described, through the lens of sexual abuse. The theme of human rights and the inequalities suffered by people who use mental health services is strong throughout the book, with a number of chapter authors exploring how stigma, discrimination and a lack of justice can be effectively overcome – but power bases, professional attitudes and culture will need a sea change to achieve these fundamental rights. Sewell (Chapter 10) outlines a series of critical issues and cultural change that is essential in order for the black population to be more confident about their expectations of more appropriate service provision. Phillips and Hughes (Chapter 8) explore the challenge posed by the cohort of service users with a dual diagnosis of serious mental illness and drug and/or alcohol addiction. A confident service response around these concerns will be essential in preventing any retrenchment into more secure psychiatric service provision. Fox and colleagues (Chapter 11) draw parallels around the need to ensure access to appropriate age-specific service provision.

This book has focused on the essential role that people who work in mental health services have in shaping services that really engage with service users in different ways and with different and more appropriate responses. There is of course a vast contribution that needs to be made by others outside of the service. McCulloch and Lawton-Smith (Chapter 1) describe how mental health services and mentally ill people are impacted by generic policies on health, welfare, housing and other issues and they note how these impacts are often more important than that of specialist policy. To appreciate the massive significance of these, the reader is directed towards Sayce (2011) for example, who reviews the importance of work and well-being and employment services as a response to assuring and maintaining mental health. Hooper (2011) picks up on the potential for personalisation to reshape the personal budgets and benefits available to service users to live their lives the way they want to, and she highlights the gaps between policy and practice that need to be addressed. Watters (2011) discusses how issues like prevention, addressing stigma and securing a coherent, modern societal understanding of mental distress remain a significant challenge.

We hope that the book will assist you in formulating an appropriate response and a stronger, better informed contribution to the part of the mental health service in which you already operate or plan to practice in the future. We will have achieved what we set out to do as editors if you find the contributions of our authors – all chosen because they are experts in their field, as well as being fantastic communicators – help you to understand more about the rapidly shifting policy and practice agendas in mental health. We hope that you will find great satisfaction in being part of a modernising movement making essential changes to our mental health services and those who use them.

References

Hooper, M. (2011) Personalisation: an ideal yet to be realised. *Open Mind,* 167: 18.
Sayce, L. (2011) *Getting in, staying in and getting on: disability employment support fit for the future.* http://www. dwp.gov.uk/docs/sayce-report.pdf.
Watters, E. (2011) *Crazy Like Us: the globalisation of the western mind.* London: Robinson.

Index

abuse: emotional 91, 93, 94; sexual *see* sexual assault/abuse
acetyl cholinesterase drugs 119
acute care pathway model 45
ADASS (Association of Directors of Adult Social Services) 120–1
Adult Placements 124
Adult Psychiatric Morbidity Survey 129, 130
age-specific service lines 116–25 *see also* dementia care; anticipatory planning, for cardiovascular disease prevention 122; developing models of care 119–22; and evaluation 123; evidence base for service effectiveness 122–3; vs needs-defined services 44; reconfiguring services for older people 117–18
aggression 72; and dual diagnosis 83–4; 'micro-aggressions' 111
AIMS-Rehab 68
alcohol misuse, co-morbidity with mental health problems *see* dual diagnosis, mental health service delivery for users with co-morbid alcohol/drug use problems
Allen, C. 76
Allen, S. 74–5
Alleyne, A. 111
All-Party Parliamentary Group on Dementia 124
Alzheimer's disease 119 *see also* dementia care; dementia, condition of
Alzheimer's Society 121
amisulpride 162
anger 72–3, 98
Annual Public Health Equity Audit 137
Annual Report of the High Commissioner for Human Rights 20
Anthony, W.A. 63
antidepressant drugs 131, 135, 161, 162
antipsychotic drugs 61, 161, 162
anxiety 62, 85, 129–32; Generalised Anxiety Disorder (GAD) 134, 135, 138; and IAPT *see* Improving Access to Psychological Therapies; measures of 135; recommended NICE interventions 135Fig.

Any Willing Provider model 40, 141, 180
AOTs *see* assertive outreach team services
Arnold, E. 110
Ashcraft, L. and Anthony, W. 18, 78, 79
Ashton, Wigan and Leigh Memory Service 121
assertive outreach team services 44, 46–7, 62
Association of Directors of Adult Social Services (ADASS) 120–1
asylums 3–4, 25, 27, 61, 64, 150
Audit Commission xvii
autonomy 20, 28, 31, 32, 63, 66, 67 *see also* control; empowerment; and self-directed support 17–18, 31–4

balance of power: changing the balance 16–21; and compulsory detention and treatment 19–21; imbalance and abuse in asylums 25; and race equality 110
Bennet, David 108–9
Bentall, R. 111, 112
Bexley Hospital 4
bipolar affective disorder 163, 164
black and minority ethnic (BME) people 105–13, 137; women 94
blame 72
blood borne viruses 162
body image 97
borderline personality disorder (BPD) 93, 98
Bracken, P. and Thomas, P. 111, 112
Brimblecombe, N. 53, 154
British National Party 104
Burns, T. 41

Callahan, C.M. *et al.* 122
Call to end violence against women and girls 94
Camden, mental health recovery centre 45–6
Cameron, David 108
Campbell, Sharon 4
Capabilities for inclusive practice 155
Caplan, G. 52
cardiovascular disease: and its causes 159, 160, 161, 164; prevention 122

care clusters 111, 174; Yorkshire 39, 43
Care in the Community 170–1 *see also* community care
care pathway approach 12, 39–47; of rehabilitation 65–6
Care Programme Approach (CPA) 6, 29–31, 33–4, 62, 94, 95
Care Quality Commission 42, 45, 67, 91, 105, 107, 181
Care Services Improvement Partnership (CSIP) 27, 84, 153; *Informed gender practice* 92
Caring for People: Community Care in the next Decade and Beyond 171
Carmichael, Stokely 104
C-BIT (Cognitive Behavioural Integrated Treatment) 86–7
CBT *see* cognitive behavioural therapy
Chamberlin, J. 14, 21
Chief Nursing Officer's review of mental health nursing 151
children: childhood abuse 91, 93, 100; mental health policy 10
cholesterol 159, 161, 163, 164, 167
Churchill, W.L.S. 17
Clark, D.M. *et al.* 138
Clark, M. 111
Clark, P. *et al.* 122
Client Satisfaction Questionnaire 55
clinical psychology 150
clozapine 161
CMHTs (community mental health teams) 42, 46, 62, 121, 151, 171
CMHTs (Community Mental Health Trusts) 119
coaching relationships 18
Coalition Government: delivering policy through outcomes 9–10; drive for choice 12; and gendered violence 94–5; localism 10, 108; mental health policy challenges 8–10; new mental health strategy 8–9, 27–8, 85, 90, 107, 110, 152, 159; NHS mantra of 'Nothing about us, without us' 11; personalisation agenda 177; public health strategy 12
Cognitive Behavioural Integrated Treatment (C-BIT) 86–7
cognitive behavioural therapy (CBT) 85, 86, 87, 152; in common mental health problems 130, 131, 132, 134, 137, 139
Coid, J. *et al.* 93
collaborative partnerships with service users 25–35, 63; Care Programme Approach 6, 29–31, 33; co-production 17, 18, 19, 32, 47, 77; direction of travel 27–8; identifying the drivers 26; and mental health staff education and training 34–5; personalisation and partnership 32–4; Wellness Recovery Action Planning 31–2
Collier, R. and Stickley, T. 35

Commissioning a Patient-led NHS 176
Commissioning for Quality and Innovation (CQUIN) 165
commissioning mental health services 170–9; challenges of 175; *Commissioning a Patient-led NHS* 176; development between the 1980s and 2010 170–3; GP commissioning responsibilities 171, 173, 176; and a new era 175–8; Payment by Results impact 172, 173–4, 176, 178; practice-based commissioning 176
common mental health problems 129–31 *see also* anxiety; depression; and diabetes 161; and IAPT *see* Improving Access to Psychological Therapies
community care: beginnings 4, 25, 27, 150; community mental health teams 42, 46; development of community mental health services 62, 150, 170–1; functional assertive community treatment model 46–7; home treatment *see* home treatment; introduction of Care in the Community 170–1; and the NHS Plan 7; social care in dementia 123–5; women-centred 91
community development workers (CDWs) 107
community mental health teams (CMHTs) 42, 46, 62, 121, 151, 171
Community Mental Health Trusts (CMHTs) 119
Community Treatment Orders (CTOs) 12, 20, 28
co-morbidity of alcohol/drug use with mental health problems *see* dual diagnosis, mental health service delivery for users with co-morbid alcohol/drug use problems
COMO trial 87
COMPASS project 86–7
compliance 15, 17; medication 83, 106
compulsion to repeat 99
compulsory powers of detention and treatment 19–21
control *see also* autonomy; balance of power; empowerment: and recovery 15, 27, 74–5; taking back control 74–5
Cook, J.A. *et al.* 31
co-production 17, 18, 19, 32, 47, 77
CPA *see* Care Programme Approach
CQUIN (Commissioning for Quality and Innovation) 165
Crenshaw, K. 104
criminal behaviour, and dual diagnosis 83–4
crisis homes/houses 45, 100–1, 166
crisis resolution teams (CRTs) 51, 52, 53–4, 55–8, 166; organisational characteristics and core components 53–4
crisis theory 52–3
CRTs *see* crisis resolution teams
CSIP *see* Care Services Improvement Partnership
CTOs (Community Treatment Orders) 12, 20, 28

Davidson, L. *et al.* 16

Dean, C. *et al.* 55

Deegan, P. 14, 16, 21, 71, 72, 74; and Drake, R. 17

Delivering Race Equality in Mental Health Care (DRE) 107, 109

dementia care 10, 44, 116–25, 181; developing models of care 119–22; and evaluation 123; evidence base for service effectiveness 122–3; and GPs 117–18, 119, 121, 122; and memory services 118, 119–20, 121, 122; National Dementia Strategy 116–17, 118, 122, 124–5; and reconfiguring services for older people 117–18; social care 123–5; and workforce redesign 122

dementia, condition of 10, 43; diagnosis of 117–18, 120

DEMoBinc study 67

denial 72–3

depression 43, 62, 72, 85, 93, 129–32; and IAPT *see* Improving Access to Psychological Therapies; measures of 135; stepped care model and recommended NICE interventions 134–5Figs

despair 72

detention, compulsory 19–21

diabetes 122, 159, 161–2

diagnostic overshadowing 163

direct payments 33, 177

disability: 1995 UK Disability Discrimination Act 21; and the environment 21; and the rights-based approach 20, 22–3; rights movement 25; UN Convention on the Rights of Persons with Disabilities (2006) 20, 22

Disability Rights Commission 163

disempowerment 19, 77

Doncaster, pilot IAPT 132, 138

drug misuse, co-morbidity with mental health problems *see* dual diagnosis, mental health service delivery for users with co-morbid alcohol/drug use problems

drugs: abuse with mental health problems *see* dual diagnosis, mental health service delivery for users with co-morbid alcohol/drug use problems; acetyl cholinesterase 119; antidepressant 131, 135, 161, 162; antipsychotic 61, 161, 162; psychotropic 51, 159, 161, 165; and weight gain 161

dual diagnosis, mental health service delivery for users with co-morbid alcohol/drug use problems 81–7; and aggression, violence and offending 83–4; development of the field 81–2; *Dual Diagnosis Good Practice Guide* 84; evidence for effective treatments 85–6; impact of dual diagnosis in mental health service settings 82–3; prevalence of co-morbidity 82; training and the workforce 86–7; UK policy response 84–5

Duffy, S. 32, 33–4

eating disorders 93, 97, 140, 175

economics: and commissioning mental health services 172, 173–4, 176, 177, 178–9; and the development of mental health services xvi–xviii, 180–1; direct payments 33, 177; GP fundholding and health promotion clinic funding 131; payment by results 44, 141, 172, 173–4, 176, 178; personal health budgets 17, 33, 125, 177; socio-economic disadvantages of BME groups 110–11

education of mental health staff *see* training/education of mental health staff

emotional intelligence 109, 113

employment 15, 135–6 *see also* unemployment

empowerment 15, 31, 39, 40, 52, 78, 91, 136, 156 *see also* autonomy; balance of power; disempowerment 19, 77

Epidemiological Catchment Area Survey (ECAS) 82

Equality Act (2010) 9, 21, 90, 105, 107

Equality and Human Rights Commission 108, 110

equality/inequality: Annual Public Health Equity Audit 137; *Equity and Excellence: Liberating the NHS* 27, 108, 141, 176; equity of access to psychological therapies 136–7; gender inequality 90–1; and language 108; race inequality 105–7, 110–11; and race in mental health care *see* race and ethnicity in mental health care

Equity and Excellence: Liberating the NHS 27, 108, 141, 176

ethnicity: compared with race 104; in mental health care *see* race and ethnicity in mental health care

ethos: of contemporary rehabilitation services 63–4; of public mental health care outcomes 152–3

explanatory models 112

FACT (functional assertive community treatment) model 46–7

Fazel, S. *et al.* 83

Fenton, F.R. *et al.* 54

Fernando, S. 112

finance *see* economics

Fortinsky, R. *et al.* 122

functional assertive community treatment (FACT) model 46–7

gender inequality 90–1

gender-specific mental health care *see* women-centred mental health care

Generalised Anxiety Disorder (GAD) 134, 135, 138

General Practice Research Database 160

General Practitioners (GPs) 7, 55, 163, 164, 167; and the care pathway approach 40, 41, 44; commissioning responsibilities 171, 173, 176; and common mental health problems 130, 131, 133; and dementia 117–18, 119, 121, 122; GP fundholding 131; GP health promotion clinic funding 131
Gilbert, P. 73
Glover, G. *et al.* 139
Good Practice Checklist for Mental Health Trusts 101
Gordon, H. and Haider, D. 83
Grad, J. and Sainsbury, P. 55
Guo, S. *et al.* 55

Hardcastle, M. 99
Harding, C. *et al.* 63
Health Act (1991) 171
Health and Social Care Bill 170, 175–6
Health and Wellbeing Boards 123
Healthcare Resource Group (HRG) 172
health care services: mental *see* mental health services; NHS *see* National Health Service; physical *see* physical health care delivery in mental health services
Health of the Nation 4
Heath, D. 53
Hertfordshire Partnership NHS Foundation Trust 120
Hewitt, Patricia 92
HIV 162
home treatment 51–8; background 51–3; and crisis theory 52–3; CRT model 52, 53–8; evidence for 54–6; fiscal conservatism 51, 52; implications for service planning and clinical practice 56–8; therapeutic radicalism 51–2
homicides, and dual diagnosis 83
hope, and recovery 15, 27, 52, 72
hopelessness 71, 72, 98–9, 100
Hoult, J.: *et al.* 55; and Nolan, F. 54
House of Commons' Committee on Public Accounts 124
HRG (Healthcare Resource Group) 172
Hughes, E. *et al.* 86
Hughes, L. 84
Hugo, M. *et al.* 55
human rights: Annual Report of the High Commissioner for 20; and compulsory detention and treatment 19–21; disability and the rights-based approach 20, 22–3; and *'No health without Mental Health'* 28
Hussein, S. *et al.* 123, 124
Hutton, John 90
hypertension 122, 159

IAPT *see* Improving Access to Psychological Therapies

ICPs (Integrated Care Pathways) *see* integrated care
Improving Access to Psychological Therapies (IAPT) 47, 129–42, 152–3; background 129–32; clinical outcome focus 142; competition 141; data reporting 140–1; and equity of access 136–7; evaluation 138–40; implications for other mental health services 141–2; and minimally qualified staff 142; payment by results 141; pilot demonstration sites 132, 138; principles 132–3; and protocolised care 142; roll-out nationally and new areas 140; service model 133–6; stepped care 132, 133, 134, 135, 139, 142; training model 137
inequality *see* equality/inequality
Informed gender practice 92
integrated care 10–11, 12; care pathway approach 12, 39–47
intersectionality 104
involuntary commitment 19–21
Islington, women's crisis house 45

Johnson, G. 79
Johnson, S.: *et al.* 55; and Needle, J. 52, 53, 54
Joint Strategic Needs Assessment 123, 136

Kemp, R. *et al.* 17
Kessler, R.C. *et al.* 130
Kikkert, M. *et al.* 111
Killaspy, H.T. *et al.* 46, 53, 63
King's Fund 107
Koontz, H. and Weihrich, H. 3

Lansley, Andrew 176
Lawrence, Stephen 104, 108
leadership 46, 57, 78, 95, 155, 176, 181
Leete, E. 75, 76
legislation, mental health *see* mental health legislation *and specific Acts*
Lewis, A. 17
Liberating the NHS: Equity and Excellence 27, 108, 141, 176
Liberman, R.P. and Kopelwicz, A. 64
lipids, abnormal 162, 163
lithium 161
localism 10, 108; and the care pathway approach 40
London Health Programmes (LHP) 177–8
Lunacy Act (1890) 12
lunatic asylums *see* asylums

MACA (Mental After Care Association) 51
MacPherson, W. 104
MAGDR (Ministerial Advisory Group on Dementia Research) 125
Mainstreaming Gender and Women's Mental Health 91, 100

Mandela, N. 21
Marks, I. *et al.* 55
Maslin, J. *et al.* 86
Masterson, A. 149
medication: compliance 83, 106; drugs *see* drugs
memory services 118, 119–20, 121, 122
Mental After Care Association (MACA) 51
Mental Capacity Act (2005) 19
Mental Health Act (1983) 4, 12, 19, 45, 105
Mental Health Act (2007) 12, 20
Mental Health Act Commission 4
mental health costs *see* economics
'Mental health in times of economic crisis' 41
mental health legislation 3, 12 *see also specific
    Mental Health Acts*; Community Treatment
    Orders 12, 20, 28; compulsory detention and
    treatment 19–21
Mental Health National Service Framework
    see National Service Framework for Mental
    Health (NSFMH)
Mental Health Policy Implementation Guide 53;
    Dual Diagnosis Good Practice Guide 84
mental health policy in the UK: from 1979 to
    1997 4; on abuse and violence 94–5; affecting
    race and ethnicity in mental health care 107–
    12; changing the balance of power 16–21;
    changing the individual and the world 21;
    children 10; Coalition Government challenges
    8–10; and community/home-based care 7,
    171; compulsory detention and treatment 19–
    21; delivering policy through outcomes 9–10;
    drivers for change regarding common mental
    health problems 131–2; and dual diagnosis
    84–5; *Equity and Excellence: Liberating the
    NHS* 27, 108, 141, 176; ethos of public mental
    health care outcomes 152–3; a framework for
    meaningful change 3–13; Health and Social
    Care Bill 170, 175–6; IAPT *see* Improving
    Access to Psychological Therapies; integrated
    care 10–11 *see also* integrated care; and
    legislation *see* mental health legislation *and
    specific Acts*; lighter touch regulation 107–8,
    113; marginalisation of mental health services
    22–3; and the meaning of 'recovery' 14–15;
    Mental Health Policy Implementation Guide 53,
    84; National Dementia Strategy 116–17, 118,
    122, 124–5; National Service Framework
    see National Service Framework for Mental
    Health (NSFMH); the nature of mental
    health policy 3; under New Labour 4–8;
    new mental health strategy 8–9, 27–8, 85, 90,
    107, 110, 152, 159; NHS plan 7–8, 9, 53, 92,
    131; *No Health without Mental Health* 27–8,
    85, 90, 107, 110, 152, 159; older people 10;
    personalisation 11; political influence as a
    lever for change 151–2; pre-IAPT policy
    regarding common mental health problems

130–2; and the purpose of services 15–16;
    recovery-focused policy 15–21, 27–8, 52,
    64; *Together we can end violence against women
    and girls: a strategy* 94; users' experiences and a
    counter-argument to 14–23; from Victorian
    times until 1979 4; wider policy picture 12;
    in women-centred mental health care 90,
    91, 92, 93, 94; *Women's mental health: into the
    mainstream* 93
mental health problem diagnosis: of common
    mental health problems 129–30; of dementia
    117–18, 120; diagnostic overshadowing 163;
    dual diagnosis *see* dual diagnosis, mental health
    service delivery for users with co-morbid
    alcohol/drug use problems; effects and shock
    of 71, 72, 73, 76
mental health services: age-specific *see* age-specific
    service lines; Any Willing Provider model 40,
    141, 180; assertive outreach team services 44,
    46–7, 62; and the balance of power *see* balance
    of power; based on self-management/direction
    17–18, 31–4; care pathway approach 12,
    39–47, 65–6; Care Programme Approach 6,
    29–31, 33–4, 62, 94, 95; CNO review 151;
    collaborative partnerships *see* collaborative
    partnerships with service users; commissioning
    see commissioning mental health services;
    community care *see* community care; crisis
    resolution and home treatment services under
    NSFMH 62; crisis resolution teams *see* crisis
    resolution teams (CRTs); delivery with dual
    diagnosis *see* dual diagnosis, mental health
    service delivery for users with co-morbid
    alcohol/drug use problems; dementia care *see*
    dementia care; early intervention services 62;
    and economics *see* economics; and ethnicity
    104–13; ethos of public mental health care
    outcomes 152–3; gender-specific *see* women-
    centred mental health care; home treatment *see*
    home treatment; IAPT *see* Improving Access
    to Psychological Therapies; incorporation into
    NHS 3; of integrated care *see* integrated care;
    leadership in *see* leadership; marginalisation
    of 22–3; multidisciplinary working in *see*
    multidisciplinary working; NHS *see* National
    Health Service; physical health care in *see*
    physical health care delivery in mental health
    services; political influence as a lever for
    change 151–2; professional boundaries and
    service delivery 149–50; professional roles
    and new service delivery 149–57; purpose
    of 15–16; and race *see* race and ethnicity in
    mental health care; recovery-focused 15–16,
    17–18, 27, 31–4, 63; rehabilitation services
    61–8; service line management 39, 40; shared
    care 178; staff *see* mental health staff; training/
    education of mental health staff; stepped

care 121, 132, 133, 134, 135, 139, 142, 156, 182; stigma 101, 112, 163, 177; training *see* training/education of mental health staff; users of *see* mental health service users; Wellness Recovery Action Planning 31–2; women-centred *see* women-centred mental health care

mental health service users: care clusters *see* care clusters; under Care Programme Approach 6, 29–31, 33–4, 94; collaborative partnerships with *see* collaborative partnerships with service users; and common mental health problems 129–31 *see also* anxiety; depression; Improving Access to Psychological Therapies (IAPT); with co-morbid alcohol/drug use problems *see* dual diagnosis, mental health service delivery for users with co-morbid alcohol/drug use problems; consumer choice/influence 26, 27, 32–3; co-production 17, 18, 19, 32, 47, 77; with dementia *see* dementia care; physical health care for *see* physical health care delivery in mental health services; recovery of *see* recovery; rehabilitation of *see* rehabilitation; self-determination of *see* autonomy; self-determination; service user movement 25–6, 27, 151, 180; social participation *see* social exclusion; social inclusion; standardised clustering of patients 111; and stigma 12, 35, 63, 76, 90, 160, 163, 166, 173, 182; UK mental health policy and the experience of 14–23; women *see* women-centred mental health care

mental health staff: change and professional role developments 151, 154–7; education and training *see* training/education of mental health staff; future-proofing the workforce 154; leadership *see* leadership; professional roles and new service delivery 149–57 *see also* professionalism; supervision 57, 84, 86–7, 92, 93, 98–9, 100, 142, 155, 181, 182; and users with drug and alcohol problems 82, 83, 86–7

Mental Health Treatment Act (1930) 12

Merson, S. *et al.* 55

Mezey, G. *et al.* 92

Michelangelo 74

MI (motivational interviewing) 86, 87

Minghella, E. *et al.* 55

Ministerial Advisory Group on Dementia Research (MAGDR) 125

mirtazepine 161

Mittelman, M. *et al.* 122

Monitor 39, 40, 181

motivational enhancement 85

motivational interviewing (MI) 86, 87

Muijen, M. *et al.* 53

multiculturalism 108

multidisciplinary working 25, 27, 29, 46, 53, 62, 65, 95, 110Fig., 111–12, 121, 123, 155

Murray-Neill, R. 27

Nadal, Rafael 18

narrative approaches 112 *see also* storytelling

National Dementia Strategy (NDS) 116–17, 118, 122, 124–5

National Dual Diagnosis Programme 84

National Health Service (NHS): climate of efficiency 165–6; commissioning mental health services *see* commissioning mental health services; competition in 141; *Equity and Excellence: Liberating the NHS* 27, 108, 141, 176; governmental mantra of 'Nothing about us, without us' 11; incorporation of mental health services into 3; mental health and NHS expenditure xvi–xviii *see also* economics; and Monitor 39, 40, 181; NHS Direct 5; NHS Outcomes Framework 9–10; NHS Plan 7–8, 9, 53, 92, 131; PCTs *see* primary care trusts; and physical health care delivery in mental health services 159, 165, 166 *see also* physical health care delivery in mental health services; *Responding to violence against women and children – the role of the NHS* 94

National Institute for Clinical Excellence (NICE) 40, 42, 85, 87, 161, 163–4; and common mental health problems 130, 131–5

National Institute for Mental Health in England (NIMHE) 52, 84, 153; National Workforce Program 153, 156

National Patient Safety Agency 91

National Service Framework for Mental Health (NSFMH) 4–8, 39, 47, 53, 62, 66, 81, 119, 131, 132, 151, 152, 171, 172, 173

National Service Framework for Older People 116, 117

National Treatment Agency 85–6

NDS (National Dementia Strategy) 116–17, 118, 122, 124–5

Newbronner, L. *et al.* 33

Newham, pilot IAPT 132, 138

New Labour: NHS Plan 7–8, 9, 53, 92, 131; NSFMH *see* National Service Framework for Mental Health

NHS *see* National Health Service

NHS Direct 5

NICE *see* National Institute for Clinical Excellence

nicotine 160

NIMHE *see* National Institute for Mental Health in England

No Health without Mental Health 27–8, 85, 90, 107, 110, 152, 159

Nolan, F. and Tang, S. 53, 57

Norfolk and Waveney NHS Foundation trust 58

NSFMH *see* National Service Framework for Mental Health

obesity 161

obligatory care planning 4
occupational therapy 64, 150
offending behaviour, and dual diagnosis 83–4
O'Gara, C. *et al.* 86
O'Hagan, M. 14, 22
olanzapine 161
older people: dementia care *see* dementia care;
   mental health policy 10
opportunity/participation, and recovery 15, 75–6
optimism: and recovery 15; therapeutic optimism
   and rehabilitation 63
Osborn, D.P. 45

Pai, S. and Kapur R.L. 55
partnerships with service users *see* collaborative
   partnerships with service users
Pasamanick, B. *et al.* 54
patient advocacy 154–5, 164
Patient Group Directions (PGDs) 57
Patient Health Questionnaire Depression Scale
   (PHQ-9) 135
Payment by Results (PbR) 44, 141, 172, 173–4,
   176, 178
PBC (practice-based commissioning) 176
PCTs *see* primary care trusts
peer support 18, 73; specialists 79; workers xviii,
   18; and WRAP 31–2
Perkins, R. 22
personal health budgets 17, 33, 125, 177
personalisation 11, 125, 177; and direct payments
   33; and partnership 32–4; personal budgets
   17, 33, 125, 177; and race equality 110
person-centred care 151, 167
Pettie, D. and Triolo, A. M. 73
phenothiazine medications 61
Phillips, P. and Johnson, S. 82
Phillips, Trevor 108
physical health care delivery in mental health
   services 159–68; acute services 165;
   assessments in settings where medical or
   nursing input is less readily accessible 165–6;
   and blood borne viruses 162; and causes
   of poor health 160–2; with diabetes and
   abnormal lipids 161–2; incentivising physical
   health monitoring in secondary care 165;
   interventions 166–7; and the mortality
   gap 159–60; with obesity 161; roles and
   responsibilities of primary and secondary
   mental health services 163–4; sexual health
   and infectious diseases 162; with smoking
   problems 160; specialist services in a climate
   of efficiency 165–6; stigma and access to 163
Physical Health Check tool 166
Pierce, C. 111
PIG (*Policy Implementation Guide*) 53
Pinquart, M. and Sorensen, S. 123
Polak, P. R. and Kirby, M. W. 54

Policy Implementation Guide (PIG) 53
Powell, Enoch 4, 151
power: balance of *see* balance of power;
   compulsory powers 19–21; histories, racism
   and 112; personal *see* autonomy; control;
   empowerment; and race equality 110, 112
practice-based commissioning (PBC) 176
Prescribing Observatory for Mental Health
   (POMH-UK) 167
primary care trusts (PCTs) 66, 136, 140, 171, 173,
   175, 176
professionalism: change and professional role
   developments 151, 154–7; professional
   boundaries and service delivery 149–50;
   professional roles and new service delivery
   149–57; professional segregation 149–50;
   and training *see* training/education of mental
   health staff
prolactin 162
psychiatry 40, 112, 150; anti-psychiatry campaigns
   25–6; post-psychiatry movement 109
psychosis 41, 42, 43, 44, 62, 64, 106, 129, 133,
   166, 167; and co-morbid alcohol/drug use
   problems 83, 85, 86, 87
psychotropic drugs 51, 159, 161, 165
Public Health Outcomes Framework 9
public mental health care ethos 152–3
*Putting People First: A Shared Vision and
   Commitment to the Transformation of Adult Social
   Care* 177

Quality and Outcomes Framework (QOF) 164
Quality Indicator for Rehabilitative Care
   (QuIRC) 67–8
Quality, Innovation, Productivity and Prevention
   (QIPP) programme xvii
Querido, A. 51, 52

race and ethnicity in mental health care
   104–13; approaches to race equality in
   the new environment 109–12; authentic
   multidisciplinary work 111–12; black and
   minority ethnic people 94, 105–13, 137;
   Delivering Race Equality in Mental Health Care
   (DRE) 107, 109; difference between race
   and ethnicity 104; environmental changes
   affecting 107–9; interpersonal factors 111;
   and the organisation 110; power, histories and
   racism 112; race inequality 105–7, 110–11;
   socio-economic factors 110–11; underlying
   factors in agenda for race equality 110–12
rape 91–2
RAWOrg (Rights and Wellbeing of Racialised
   Groups) 109
REACT trial 46
recovery 14–15, 27, 32, 52, 63–4, 71–9; and
   control 15, 27, 74–5; and hope 15, 27, 52,

72; and opportunity/participation 15, 75–6; plans 18, 27; promoting 76–9; recovery-focused policy 15–21, 27–8, 52, 64; recovery-focused services 15–16, 17–18, 27, 31–4, 63; rehabilitation *see* rehabilitation; Wellness Recovery Action Planning 31–2

Recovery Innovations 77–8

rehabilitation 61–8; care pathway 65–6; disinvestment in services and the use of out of area placements 66–7; ethos of contemporary rehabilitation services 63–4; interventions and skills 64–5; quality and effectiveness of services 67–8; remodelling of 61

Rehabilitation Effectiveness for Activities for Life study 68

repetition compulsion 99

Repper, J. and Perkins, R. 52, 72

resentment 72

Responding to violence against women and children – the role of the NHS 94

Rethink 163, 166

Richards, D.A. and Suckling, R. 138

Rights and Wellbeing of Racialised Groups (RAWOrg) 109

risperidone 162

Roberts, D. *et al.* 64

Roberts, L. *et al.* 163

Romme, M. *et al.* 112

Rosen, A. 52

Royal College of Psychiatrists (RCPsych) 27

Sainsbury Centre for Mental Health 4, 19, 53

schizophrenia 16, 62–3, 64, 74, 159, 161, 163–4; and diabetes 161–2

SCIE (Social Care Institute for Excellence) 27, 33

self-determination *see also* control; empowerment: autonomy *see* autonomy; psychological theory of 31; self-directed support 17–18, 31–4

self-worth/self-esteem 12, 61, 75; loss of 71

Service Development and Organisation (SDO) Research Programme 138

service users *see* mental health service users

sexual assault/abuse 91–2; childhood 91, 93, 100; and mixed sex acute wards 97–9; and the therapeutic relationship 97–9; UK policy on abuse and violence 94–5

Sexual boundary issues in psychiatric settings 99

sexual health 162

sexuality, women's 96

SGAs (second generation antipsychotics) 161, 162

shared care 178

Shared Lives 124

Siddiqui, H. and Patel, M. 94

Siegfried, N. *et al.* 86

smoking 160

social capital 111

social care in dementia 123–5

Social Care Institute for Excellence (SCIE) 27, 33

Social Care Outcomes Framework 9

social deprivation 84, 162

social exclusion 5, 20, 21, 22, 63, 71, 84

social inclusion 5, 22, 23, 52, 53, 63, 64, 154–5

South East Strategic Health Authority 121

South London and Maudsley NHS Foundation Trust 28, 39–40

South Staffordshire dementia care 119–20

South West London and St George's Mental Health NHS Trust 28

Spaniol, L. and Koehler, M. 72–3

staff *see* mental health staff; professionalism; training/education of mental health staff

Stein, L. I. and Test, M.A. 52–3, 54–5

stigma 12, 35, 63, 76, 81, 82, 90, 101, 112, 136, 154, 160, 163, 166, 173, 177, 182, 183

Stone, R.I. 124

storytelling 73; narrative approaches 112

substance misuse, co-morbidity with mental health problems *see* dual diagnosis, mental health service delivery for users with co-morbid alcohol/drug use problems

suicide 5, 6, 7, 8, 56, 83, 85

supervision 57, 84, 86–7, 92, 93, 98–9, 100, 142, 155, 181, 182

Supporting into the mainstream 101

Sussex Dementia Partnership 121

Sussex Partnership Trust 121

Szmukler G. *et al.* 20

Talking therapies: a four year plan of action 140

Team for the Assessment of Psychiatric Services (TAPS) 61

A Template for Rehabilitation Services 65

therapeutic optimism 63

therapeutic relationship 97–9; vs coaching relationship 18; Toxic Interaction Theory 111

Time to Change campaign 136, 163

Together we can end violence against women and girls: a strategy 94

Toxic Interaction Theory 111

training/education of mental health staff: and dual diagnosis 86–7; future-proofing the workforce 154; and partnership 34–5; and professional segregation 149–50; in women-centred mental health care 93, 95–9

transference 98

Trust Acute Care Forums 58

Tuke, William 64

Tyrer, P. *et al.* 55

unemployment xvii, 135–6

United Nations Convention on the Rights of Persons with Disabilities (2006) 20, 22

valproate 161

Vickrey, B.G. *et al.* 122
viruses, blood borne 162

Warner, R. 15, 16
weight gain 161, 164
Wellin, C. and Jaffe, D.J. 124
Wellness Recovery Action Planning (WRAP)
    31–2
Wing, J.K. 61
Wirral Memory Service 121
women-centred mental health care 90–101;
    acute impatient care 92; black and minority
    ethnic women 94; and body image 97; and
    childhood sexual abuse 91, 93; and crisis
    homes 100–1; and gendered violence 94–5,
    96–7, 100–1; and mixed sex acute wards 97–9;

and sexual expression 96; staff education
    and training 93, 95–9; and the therapeutic
    relationship 97–9
Women's mental health: into the mainstream 93
Women's National Commission 94
Work and Social Adjustment Scale (WASAS) 135
WRAP (Wellness Recovery Action Planning)
    31–2
With safety in mind 91

Zimmerman, S. *et al.* 124

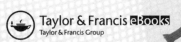